Atlas of
Abdominal Wall Reconstruction

Atlas of Abdominal Wall Reconstruction

Michael J. Rosen, MD, FACS
Associate Professor of Surgery
Chief, Division of GI and General Surgery
Case Western Reserve University
Case Medical Center
Cleveland, Ohio, USA

ELSEVIER
SAUNDERS

1600 John F. Kennedy Blvd.
Ste 1800
Philadelphia, PA 19103-2899

ATLAS OF ABDOMINAL WALL RECONSTRUCTION

Copyright © 2012 by Saunders, an imprint of Elsevier Inc.

ISBN: 978-1-4377-2751-7

No part of this publication may be reproduced or transmitted in any form or by any means, electronic or mechanical, including photocopying, recording, or any information storage and retrieval system, without permission in writing from the publisher. Details on how to seek permission, further information about the Publisher's permissions policies and our arrangements with organizations such as the Copyright Clearance Center and the Copyright Licensing Agency, can be found at our website: www.elsevier.com/permissions.

This book and the individual contributions contained in it are protected under copyright by the Publisher (other than as may be noted herein).

Notice

Knowledge and best practice in this field are constantly changing. As new research and experience broaden our understanding, changes in research methods, professional practices, or medical treatment may become necessary.

Practitioners and researchers must always rely on their own experience and knowledge in evaluating and using any information, methods, compounds, or experiments described herein. In using such information or methods they should be mindful of their own safety and the safety of others, including parties for whom they have a professional responsibility.

With respect to any drug or pharmaceutical products identified, readers are advised to check the most current information provided (i) on procedures featured or (ii) by the manufacturer of each product to be administered, to verify the recommended dose or formula, the method and duration of administration, and contraindications. It is the responsibility of practitioners, relying on their own experience and knowledge of their patients, to make diagnoses, to determine dosages and the best treatment for each individual patient, and to take all appropriate safety precautions.

To the fullest extent of the law, neither the Publisher nor the authors, contributors, or editors, assume any liability for any injury and/or damage to persons or property as a matter of products liability, negligence or otherwise, or from any use or operation of any methods, products, instructions, or ideas contained in the material herein.

Library of Congress Cataloging-in-Publication Data

Atlas of abdominal wall reconstruction / [edited by] Michael J. Rosen. -- 1st ed.
  p. ; cm.
  Includes bibliographical references and index.
  ISBN 978-1-4377-2751-7 (hardcover : alk. paper)
  1. Hernia--Surgery--Atlases. 2. Abdominal wall--Surgery--Atlases. I. Rosen, Michael J., MD.
  [DNLM: 1. Hernia, Ventral--surgery--Atlases. 2. Abdominal Wall--surgery--Atlases.
3. Laparoscopy--methods--Atlases. WI 17]
  RD621.A85 2012
  617.5'59059--dc23

2011014084

Acquisitions Editor: Judith Fletcher
Developmental Editor: Roxanne Halpine Ward
Publishing Services Manager: Jeff Patterson
Project Manager: Bill Drone
Design Direction: Steve Stave

Printed in the U.S.A.

Last digit is the print number: 9 8 7 6 5 4 3 2

Working together to grow
libraries in developing countries

www.elsevier.com | www.bookaid.org | www.sabre.org

ELSEVIER   BOOK AID International   Sabre Foundation

I would like to dedicate this atlas to my wife Deb, my lovely children Samantha, Alexandra, and Zachary who have always supported my endeavors as a surgeon, and to all of the surgeons who have so graciously participated in my training throughout the years.

Contributors

Charles E. Butler, MD
Professor
Department of Plastic Surgery
The University of Texas M.D. Anderson Cancer Center
Houston, Texas, USA
Modified Minimally Invasive Component Separation

Alfredo M. Carbonell, DO, FACS, FACOS
Associate Professor of Clinical Surgery
The Hernia Center and Division of Minimal Access
 and Bariatric Surgery
Greenville Hospital System
University Medical Center
University of South Carolina School of Medicine -
 Greenville
Greenville, South Carolina, USA
Progressive Preoperative Pneumoperitoneum for Hernias with Loss of Abdominal Domain

Harvey Chim, MD
Resident
Department of Plastic Surgery
Case Western Reserve University
Cleveland, Ohio, USA
Abdominal Wall Anatomy and Vascular Supply

William S. Cobb IV, MD
Associate Professor of Clinical Surgery
Department of Surgery
University of South Carolina School of Medicine
Director, Division of Minimal Access and Bariatric
 Surgery, and Co-Director, The Hernia Center
Department of Surgery
Greenville Hospital System University Medical
 Group
Greenville, South Carolina, USA
Laparoscopic Ventral Hernia Repair-Standard

George DeNoto III, MD, FACS
Associate Professor of Surgery
Hofstra North Shore-LIJ School of Medicine
Chief, Division of Minimally Invasive Surgery
North Shore University Hospital at Manhasset
Director
North Shore-LIJ Minimally Invasive Surgery
 Fellowship
North Shore Long Island Jewish Health System
Manhasset, New York, USA
Periumbilical Perforator Sparing Components Separation

Karen Kim Evans, MD
Chief of Plastic Surgery
Department of Surgery
Veterans Affairs Medical Center
Assistant Professor
Department of Plastic Surgery
Georgetown University Medical Center
Washington, District of Columbia, USA
Abdominal Wall Anatomy and Vascular Supply

Michael G. Franz, MD
Associate Professor of Surgery
Chief, Division of Minimally Invasive Surgery
Department of Surgery
University of Michigan
Ann Arbor, Michigan, USA
Biologic Mesh Choices for Surgical Repair

Ron Israeli, MD, FACS
Clinical Assistant Professor
Department of Surgery
Division of Plastic Surgery
Hofstra University School of Medicine in partnership
 with the North Shore LIJ Health System
Hempstead, New York, USA
Periumbilical Perforator Sparing Components Separation

Arjun Khosla, MD
Postdoctoral Research Fellow
Department of Surgery
Division of Pediatric Surgery
Rainbow Babies and Children's Hospital
University Hospitals Case Medical Center
Cleveland, Ohio, USA
Managing Pediatric and Neonatal Abdominal Wall Defects

Samir Mardini, MD
Professor of Surgery
Mayo Clinic College of Medicine
Program Director
Division of Plastic Surgery
Department of Surgery
Mayo Clinic
Rochester, Minnesota, USA
Abdominal Wall Anatomy and Vascular Supply

Daniel A. Medalie, MD
Assistant Professor of Surgery
Case Western Reserve and MetroHealth Medical Center
Department of Plastic Surgery, MetroHealth Medical Center
Case Western Reserve Medical School
Assistant Professor of Plastic Surgery
Department of Surgery, MetroHealth Medical Center
Assistant Professor of Plastic Surgery
Department of Surgery
University Hospital
Cleveland, Ohio, USA
Tissue and Fascial Expansion of the Abdominal Wall

Maurice Y. Nahabedian, MD, FACS
Associate Professor of Plastic Surgery
Department of Plastic Surgery
Georgetown University Hospital
Johns Hopkins University
Washington, District of Columbia, USA
Panniculectomy and Abdominal Wall Reconstruction

Yuri W. Novitsky, MD, FACS
Assistant Professor
Department of Surgery
Director, Connecticut Comprehensive Center for Hernia Repair
University of Connecticut Health Center
Farmington, Connecticut, USA
Open Retromuscular Ventral Hernia Repair; Synthetic Mesh Choices for Surgical Repair

Sean B. Orenstein, MD
General Surgery Resident
Department of Surgery
University of Connecticut School of Medicine
Farmington, Connecticut, USA
Synthetic Mesh Choices for Surgical Repair

Melissa S. Phillips, MD
Laparoendoscopic Clinical Fellow
Department of Surgery
University Hospitals Case Medical Center
Cleveland, Ohio, USA
Open Flank Hernia Repair

Todd A. Ponsky, MD
Assistant Professor
Department of Surgery
Division of Pediatric Surgery
Rainbow Babies and Children's Hospital
University Hospitals Case Medical Center
Cleveland, Ohio, USA
Managing Pediatric and Neonatal Abdominal Wall Defects

Benjamin K. Poulose, MD, MPH
Assistant Professor
Division of Surgery
Vanderbilt University School of Medicine
Vanderbilt University Medical Center
Nashville, Tennessee, USA
Laparoscopic Repair of Atypical Hernias: Suprapubic, Subxyphoid, and Lumbar

Harry L. Reynolds Jr., MD, FACS, FASCRS
Associate Professor of Surgery
Department of Surgery
Division of Colon and Rectal Surgery
Case Western Reserve University
Cleveland, Ohio, USA
Open Repair of Parastomal Hernias

Michael J. Rosen, MD, FACS
Associate Professor of Surgery
Chief, Division of GI and General Surgery
Case Western Reserve University
Case Medical Center
Cleveland, Ohio, USA
Open Flank Hernia Repair; Endoscopic Component Separation

Alan A. Saber, MD, FACS
Associate Professor
Department of Surgery
Case Western Reserve University
Cleveland, Ohio, USA
Laparoscopic Repair of Parastomal Hernias

Christopher J. Salgado, MD
Associate Professor of Surgery
Department of Surgery
University of Miami/Miller School of Medicine
Miami, Florida, USA
Abdominal Wall Anatomy and Vascular Supply

Ronald P. Silverman, MD, FACS
Associate Professor of Surgery
Division of Plastic Surgery
University of Maryland School of Medicine
Adjunct Professor of Plastic Surgery
Department of Plastic Surgery
Johns Hopkins School of Medicine
Baltimore, Maryland, USA
Open Component Separation

Hooman Soltanian, MD, FACS
Assistant Professor
Division Chief, Breast Plastic Surgery
Department of Plastic Surgery
Case Medical Center
Cleveland, Ohio, USA
Rotational and Free Flap Closure of the Abdominal Wall

Daniel Vargo, MD
Program Director, Surgery
Associate Professor
Department of Surgery
University of Utah School of Medicine
Salt Lake City, Utah, USA
Managing the Open Abdomen

Christopher G. Zochowski, MD
Department of Plastic and Reconstructive Surgery
Case Western Reserve University
Cleveland, Ohio, USA
Rotational and Free Flap Closure of the Abdominal Wall

Introduction

Abdominal wall reconstruction represents a broad spectrum of patients, defect characteristics and surgical options. Several innovative minimally invasive reconstructive techniques and the exponential growth of bioprosthetics have revolutionized abdominal wall reconstruction. The surgical approaches to these problems have evolved from simply patching the defect to reconstructing functional dynamic abdominal walls. It is important to point out that the reconstructive surgeon must individualize his or her approach to abdominal wall reconstruction. It is likely no single technique or prosthetic will accomplish the goals for all repairs. As this field has continued to expand, it now represents a collaborative effort among general surgeons, plastic surgeons, trauma surgeons, and herniologists. This atlas represents the compilation of these efforts and, like reconstructive surgery, would not be possible without each of their respective contributions.

The *Atlas of Abdominal Wall Reconstruction* focuses on many of the technical aspects of ventral hernia repair. We have paid particular attention to key anatomic planes in each of these procedures, as well as preserving the neurovascular anatomy when reconstructing the abdominal wall. Each of these procedures has been described in detail, with particular attention to avoiding common surgical pitfalls and employing strategies to deal with technical challenges once they are encountered. In addition, each chapter is accompanied by a representative video of the reconstructive approach to guide the surgeon in the technical nuances of the procedure. In this textbook, three approaches are described: laparoscopic, open, and hybrid. This atlas will provide the surgeon with the skills necessary to repair not only straightforward defects but also some of the most complex reconstructive challenges, including loss of domain, contaminated ventral hernia repair, and dealing with reconstruction in the setting of major tissue loss.

While there are often many ways to repair an abdominal wall defect, this atlas describes a multitude of safe and effective strategies to deal with these challenging problems across the entire spectrum of ventral hernia repair as described by experts in the field. In addition, a clear and clinically relevant summary of the available synthetic and biologic grafts will aid the surgeon in appropriate prosthetic selection. I hope that this atlas provides the practicing surgeon with a useful guide to optimize outcomes for their patients.

CONTENTS

Section I ANATOMY

Chapter 1 ABDOMINAL WALL ANATOMY AND VASCULAR SUPPLY 2
Harvey Chim, Karen Kim Evans, Christopher J. Salgado and Samir Mardini

Section II LAPAROSCOPIC REPAIRS

Chapter 2 LAPAROSCOPIC VENTRAL HERNIA REPAIR–STANDARD 22
William S. Cobb IV

Chapter 3 LAPAROSCOPIC REPAIR OF ATYPICAL HERNIAS: SUPRAPUBIC, SUBXIPHOID, AND LUMBAR 42
Benjamin K. Poulose

Chapter 4 LAPAROSCOPIC REPAIR OF PARASTOMAL HERNIAS 60
Alan A. Saber

Section III OPEN REPAIRS

Chapter 5 OPEN RETROMUSCULAR VENTRAL HERNIA REPAIR 74
Yuri W. Novitsky

Chapter 6 OPEN FLANK HERNIA REPAIR 97
Melissa S. Phillips and Michael J. Rosen

Chapter 7 OPEN REPAIR OF PARASTOMAL HERNIAS 110
Harry L. Reynolds, Jr.

Section IV COMPONENT SEPARATION

Chapter 8 OPEN COMPONENT SEPARATION 131
Ronald P. Silverman

Chapter 9 PERIUMBILICAL PERFORATOR SPARING COMPONENTS SEPARATION 139
George DeNoto III and Ron Israeli

Chapter 10 MODIFIED MINIMALLY INVASIVE COMPONENT SEPARATION 171
Charles E. Butler

Chapter 11 ENDOSCOPIC COMPONENT SEPARATION 185
Michael J. Rosen

Section V OTHER ABDOMINAL WALL PROCEDURES

Chapter 12 PANNICULECTOMY AND ABDOMINAL WALL RECONSTRUCTION 204
Maurice Y. Nahabedian

Chapter 13 TISSUE AND FASCIAL EXPANSION OF THE ABDOMINAL WALL 224
Daniel A. Medalie

Chapter 14 PROGRESSIVE PREOPERATIVE PNEUMOPERITONEUM FOR HERNIAS WITH LOSS OF ABDOMINAL DOMAIN   244
Alfredo M. Carbonell

Chapter 15 ROTATIONAL AND FREE FLAP CLOSURE OF THE ABDOMINAL WALL   259
Christopher G. Zochowski and Hooman Soltanian

Chapter 16 MANAGING THE OPEN ABDOMEN   290
Daniel Vargo

Chapter 17 MANAGING PEDIATRIC AND NEONATAL ABDOMINAL WALL DEFECTS   302
Arjun Khosla and Todd A. Ponsky

Section VI MESH CHOICES

Chapter 18 BIOLOGIC MESH CHOICES FOR SURGICAL REPAIR   316
Michael G. Franz

Chapter 19 SYNTHETIC MESH CHOICES FOR SURGICAL REPAIR   322
Sean B. Orenstein and Yuri W. Novitsky

INDEX   330

Video Contents

 This icon appears throughout the book to indicate chapters with accompanying video, available on Expertconsult.com.

Section II Laparoscopic Repairs

Chapter 2 Laparoscopic Ventral Hernia Repair–Standard
  Video 2 Laparoscopic Ventral Hernia Repair: A Systematic Technique
  William S. Cobb IV

Chapter 3 Laparoscopic Repair of Atypical Hernias: Suprapubic, Subxiphoid, and Lumbar
  Video 3.1 Laparoscopic Grynfeltt Repair of Lumbar Hernias
  K. Harth and Michael J. Rosen
  Video 3.2 Laparoscopic Repair of a Subxyphoid Hernia
  Benjamin K. Poulose
  Video 3.3 Laparoscopic Repair of Suprapubic Hernia
  Benjamin K. Poulose

Chapter 4 Laparoscopic Repair of Parastomal Hernias
  Video 4.1 Laparoscopic Paracolostomy Hernia Repair
  Alan A. Saber
  Video 4.2 Laparoscopic Sugarbaker Technique
  Alan A. Saber

Section III Open Repairs

Chapter 5 Open Retromuscular Ventral Hernia Repair
  Video 5 Posterior Component Separation Using Transversus Abdominis Muscle Release (TAR) Technique
  Yuri W. Novitsky

Chapter 6 Open Flank Hernia Repair
  Video 6 Open, Pre-Peritoneal Repair of Recurrent Flank Hernia with Iliac Bone Fixation
  Melissa S. Phillips, Jeffrey A. Blatnik, and Michael J. Rosen

Chapter 7 Open Repair of Parastomal Hernias
  Video 7 Open Parastomal Hernia Repair
  Harry L. Reynolds, Jr.

Section IV Component Separation

Chapter 8 Open Component Separation
  Video 8.1 Open Component Separation*
  Ronald P. Silverman
  Video 8.2 Advanced Open Component Separation*
  Ronald P. Silverman

Chapter 9 Periumbilical Perforator Sparing Components Separation
  Video 9 Open Periumbilical Perforator Sparing Components Separation
  George DeNoto III and Ron Israeli

---

*Video courtesy of LifeCell Corporation, makers of AlloDerm™ Regenerative Tissue Matrix and Strattice™ Reconstructive Tissue Matrix.

Chapter 10 MODIFIED MINIMALLY INVASIVE COMPONENT SEPARATION
Video 10 Modified Minimally Invasive Component Separation
Charles E. Butler

Chapter 11 ENDOSCOPIC COMPONENT SEPARATION
Video 11 Endoscopic Component Separation and Complex Abdominal Wall Reconstruction
Michael J. Rosen

Section V OTHER ABDOMINAL WALL PROCEDURES

Chapter 12 PANNICULECTOMY AND ABDOMINAL WALL RECONSTRUCTION
Video 12 Panniculectomy
Maurice Y. Nahabedian

Chapter 13 TISSUE AND FASCIAL EXPANSION OF THE ABDOMINAL WALL
Video 13 Tissue Expansion
Daniel A. Medalie

Chapter 14 PROGRESSIVE PREOPERATIVE PNEUMOPERITONEUM FOR HERNIAS WITH LOSS OF ABDOMINAL DOMAIN
Video 14 Preoperative Pneumoperitoneum
Alfredo M. Carbonell

Chapter 15 ROTATIONAL AND FREE FLAP CLOSURE OF THE ABDOMINAL WALL
Video 15 Complex Abdominal Wall Reconstruction with Pedicle Latissimus Dorsi Flap
Jeffrey A. Blatnik, Hooman Soltanian, and Michael J. Rosen

Chapter 17 MANAGING PEDIATRIC AND NEONATAL ABDOMINAL WALL DEFECTS
Video 17 Gastroschisis: A Sutureless Approach to Repair
Daniel Kelmenson, Anthony Sandler, and Todd A. Ponsky

SECTION I

Anatomy

CHAPTER 1

Abdominal Wall Anatomy and Vascular Supply

Harvey Chim, MD, Karen Kim Evans, MD, Christopher J. Salgado, MD, and Samir Mardini, MD

1. Clinical Anatomy

1. Overview

- ▲ The anterior abdominal wall (Figs. 1-1 to 1-3) is a hexagonal area defined superiorly by the costal margin and xiphoid process; laterally by the midaxillary line; and inferiorly by the symphysis pubis, pubic tubercle, inguinal ligament, anterior superior iliac spine, and iliac crest.
- ▲ Layers of the anterior abdominal wall include skin, subcutaneous tissue, superficial fascia, deep fascia, muscle, extraperitoneal fascia, and peritoneum.

2. Superficial Fascial Layers (see Figs. 1-1 and 1-2)

- ▲ The superficial fascia of the abdominal wall consists of a single layer above the umbilicus, consisting of the fused Camper and Scarpa fasciae.
- ▲ Below the umbilicus the superficial fascia consists of a fatty outer layer (Camper fascia) and a membranous inner layer (Scarpa fascia).
- ▲ Camper fascia is continuous inferiorly with the superficial thigh fascia and extends inferiorly to the scrotum in males and labia majora in females.
- ▲ Scarpa fascia fuses inferiorly with the fascia lata of the thigh and continues posteriorly to the perineum, where it is called Colles fascia.

Chapter 1 • Abdominal Wall Anatomy and Vascular Supply

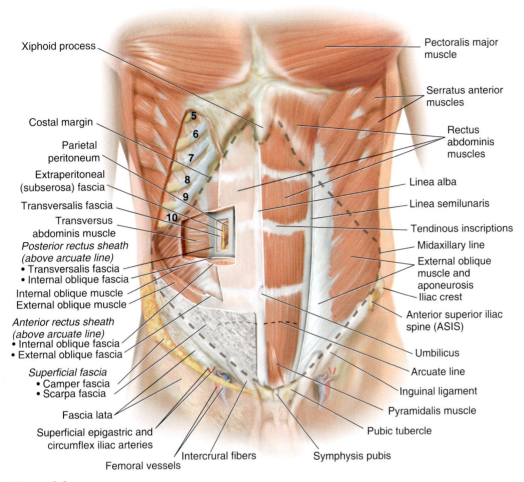

Figure 1-1.

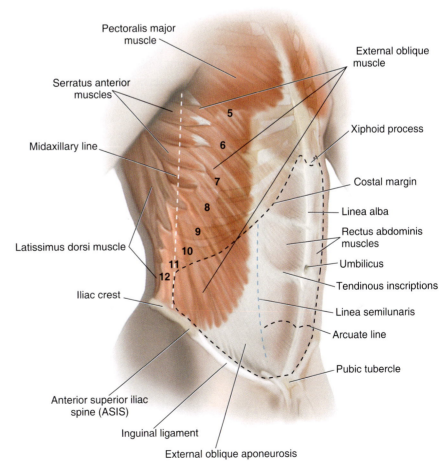

Figure 1-2.

▲ *Pearls and Pitfalls*

Scarpa fascia is usually a visible and durable structure and is closed separately during various surgeries on the abdominal wall to achieve optimal scar result.

3. Deep Fascial Layers (see Figs. 1-1 and 1-2)

- ▲ The rectus sheath is found in the midline.
- ▲ Laterally, layers of the abdominal wall deep to superficial fascia include external oblique, internal oblique, transversus abdominis, and parietal peritoneum.
- ▲ The arcuate line (see Fig. 1-3) is located midway between the umbilicus and symphysis pubis and is a transition point where the posterior rectus sheath transitions from being the fusion of part of internal oblique fascia and transversalis fascia superiorly to only transversalis fascia inferiorly.
- ▲ Above the arcuate line, the anterior rectus sheath consists of external oblique fascia and part of internal oblique fascia. The posterior rectus sheath consists of internal oblique fascia and transversalis fascia. The anterior and posterior layers of the rectus fascia therefore invest the rectus abdominis muscles.
- ▲ Below the arcuate line, the external oblique and internal oblique fasciae merge to form the anterior rectus sheath. The posterior rectus sheath consists of transversus abdominis fascia, making this only a thin layer with minimal strength.

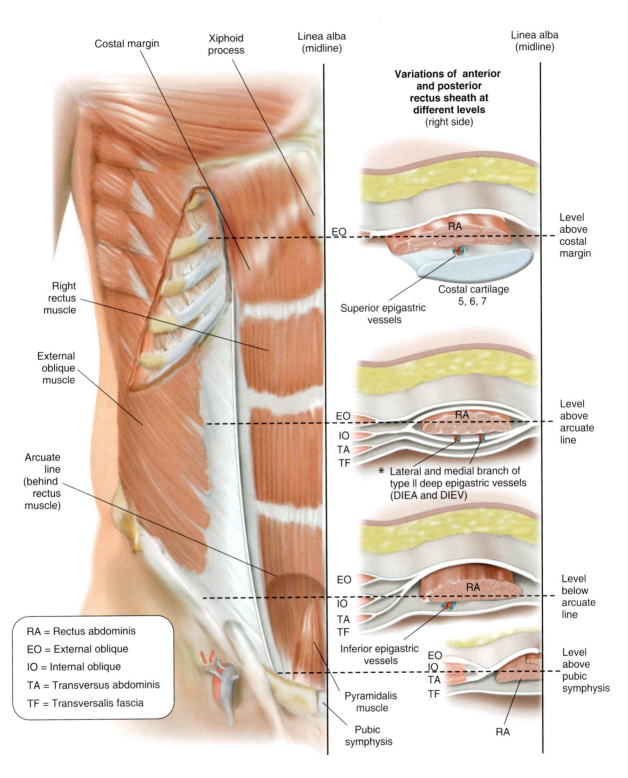

Figure 1-3.

▲ The linea alba results from fusion of the anterior and posterior rectus sheaths and lies in the midline, extending cranially from the xiphoid process to the pubic symphysis caudally Figure 1-4 shows the anterior wall fascia after dissection of the abdominal wall skin and subcutaneous tissue, showing the linea alba and linea semilunaris.

▲ *Pearls and Pitfalls*

Incision, release, and dissection of the anterior external oblique fascia can be done for repair of ventral hernias. This technique is called the components separation (Fig. 1-5). The incision in the external oblique fascia is made 1 to 2 cm lateral to the linea semilunaris, and the fascia is released to attain primary closure. Incisions also can be made in the posterior rectus sheath to gain additional length.

4. **Abdominal Wall Musculature (see Figs. 1-1 to 1-3)**

▲ The paired rectus abdominis muscles are the principal flexors of the anterior abdominal wall. They function to stabilize the pelvis while walking. They also protect the abdominal organs and help in forced expiration.
▲ The rectus abdominis muscles originate from the pubic symphysis and pubic crest and insert on the anterior surfaces of the fifth, sixth, and seventh costal cartilages and the xiphoid processes. Laterally, the rectus sheath merges with the aponeurosis of the external oblique muscles to form the linea semilunaris (Fig. 1-4).
▲ Three to four tendinous inscriptions, which are adherent to the anterior rectus sheath, interrupt the rectus abdominis along its length (Fig. 1-6).
▲ The external oblique muscle is the most superficial and thickest of the three lateral abdominal wall muscles. It originates from the lower eight ribs and courses in an inferomedial direction. Inferiorly it folds back on itself and forms the inguinal ligament, which extends between the anterior superior iliac spine and pubic tubercle. It is attached medially to the pubic crest.
▲ The internal oblique muscle is deep to the external oblique muscle, and its aponeurosis splits medially above the arcuate line to form part of the anterior rectus sheath and part of the posterior rectus sheath. Below the arcuate line, the inferior oblique aponeurosis does not split and fuses with the external oblique fascia to form the anterior rectus sheath. The internal oblique muscle runs in a superomedial direction, perpendicular to the external oblique muscle. It originates from the thoracolumbar fascia, anterior two thirds of the iliac crest, and lateral half of the inguinal ligament. It inserts on the inferior and posterior borders of the tenth through twelfth ribs superiorly. Inferiorly, the internal oblique inserts on the pectineal line with fibers from the transversus abdominis, forming the conjoint tendon, which inserts on the pubic crest.
▲ The transversus abdominis muscle is the deepest of the three lateral abdominal wall muscles and courses in a horizontal direction. It originates from the anterior three fourths of the iliac crest; lateral third of the inguinal ligament; and inner surface of the lower six costal cartilages, interdigitating with fibers of the diaphragm. The muscle ends medially in a broad flat aponeurosis, merging above the arcuate line with the posterior lamella of the internal oblique aponeurosis and the linea alba. Below the arcuate line, it inserts into the pubic crest and pectineal line, forming the conjoint tendon with the internal oblique.

Chapter 1 • Abdominal Wall Anatomy and Vascular Supply 7

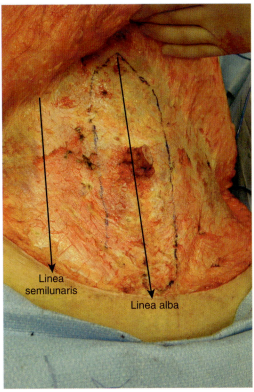

Figure 1-4.

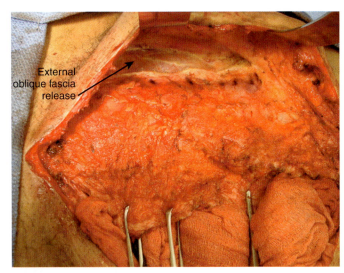

Figure 1-5.

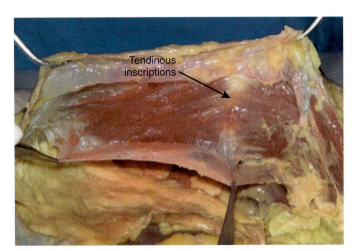

Figure 1-6.

- ▲ The pyramidalis is a small triangular muscle found anterior to the inferior aspect of the rectus abdominis; it is absent in about 20% of the population. It originates from the body of the pubis and inserts into the linea alba inferior to the umbilicus.
- ▲ The semilunar lines are formed by fusion of the external oblique, internal oblique, and transversus abdominis aponeuroses at the lateral border of the rectus abdominis.

▲ Pearls and Pitfalls

Of all the muscles in the abdominal wall, the rectus abdominis muscle is the most versatile and useful for flap procedures. The rectus muscle can be harvested as a free flap for microsurgical transfer of tissue to various defects. It also can be harvested as a pedicled flap, based on the superior or inferior epigastric arteries and rotated to fill groin, chest wall, mastectomy defects, vaginal, and perianal wounds.

It is also important to note the functional loss that results if the rectus abdominis muscle is harvested. Using isometric dynamometry, studies have shown that there is at least a 20% functional loss in trunk flexion. Bilateral harvest of the rectus abdominis muscles can be debilitating for patients who are very active because there is a 40% functional loss in trunk flexion, which may infringe upon activities of daily living.

5. Neurovascular Supply of the Abdominal Wall

▲ Pearls and Pitfalls

- ▲ The blood supply of the abdominal wall can be divided into three zones (Huger, 1979).
- ▲ Zone I consists of the upper and midcentral abdominal walls and is supplied by the vertically oriented deep superior (Fig. 1-7, A).and deep inferior epigastric arteries (Fig. 1-7, B).
- ▲ Zone II consists of the lower abdominal wall and is supplied by the epigastric arcade, superficial inferior epigastric, superficial external pudendal, and superficial circumflex iliac arteries. Perforators from the deep circumflex iliac arteries also supply a region of skin posterior and cephalad to the anterior superior iliac spine along the axis of the iliac crest.

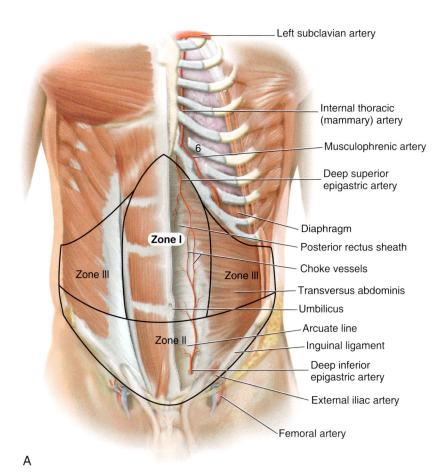

A

Figure 1-7.

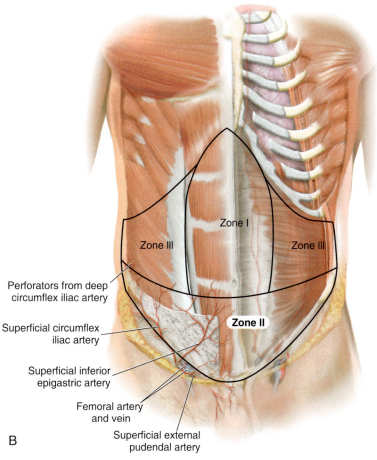

B

Figure 1-7—Cont'd.

- ▲ Zone III consists of the lateral abdominal wall (flank region) and is supplied by the musculophrenic, lower intercostals (Fig. 1-8, *A*), and lumbar arteries (Fig. 1-8, *B*).

▲ *Vascular Supply*

- ▲ Knowledge of these zones of blood supply to the anterior abdominal wall is important when planning incisions for surgical procedures. A previous subcostal incision can compromise the circulation to Huger's zone III of the abdominal wall. In transverse rectus abdominis myocutaneous (TRAM) flap harvest, the presence of a subcostal scar was found to increase donor site complications, with a significantly higher incidence of abdominal wall skin necrosis (25%) compared with patients without abdominal wall scars (5%).
- ▲ The superior epigastric artery and deep inferior epigastric arteries lie on the posterior aspect of the rectus abdominis muscles and supply the muscle and overlying skin and subcutaneous tissue through musculocutaneous perforators (Fig. 1-9).
- ▲ A study by Saber et al. (2004) provides guidelines for location of the epigastric vessels based on computed tomography (CT) scan data in 100 patients. At the xiphoid process, the superior epigastric arteries (SEA) were 4.41 ± 0.13 cm from the midline on the right and 4.53 ± 0.14 cm from the left. Midway between xiphoid and umbilicus, the SEA was 5.50 ± 0.16 cm on right of midline and 5.36 ± 0.16 cm on the left. At the umbilicus, the epigastric vessels were 5.88 ± 0.14 cm on the right and 5.55 ± 0.13 on left of midline. Midway between umbilicus and symphysis pubis, the inferior epigastric arteries (IEA) were 5.32 ± 0.12 cm on right and 5.25 ± 0.11 cm on left of midline. While at the symphysis pubis, the IEA were 7.47 ± 0.10 cm from the midline on the right and 7.49 ± 0.09 cm from midline on the left side.
- ▲ The deep inferior epigastric artery is dominant in the vascular supply of the abdominal compared with the superior epigastric artery. The two arborizing vascular systems converge within the rectus abdominis muscle at a point in between the xiphoid process and umbilicus. In a study by Taylor et al. (2003), the mean diameter of the deep inferior epigastric artery at its point of origin was 3.4 mm, compared to 1.6 mm for the superior epigastric artery, perhaps explaining the dominant arterial supply of the deep inferior epigastric artery.
- ▲ The deep inferior epigastric artery arises from the medial aspect of the external iliac artery opposite the origin of the deep circumflex iliac artery, approximately 1 cm above the inguinal ligament. It passes superomedially behind the transversalis fascia and towards the lateral border of the rectus abdominis muscle. It then enters the rectus sheath, passing anterior to the arcuate line, midway between pubis and umbilicus.
- ▲ The superior epigastric artery originates at the bifurcation of the internal mammary artery into the musculophrenic artery and deep superior epigastric artery, around the region of the sixth costal cartilage. It subsequently passes inferolaterally and pierces the posterior rectus sheath to lie on the posterior surface of the abdominal muscle. It then gives off two or more branches before anastomosing with the branches of the deep inferior epigastric artery.
- ▲ The superior epigastric artery, when described, refers in general to the deep superior epigastric artery. A superficial superior epigastric artery has been noted in anatomic studies, but it is not clinically significant.

Chapter 1 • Abdominal Wall Anatomy and Vascular Supply

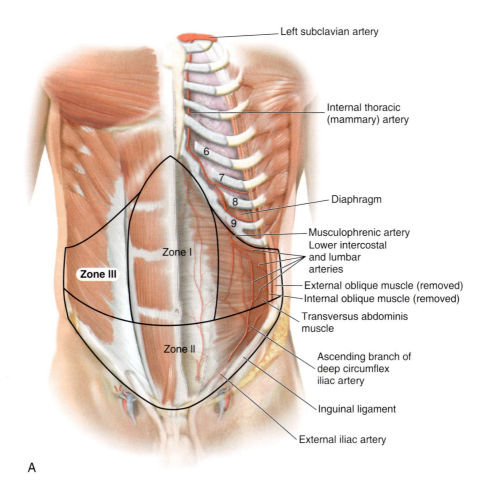

A

Figure 1-8.

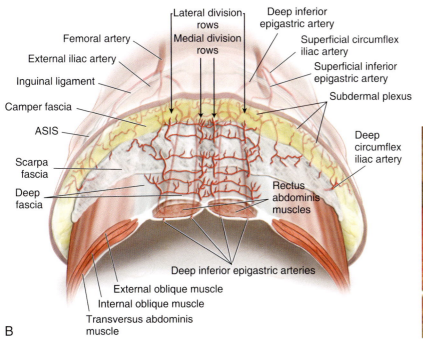

B

Figure 1-8—cont'd.

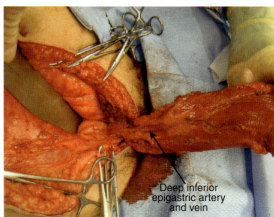

Figure 1-9.

- The musculophrenic artery passes inferolaterally behind the seventh, eighth, and ninth costal cartilages and provides large branches to the intercostal spaces, which become continuous with the posterior intercostal vessels. Together with the lumbar arteries, it supplies the lateral part of the abdominal wall. The musculophrenic artery provides an alternative vascular supply for a pedicled TRAM flap when the proximal portion of the internal mammary artery has been divided or is obstructed.
- Three patterns of blood supply of the rectus abdominis muscle were described by Taylor et al. (2003), based on divisions of the deep inferior epigastric artery (DIEA) at the level of the arcuate line. In type 1 (29%), there was a single intramuscular artery. In type 2 (57%), the DIEA divided at the arcuate line into two major intramuscular vessels. In type 3 (14%) the DIEA divided into three branches at the arcuate line.
- Musculocutaneous perforators arise from the deep inferior epigastric artery and lie in a medial and lateral subdivision in the form of longitudinal rows of perforators parallel to the sagittal plane.
- Medial row perforators, in general, tend to have a vascular territory that is larger and crosses the midline, well perfusing Hartrampf zones I and II.
- Lateral row perforators tend to have a zone of perfusion that is localized to a hemiabdomen and may be used preferentially when a smaller flap is required.
- A study by Chowdhry et al. (2010) reported that the DIEA encountered the lateral border of the rectus abdominis at a mean distance of 10.45 ± 1.58 cm from the umbilicus, with the first perforator transversing the rectus abdominis muscle around 7.4 ± 1.64 cm from the umbilicus.
- Veins draining the anterior abdominal wall (Fig. 1-10) run as venae comitantes, accompanying the perforators and subsequently main arteries of the deep inferior and superior epigastric arteries. These ultimately drain into the azygos system and external iliac veins.
- The superficial inferior epigastric artery (SIEA) arises from the external iliac artery or superficial circumflex iliac artery, and together with its accompanying vein, lies in the plane between the Camper and Scarpa fasciae on each side, lateral to the rectus abdominis muscles. These provide an accessory blood supply to the anterior abdominal wall, which may be used in the harvesting of flaps.
- The SIEA was reported to have a mean diameter of 0.6 mm, with a diameter >1.5 mm only in 24% of patients. Location of the SIEA is highly variable, with a mean position 2 cm lateral to the linea semilunaris (range 0 to 8 cm).
- The location of the superficial inferior epigastric vein (SIEV) is highly variable compared with the SIEA, with the distance between SIEA and SIEV ranging from 0.3 to 8.5 cm apart. Unlike the veins accompanying the other arteries supplying the anterior abdominal wall, the SIEV often runs a distance away from its corresponding artery, the SIEA.
- The lower intercostals and lumbar arteries supplying the abdominal wall lie in the plane between the internal oblique and transversalis muscles.

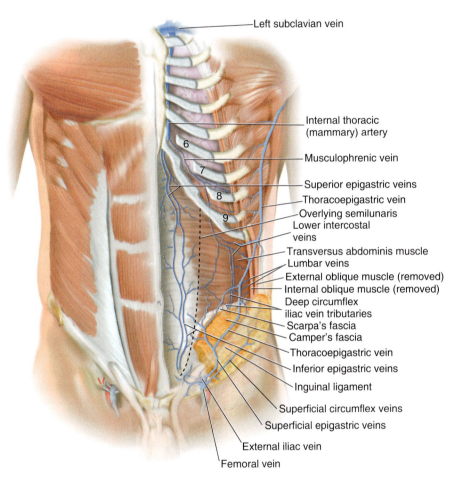

Figure 1-10.

▲ Nerve Supply (Fig. 1-11)

- ▲ Sensory innervation of the abdominal wall is derived from the anterior branches of the intercostals and subcostal nerves, from T7 to L1. These nerves run together with the intercostal and lumbar arteries in the plane between the internal oblique and transversalis muscles. Figure 1-12 shows the motor nerves to the rectus abdominis muscle. The internal oblique muscle has been divided, showing the nerve deep to the internal oblique muscle and superficial to the transversus abdominis muscle.
- ▲ T7 to T9 supply skin superior to the umbilicus.
- ▲ T10 supplies area of skin around the umbilicus.
- ▲ T11 to L1 supply skin inferior to the umbilicus.
- ▲ Lateral cutaneous branches of the intercostal nerves supply the lateral areas of the abdominal wall.
- ▲ Motor innervation is supplied by the seventh through twelfth intercostal nerves, iliohypogastric, and ilioinguinal nerves.
- ▲ The rectus abdominis muscle is innervated segmentally by ventral rami of the lower six intercostal nerves.
- ▲ The external oblique is innervated by the lower six thoracic and upper two lumbar anterior rami.
- ▲ The internal oblique is innervated by the lower thoracic intercostal nerves (T6 to T12) and the iliohypogastric and ilioinguinal nerves.
- ▲ The transversus abdominis muscle is innervated by the lower intercostal nerves (T7 to T12) and the iliohypogastric and ilioinguinal nerves.

▲ Pearls and Pitfalls

Knowledge of the anatomy and course of abdominal wall nerves is important. Painful neuromas of the ilioinguinal and iliohypogastric nerves have been well documented following anterior abdominal wall incisions for herniorrhaphy, iliac bone crest harvest, laparoscopic port placement, and appendectomy. Surrounding scar tissue usually entraps the nerve leading to the development of a neuroma, which causes severe pain, point tenderness, and pain radiating to the groin. Surgery involving neuroma resection and scar division usually treats the pain.

2. Abdominal Wall Physiology

1. Function in Respiration

- ▲ The abdominal wall plays an accessory role to the intercostal muscles, thorax, and diaphragm in respiration.
- ▲ The diaphragm maintains a constant positive pressure differential between the abdomen and thorax, increasing the volume of the thorax in inspiration and decreasing the volume of the thorax in expiration.

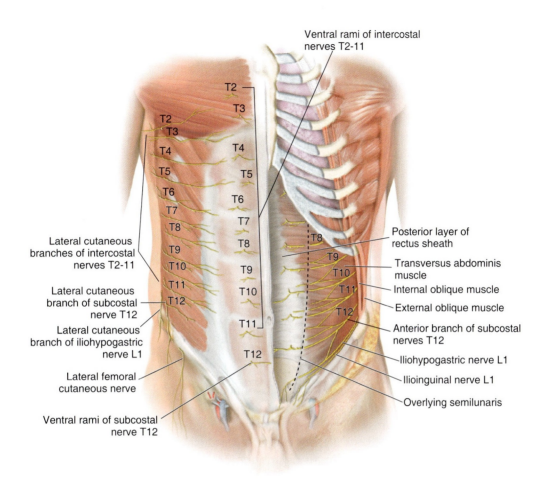

Figure 1-11.

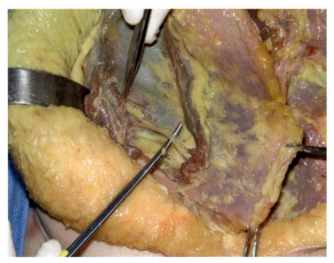

Figure 1-12.

- ▲ The abdominal wall primarily functions in expiration, whereas the transversus abdominis and external and internal obliques raise intraabdominal pressure to meet increased demands of breathing during exercise. This increase in intraabdominal pressure is transmitted through the diaphragm to the thorax and forces air from the lungs.
- ▲ In the absence of exertion or exercise, expiration is largely passive, and relies on relaxation of the intercostal muscles and diaphragm.
- ▲ In inspiration, the abdominal wall provides anterior support for the abdominal cavity, allowing for generation of a pressure differential between the abdomen and thorax through the diaphragm.
- ▲ The large mass of the intraabdominal contents hydraulically transmits a negative pressure to the thorax at steady state, through gravity, when a person is upright. When a person is supine, this effect is diminished, therefore resulting in a decrease of functional respiratory capacity of the lungs by around 15% to 20% of vital capacity.

2. Muscle Function

- ▲ The musculature of the anterior abdominal wall works in a synkinetic fashion to protect intraabdominal contents and also increase abdominal pressure where required.
- ▲ An increase in intraabdominal pressure facilitates expiration, micturition, defecation, and even parturition.
- ▲ The rectus abdominis muscle tenses the abdominal wall and flexes the vertebral column.
- ▲ The diaphragm interdigitates with the abdominal wall.
- ▲ The diaphragm, iliopsoas, and quadratus lumborum muscle form a kinetic chain that integrates upper and lower body activity, allowing coordinated movement and weight shifts.
- ▲ Together with this kinetic chain, the rectus abdominis muscle stabilizes the pelvis during walking, running, and jumping.
- ▲ A number of studies have been performed to evaluate function of the abdominal wall after bilateral TRAM flaps for breast reconstruction. Although results are highly variable, it is generally agreed that loss of both rectus muscles results in some degree of pain, back pain, and decreased flexor strength of the anterior abdominal wall.

3. Abdominal Wall Disruption Relevant to Anatomy

1. Rectus Diastasis

- ▲ Diastasis of the rectus abdominis muscles is defined as separation of the paired recti at the midline (Fig. 1-13).
- ▲ This occurs physiologically in newborns and pregnant women.
- ▲ The inter-recti distance (IRD) has been reported to be up to 58 mm in the antenatal period, with a continuing increase in IRD up to four times in the postpartum period.
- ▲ Severe cases in adults, typically in postpartum women, can be treated by plication of the rectus abdominis muscles.
- ▲ Another reported association with diastasis recti is abdominal aortic aneurysm, particularly in males.

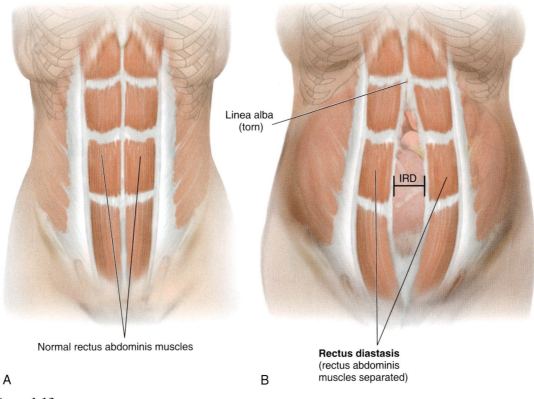

Figure 1-13.

▲ Human immunodeficiency virus (HIV)-associated lipodystrophy has been reported to be associated with diastasis recti.
▲ A rare congenital cause is Beckwith-Wiedemann syndrome.

2. Ventral Hernia

▲ Ventral hernia typically develops as an incisional hernia, following a midline laparotomy through the linea alba; it is due to incomplete healing that results in a fascial defect.
▲ Greater than 10% of patients undergoing abdominal surgical procedures develop incisional hernias (>150,000 incisional hernias per year).
▲ Risk factors for developing an incisional hernia are obesity, smoking, aneurysmal disease, malnourishment, steroid dependency, renal disease, and malignancy.
▲ Patients present with a mass protruding through the fascia defect and causing localized protuberance of the anterior abdominal wall (Fig. 1-14).
▲ Possible complications include incarceration and strangulation.
▲ Repair can be achieved with laparoscopic or open ventral hernia repairs with or without mesh or components separation techniques.
▲ Optimization of nutrition is essential for wound healing after reconstructive surgery in the anterior abdominal wall. During closure, it is important to ensure proper alignment of layers of the abdominal wall and tension-free closure. Meticulous surgical technique and avoidance of smoking in patients before and after surgery minimize the incidence of abdominal wall complications.

3. Physiology of Ventral Hernia Formation

▲ Most incisional hernias resulting from disruption of laparotomy wounds begin forming within 30 days after surgery.
▲ In mechanical failure of the midline laparotomy wound, fibrosis, myopathic disuse atrophy, and change in muscle fiber type occur in abdominal wall musculature.
▲ Abnormal load signaling, together with the above pathologic changes, results in reduced abdominal wall compliance.
▲ Animal studies confirm lateral abdominal wall shortening and atrophy of internal oblique muscles, leading to decreased extensibility and increased stiffness of the abdominal wall. This results in persistent mechanical disruption of the hernia at a lower force compared with nonherniated abdominal walls.
▲ Biologic changes resulting from mechanical failure of the abdominal wall include decreased fibroblast contraction, decreased extracellular matrix formation, and collagen deposition.
▲ The incisional hernia is a chronic wound with abnormal tissue repair pathways and is therefore prone to fail in the presence of a lower mechanical disruptive force compared with a normal physiologic abdominal wall.

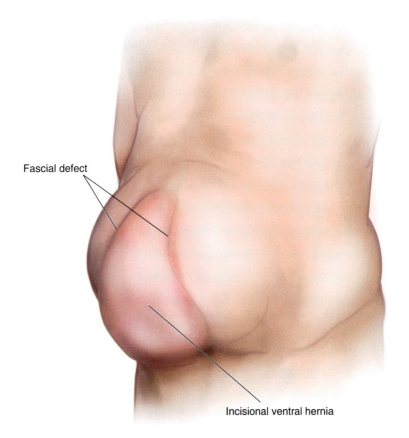

Figure 1-14.

4. Congenital Abnormalities

▲ Defects in abdominal wall closure during embryogenesis include omphalocele and gastroschisis.
▲ Omphalocele is the protrusion of abdominal wall contents from a midline defect in the abdominal wall at the base of the umbilicus. The herniated contents are covered by a very thin membrane of tissue and can become dry and necrotic after birth. In infants with omphalocele, the incidence of other congenital anomalies, such as bowel atresia, chromosomal abnormalities, and cardiac and renal anomalies, is very high (up to 70%).
▲ Gastroschisis is the protrusion of abdominal wall contents through a defect in the abdominal wall that is NOT midline, usually to the right of the umbilicus. No membrane covers the abdominal wall contents, and the bowel is usually very edematous and inflamed. There are no associated congenital anomalies in these infants.

Selected References

Atisha D, Alderman AK: A systematic review of abdominal wall function following abdominal flaps for post mastectomy breast reconstruction, *Ann Plast Surg* 63:222–230, 2009.
Blanchard PD: Diastasis recti abdominis in HIV-infected men with lipodystrophy, *HIV Med* 6:54–56, 2005.
Boyd JB, Taylor GI, Corlett R: The vascular territories of the superior epigastric and the deep inferior epigastric systems, *Plast Reconstr Surg* 73:1–16, 1984.
Chowdhry S, Hazani R, Collis P, Wilhelmi BJ: Anatomical landmarks for safe elevation of the deep inferior epigastric perforator flap: a cadaveric study, *Eplasty* 10:e41, 2010.
DuBay DA, Choi W, Urbanchek MG, et al: Incisional herniation induces decreased abdominal wall compliance via oblique muscle atrophy and fibrosis, *Ann Surg* 245:140–146, 2007.
Ducic I, Moxley M, Al-Attar A: Algorithm for treatment of postoperative incisional groin pain after cesarean delivery or hysterectomy, *Obstet Gynecol* 108:27–31, 2006.
El-Mrakby HH, Milner RH: The vascular anatomy of the lower anterior abdominal wall: a microdissection study on the deep inferior epigastric vessels and the perforator branches, *Plast Reconstr Surg* 109:539–543, 2002.
Franz MG: The biology of hernia formation, *Surg Clin North Am* 88:1–15, 2008.
Hartrampf CR, Scheflan M, Black PW: Breast reconstruction with a transverse abdominal island flap, *Plast Reconstr Surg* 69:216–225, 1982.
Hsia M, Jones S: Natural resolution of rectus abdominis diastasis. Two single case studies, *Aust J Physiother* 46:301–307, 2000.
Huger WE Jr: The anatomic rationale for abdominal lipectomy, *Am Surg* 45:612–617, 1979.
Losken A, Carlson GW, Jones GE, Culbertson JH, Schoemann M, Bostwick J 3rd: Importance of right subcostal incisions in patients undergoing TRAM flap breast reconstruction, *Ann Plast Surg* 49:115–119, 2002.
Moesbergen T, Law A, Roake J, Lewis DR: Diastasis recti and abdominal aortic aneurysm, *Vascular* 17:325–329, 2009.
Moon HK, Taylor GI: The vascular anatomy of rectus abdominis musculocutaneous flaps based on the deep superior epigastric system, *Plast Reconstr Surg* 82:815–832, 1988.
Ramirez OM, Ruas E, Dellon AL: "Components separation" method for closure of abdominal-wall defects: an anatomic and clinical study, *Plast Reconstr Surg* 86:519–526, 1990.
Rozen WM, Chubb D, Grinsell D, Ashton MW: The variability of the superficial inferior epigastric artery (SIEA) and its angiosome: A clinical anatomical study, *Microsurgery* , 2010 Jan 7:[Epub ahead of print].
Saber AA, Meslemani AM, Davis R, Pimental R: Safety zones for anterior abdominal wall entry during laparoscopy: a CT scan mapping of epigastric vessels, *Ann Surg* 239:182–185, 2004.
Schneid H, Vazquez MP, Vacher C, Gormelen M, Cabrol S, Le Bouc Y: The Beckwith-Wiedemann syndrome phenotype and the risk of cancer, *Med Pediatr Oncol* 28:411–415, 1997.
Taylor GI: The angiosomes of the body and their supply to perforator flaps, *Clin Plast Surg* 30:331–342, 2003.
Wong C, Saint-Cyr M, Mojallal A, et al: Perforasomes of the DIEP flap: vascular anatomy of the lateral versus medial row perforators and clinical implications, *Plast Reconstr Surg* 125:772–782, 2010.

SECTION II

Laparoscopic Repairs

CHAPTER 2

Laparoscopic Ventral Hernia Repair—Standard

William S. Cobb IV, MD

1. Surgical Anatomy

- ▲ The laparoscopic repair of ventral hernia borrows from the open technique espoused by Rives and Stoppa. It maintains the tenets of large mesh overlap with transabdominal fixation of the prosthetic. In a standard laparoscopic ventral herniorrhaphy, the biomaterial is placed intraabdominally in juxtaposition to the underlying viscera; therefore, a tissue-separating mesh is required. Traditionally, the hernia defect is bridged with mesh; however, some authors have described reapproximating the midline by closing the defect with transabdominal sutures.
- ▲ The amount of mesh overlap required for a durable ventral hernia repair is unknown. Based on Pascal's principle, the intraabdominal pressure is evenly distributed over a large surface area of mesh. The initial experience with laparoscopic ventral herniorrhaphy reported a 3-cm overlap of mesh, but the current recommendation is at least a 4- to 5-cm margin. The amount of overlap depends on the diameter of the largest hernia defect and the thickness of the patient's abdominal wall. One large defect deserves at least 5 cm, whereas numerous small defects (i.e., Swiss cheese hernia) may only require 4 cm of additional mesh.
- ▲ In a laparoscopic ventral hernia repair, the mesh is placed in an insufflated abdominal cavity. Ideally, there is a slight degree of tension on the mesh at the completion of the repair. The mesh does not lie flush against the underside of the abdominal wall. Rather, it transects the abdominal space, so that when the abdominal cavity is desufflated, the mesh will not occupy the hernia sac (Fig. 2-1).
- ▲ There has been a lot of debate in the literature regarding the approach for ventral herniorrhaphy. Length of stay, postoperative pain, and operative times are essentially similar between the open and laparoscopic techniques in experienced hands. However, the laparoscopic technique consistently demonstrates significant reductions in wound and mesh infections. For this reason alone, the laparoscopic repair of ventral hernias should be the preferred approach when applicable.

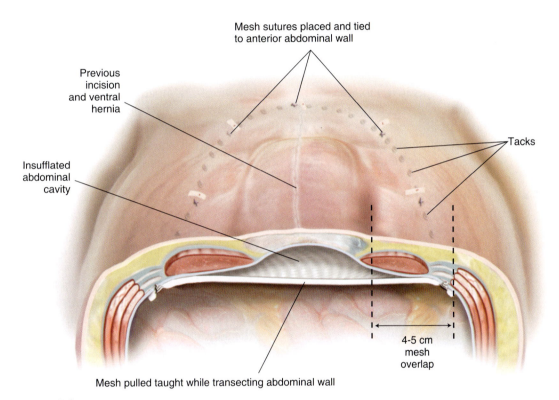

Figure 2-1.

2. Preoperative Considerations

- When considering who is a candidate for a laparoscopic ventral hernia repair, certain patient characteristics must be considered. Contraindications include:
  Inability to tolerate general anesthesia
  Hypercoagulability
  Active infection
  Loss of domain
  Poor skin quality overlying hernia (ulceration, skin graft)
  Patient expectations (scar revision or panniculectomy desired)
- Surgeon skill, particularly in the area of adhesiolysis, needs to be factored in when making the choice for a laparoscopic ventral hernia repair. Factors that portend a more difficult case requiring experience with the technique include:
  Multiple previous laparotomies
  Previous intraabdominal mesh
  History of peritonitis
  Atypical location of hernia (suprapubic, subxiphoid, flank)
- The preoperative consultation is critical in the patient undergoing laparoscopic ventral herniorrhaphy. The procedure is painful and not much different from an open repair in terms of postoperative discomfort. The real benefit of the laparoscopic approach is the well-documented reduction in wound- and mesh-related infectious complications. The likelihood of postoperative seroma formation should be discussed. The need for conversion to an open repair and the possibility of an enterotomy should be considered as well. The anticipated options if an enterotomy occurs should be explained to include not repairing the hernia defect at all.
- Ventral hernias usually can be identified on physical exam, and no further work up is required. Computed tomography (CT) of the abdominal wall can be helpful in the patient who is morbidly obese, has a recurrent hernia (particularly with intraabdominal mesh), demonstrates a defect in proximity to a bony structure (i.e. suprapubic, subxiphoid, flank defects), or has concern for loss of domain.
- Patients who have previous failed attempts at repair can be difficult. The reasons for recurrence are usually not known, but certainly, efforts should be made not to repeat errors of the past. Every effort to obtain all operative reports that pertain to prior hernia repairs should be made. Before embarking on a recurrent defect, the surgeon should feel extremely confident with adhesiolysis and have a low threshold to convert to open. Patients who have had previous mesh infections that required removal of the prosthesis pose an extremely difficult challenge.
- The preoperative orders consist of antibiotic and deep venous thrombosis prophylaxis. A first-generation cephalosporin is typically given, and the dose is adjusted for the morbidly obese. Because the ventral hernia patient is frequently obese, will be immobile postoperatively, and will experience increased intraabdominal pressure from pneumoperitoneum, sequential compression devices and subcutaneous heparin are employed preoperatively.

3. Operative Steps

1. Patient Positioning

- For the majority of patients with defects in the midline, supine positioning with the arms tucked works well. The pressure points at the elbow and wrist should be padded (Fig. 2-2). For larger patients, the arm sleds may be required. In patients with defects off the midline or lumbar defects, a bump may be placed under the hip on the side of the hernia, or a true lateral position may be necessary with the aid of a bean bag.

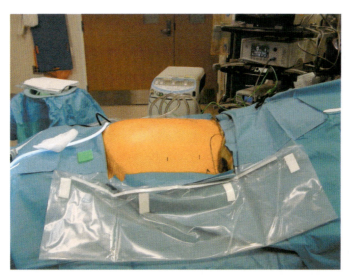

Figure 2-2.

- ▲ A Foley catheter is placed for bladder decompression and may be used to insufflate the bladder for identification in the repair of suprapubic defects. Gastric decompression is usually reserved for the patient requiring a difficult orotracheal intubation and may be achieved with orogastric tube decompression.
- ▲ An iodine-impregnated adhesive drape is applied to the skin of the prepped and draped patient. This protects the biomaterial from the patient's skin flora.

2. Gaining Abdominal Access

- ▲ Abdominal entry can be the most difficult step in the patient who has undergone multiple abdominal operations. Selecting the location for entry can be challenging because many of these patients have had numerous abdominal incisions. The upper quadrant at the tip of the eleventh rib is generally a safe place to gain access even in such cases. The side of entry should avoid previous incisions. For example, in the patient with an open cholecystectomy incision, the left upper quadrant should be chosen.
- ▲ Several safe methods for initial access have been described. A cut-down technique works very well. Through a small incision in the upper quadrant, each layer of the abdominal wall is divided down to the peritoneum. The peritoneum can be sharply entered with a scalpel or bluntly penetrated with the finger to gain safe access to the abdominal cavity. The optical trocar can be used safely in the upper quadrant just below the rib line as well. Some surgeons prefer the Veress needle. The best technique is the one the surgeon is most comfortable and familiar with.
- ▲ Once initial entry into the abdominal cavity is achieved, at least one and preferably two additional trocars are placed laterally on the side of entry. Typically one can be placed above the initial site once pneumoperitoneum has been initiated, and an additional one can be inserted inferiorly with care not to be too close to the iliac crest. Two trocars are placed on the opposite side to provide additional viewing perspective for adhesiolysis and aid in retraction (Fig. 2-3).

3. Adhesiolysis

- ▲ The Achilles' heel of the laparoscopic ventral hernia repair is the lysis of adhesions. This step can be the most time consuming and usually determines the length and complexity of the case.
- ▲ A 30-degree laparoscope is mandatory to adequately visualize the anterior abdominal wall. A 5-mm laparoscope provides more flexibility in moving the camera; however, if the visual clarity is poor, a 10-mm scope should be used.
- ▲ Energy sources should be avoided during adhesiolysis. Ultrasonic energy sources or bipolar coagulating shears should not be used. Thermal injuries seal at the time of dissection and may not be apparent for 3 to 5 days postoperatively. Sharp, cold, endoscopic scissor dissection should dominate the dissection. Blunt bowel graspers are crucial to aid in retraction of the viscera and can be used to provide gentle blunt dissection as well. Typically, during lysis of adhesions, the outer rind of adhesions may be sharply cut, giving way to a "cotton candy" appearance to the loose areolar tissue that comprises most of the adhesions (Fig. 2-4). Blunt dissection with gentle, short sweeps is very effective in this situation.

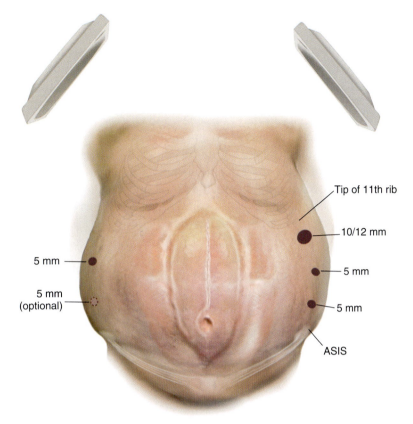

Figure 2-3.

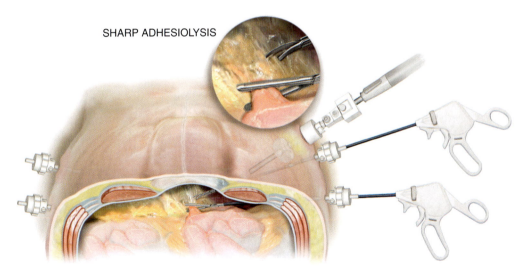

Figure 2-4.

- ▲ External pressure applied on the abdominal wall by the assistant provides help during adhesiolysis. This move can be critical in the morbidly obese patient or in the situation where adhesions are up in the hernia sac. By bringing the dissection into the abdomen with pressure, visualization of the proper tissue planes is made possible.
- ▲ Previous intraabdominal mesh can pose a real hazard to performing adhesiolysis. If the previous mesh contains a polypropylene or polyester component that becomes directly exposed to the bowel, there is not a plane of dissection. Attempts to mobilize the bowel off the adherent mesh will result in an enterotomy. In this situation, the mesh should be cut down off of the abdominal wall, leaving a swatch of prosthetic attached to the bowel (Fig. 2-5). Certainly, conversion to open is mandatory, if there is any concern for a bowel injury. Some cases of intense adhesion formation to the prosthetic may require a bowel resection.
- ▲ Bleeding during adhesiolysis can be very problematic. Slight oozing that typically occurs should be largely ignored. It rarely continues, and chasing it, especially with cautery, may lead to a bowel injury. If the area of oozing can be isolated from viscera, judicious monopolar cautery may be used. An oozing area of adipose tissue can be lifted away from underlying bowel and cauterized. Endoscopic hemoclip appliers can be extremely helpful in controlling bleeding in areas adjacent to bowel or where the location of bowel is unknown. Endoscopic pretied suture loops assist with bleeding sections of omentum or mesenteric fat. Be careful not to secure around a loop of bowel.
- ▲ Clearing the abdominal wall of all adhesions for the entire extent of the prior surgical incision is imperative. "Swiss cheese" defects not apparent preoperatively may become evident at this time. Extra time in this step is worthwhile to avoid the "early recurrence"—actually a defect missed at the initial repair.
- ▲ For defects above the umbilicus, the falciform ligament will have to be taken down to allow for flush placement of mesh against the abdominal wall. This move is best performed with electrocautery attached to the endoshears. The falciform is divided just below its insertion to the underside of the abdominal wall fascia.

4. Sizing the Hernia Defect

- ▲ Measuring the defect is a critical step in the procedure. Many times, particularly following a lengthy adhesiolysis, this step may not be given much attention. A durable repair relies on adequate mesh overlap with proper placement, which are both directly a result of accurately measuring the defect.
- ▲ The edges of the hernia defect are best delineated with the aid of 3.5-in, 20-gauge spinal needles placed at each edge of the defect. Insert the needle into the abdominal wall at a 90-degree angle to the floor, so the needle can emerge at the defect edge within the abdomen. Use a metric ruler to measure the vertical and horizontal dimensions of the defect between the needles. For multiple defects, place the needles to encompass all fascial defects, measuring them as one large defect.
- ▲ Three techniques have been described for measuring the defect: (1) externally with abdomen insufflated, (2) externally with abdomen desufflated, and (3) internally with abdomen insufflated. Because the mesh is being placed intracorporeally, it makes sense to make all measurements internally. The external measuring techniques overestimate the defect, which is more pronounced in larger defects and obese patients with thick anterior abdominal walls.
- ▲ Measure the defect internally under pneumoperitoneum. A plastic metric ruler is cut in half lengthwise and introduced via a 5-mm trocar. Two Maryland graspers manipulate the ruler and measure the defect between the spinal needles in the abdomen (Fig. 2-6). If the defect is longer than the ruler, insert another spinal needle along the axis of the defect within the length of the ruler. The sum of the two is the true measurement.

Chapter 2 • Laparoscopic Ventral Hernia Repair—Standard

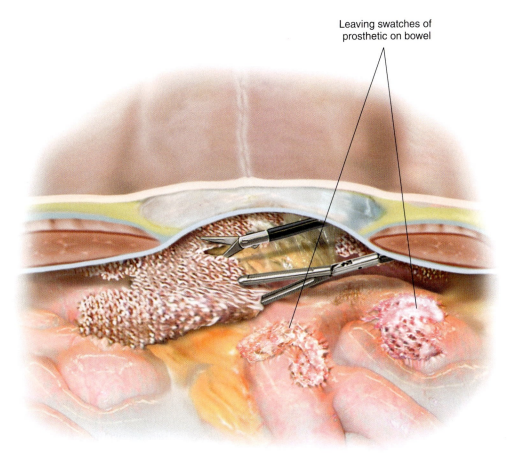

CUTTING DOWN PREVIOUS MESH

Figure 2-5.

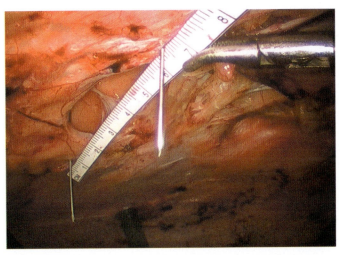

Figure 2-6.

5. Mesh Introduction and Orientation

- ▲ Not all hernia defects are perfectly circular, nor are they located exactly in the midline of the abdomen. In order to ensure that the mesh will be centered reliably over the defect every time, it is necessary to draw a grid of the x- and y-axes of the hernia defect on the external abdominal wall (Fig. 2-7).
- ▲ With a ruler outside the abdomen, measure the distance halfway between the most superior and most inferior spinal needle. This determines the x-axis, the horizontal midpoint of the hernia. Half the horizontal distance between the lateral most spinal needles marks the y-axis, or the vertical midpoint. Draw both axes on the skin with a permanent marker to grid the abdomen and mark the center of the hernia defect. Once the mesh is brought into the abdomen, any attempt to retrieve one of the vertical or lateral cardinal sutures should be done along the corresponding x- or y-axis line. This will align the mesh over the defect and ensure the most accurate placement to achieve desired overlap (Fig. 2-8).
- ▲ The type of mesh chosen for repair should have a favorable adhesion profile. Expanded polytetrafluoroethylene (ePTFE) has an excellent antiadhesion profile and works well for intraabdominal placement. Various absorbable barriers that coat polypropylene or polyester have been shown to provide reduction in adhesions as well. The infection profile of the biomaterial also should be considered.
- ▲ Before introducing the mesh into the abdomen, simply fold the sheet in half vertically and horizontally. Mark the midpoint of each mesh edge. Then place the cardinal sutures at the 4 midpoints, taking a 1-cm bite in from the edge. PTFE suture works well because it has less memory and recoil. Tuck in the tails of the cardinal sutures and roll the mesh from both ends toward the middle like a scroll along the horizontal axis.
- ▲ Once rolled, ePTFE mesh can be compressed and twisted to expunge air. Other tissue-separating meshes are soaked in saline and their slick texture makes them easier to introduce through a trocar. The rolled mesh may be passed directly through a 12-mm or 15-mm trocar (Fig. 2-9). Very large pieces of mesh can be dragged into the abdomen by passing

Chapter 2 • Laparoscopic Ventral Hernia Repair—Standard 31

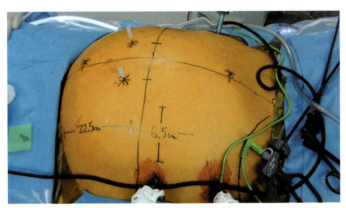

Figure 2-7.

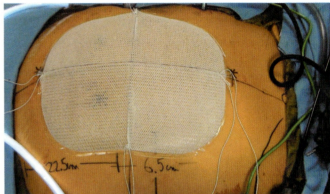

Figure 2-8.

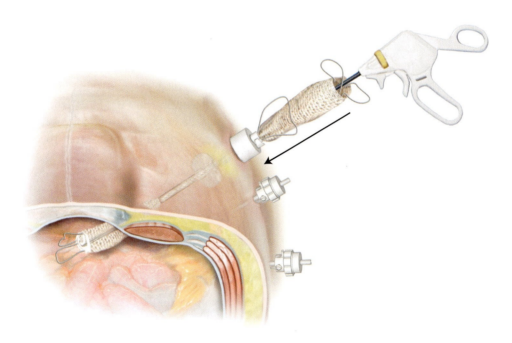

MESH ROLLED AROUND GRASPER AND
PASSED THROUGH 10+ MM TROCAR

Figure 2-9.

a heavy grasper across the abdomen through a 5-mm trocar and out the contralateral side trocar. The cap of the trocar is removed, and the mesh is pulled into the abdominal cavity (Fig. 2-10). Every effort should be made to introduce the mesh through the trocar. This maneuver avoids contact with the patient's skin.
▲ Once inside the abdominal cavity, the mesh is unfurled. A grasper holds one end of the rolled mesh while the Maryland grasper uncoils the mesh (Fig. 2-11). It is important to maintain the proper orientation of the mesh. It may be helpful with larger pieces to mark a line across the horizontal axis of the mesh before insertion to ensure that the line runs from side-to-side.

Chapter 2 • Laparoscopic Ventral Hernia Repair—Standard

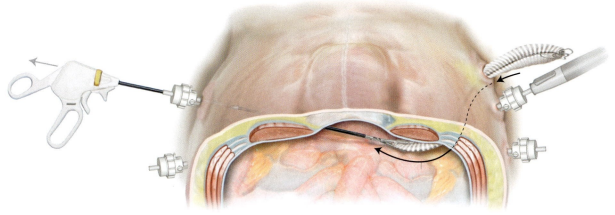

LARGE MESH PULLED THROUGH FROM CONTRALATERAL SIDE GRASPER

Figure 2-10.

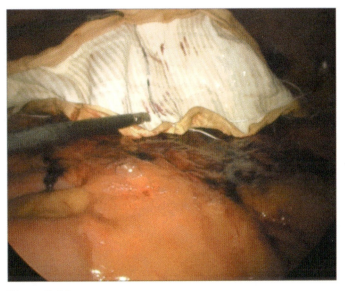

Figure 2-11.

6. Securing the Mesh

- ▲ After unrolling the mesh, retrieve the cardinal suture at the vertical site where there is the least amount adjustment first. For example, if the defect is in the lower abdomen, the inferior suture should be placed initially to avoid having to move its location caudally towards the bladder when stretching the mesh. Likewise, if the defect approximates the xiphoid, the superior suture is placed first. Mark the edge of the defect at the site of cardinal suture placement with the spinal needle. An additional spinal needle is "walked out" the axis line for a distance of 5-cm to ensure overlap (Fig. 2-12). This measured spot is injected with local anesthesia, and a stab incision is made through which the suture passer is introduced. The suture passer retrieves each tail of the initial cardinal suture through the same small incision but at a different angle to achieve a separate fascial bite. Tag both suture tails but leave them untied.
- ▲ Retrieve the lateral suture farthest from the camera. Measure a 5-cm overlap and mark the point for suture retrieval with an additional spinal needle placed along the x-axis. Bring this suture out of the abdomen, tag it, and leave it untied.
- ▲ The assistant pulls on the tagged sutures to bring the mesh against the abdominal wall. The surgeon pulls the site in the vertical axis that is free along the y-axis. Advance a spinal needle through the abdominal wall along the axis. This guides where the suture will be retrieved, ensuring the mesh will be taut (Fig. 2-13). During this maneuver, avoid grasping the suture or the knot as this can weaken it. Measuring the overlap at this point is unnecessary because most prosthetic meshes stretch.
- ▲ The three cardinal sutures are pulled up to approximate the mesh to the underside of the abdominal wall. If the mesh appears to be centered over the defect and is taut, the sutures are secured.

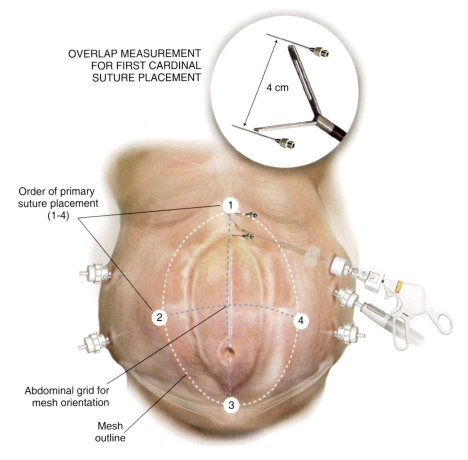

Figure 2-12.

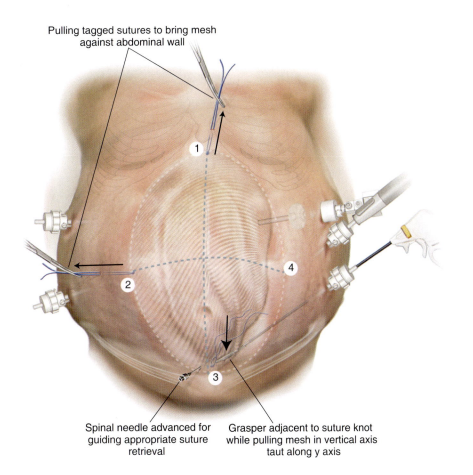

Figure 2-13.

▲ The mesh at the final suture site is grasped adjacent to the knot and stretched along the x-axis. A spinal needle passed along the x-axis marks the spot for final cardinal suture retrieval, just as was done when placing the third suture. The suture passer retrieves the suture tails, and they are secured. Placing a hemostat into the small skin incision and lifting it allows the knot to fall below Scarpa fascia and not dimple the skin (Fig. 2-14).

▲ Once the mesh is secured and overlap ensured, a tacking device is used to fixate the edges of the mesh circumferentially (Fig. 2-15). The purpose of the tacks is not to provide strength to the repair, but rather, to prevent bowel or mesenteric fat from creeping over the top of the mesh, exposing it to the ingrowth side. Fixation devices are both permanent and absorbable.

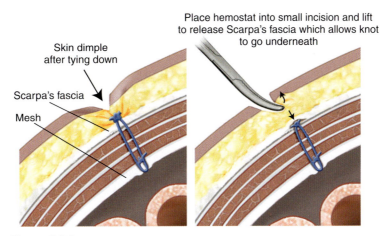

Figure 2-14.

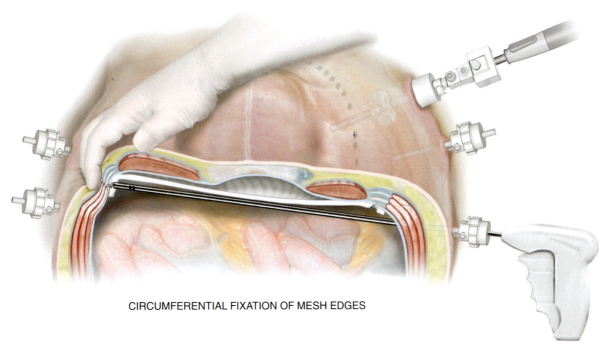

CIRCUMFERENTIAL FIXATION OF MESH EDGES

Figure 2-15.

- ▲ The strength of the repair is the transabdominal fixation that the permanent sutures provide. After tack fixation at the periphery of the mesh, additional permanent, monofilament sutures are placed every 5 to 7 cm around the circumference of the mesh (Fig. 2-16). Large defects require more frequent sutures; smaller, "Swiss cheese"–type defects may need fewer.
- ▲ Before completion of the case, one last inspection of the abdominal cavity is performed to rule out continued bleeding. The fascia at trocars larger than 5 mm should be closed with suture in this hernia-prone population. The skin at the trocar sites is closed with subcuticular stitches, followed by skin tapes or tissue cyanoacrylate.
- ▲ An abdominal binder may be placed for patient comfort. The role of binders in seroma reduction is unclear.

4. Postoperative Care

1. **Perioperative Concerns**

- ▲ Appropriate pain management is vital in the immediate postoperative period. Apart from the 2- to 3-cm umbilical defect or trocar-site hernia, all patients undergoing laparoscopic ventral herniorrhaphy are admitted. Patient-controlled analgesia is very effective, especially in the first 24 to 48 hours after surgery. Scheduled intravenous ketorolac is a useful adjunct.
- ▲ The postoperative diet depends on the degree of adhesiolysis. Following procedures where there is a lengthy lysis of adhesions or when bowel is densely involved, the patient is kept NPO. The diet may be advanced when abdominal distention has resolved, and the patient is without nausea.
- ▲ Hospitalization in the immediate postoperative period also allows the surgeon to monitor for any signs of missed enterotomy. There should always be an index of suspicion, particularly in difficult cases. Any unexplained tachycardia, leukocytosis, or persistent fever should be evaluated to rule out the presence of a bowel injury. Plane abdominal films or computed tomography can be used; however, if there is any concern, the patient should be returned to the operating room for diagnostic laparoscopy or laparotomy.

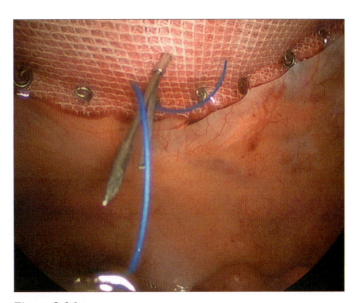

Figure 2-16.

2. Long-term Issues

- ▲ Nearly all patients undergoing laparoscopic ventral hernia repair develop some degree of seroma at the previous hernia site. Patients should be educated about this possibility in the preoperative evaluation. Seromas rarely, if ever, require drainage or aspiration. The risk of contaminating the mesh with drainage should be weighed against the benefits of relieving the fluid. Indications for aspiration include failure to resolve after 6 months, significant patient discomfort, or pressure on the skin causing excoriation or necrosis.
- ▲ Persistent pain can be seen beyond 6 weeks following laparoscopic ventral herniorrhaphy. The pain almost always occurs at suture sites. Patients describe a burning or pulling sensation with movement. These suture sites can be injected with 30 mL of a mixture of lidocaine and bupivacaine; however, this treatment is rarely required.
- ▲ Mesh infection is the bane of all hernia surgeons' existence. Fortunately, the incidence of mesh infection is low; however, the consequences are grave. The management of mesh contamination is extensive and many times requires mesh removal. In patients that present with erythema of the abdominal wall or delayed abdominal pain over the mesh, CT imaging of the abdomen should be obtained. Fluid collection above or deep to the prosthetic that contains air is a mesh infection and is treated as such. The fluid may be aspirated and sent for gram stain and culture. The mesh should be removed if it has a component of ePTFE. Attempts to salvage the prosthetic should involve open drainage of the fluid collection with negative pressure vacuum therapy. This maneuver may be successful with lightweight polypropylene materials but is less so with polyester-based materials.
- ▲ Follow-up in patients after laparoscopic ventral hernia repair has historically been very poor in the literature. The postoperative schedule should include appointments at 2 weeks, 6 weeks, 6 months, 1 year, and yearly thereafter. Ideally, hernia patients should be examined at least up to 1 year for complications of seroma, persistent pain, and recurrence.

5. Pearls/Pitfalls

- ▲ Patients with poor skin quality should not be offered a laparoscopic ventral hernia repair. Many times the adhesions to the underlying fat or viscera provide blood supply to the compromised skin. Skin loss may result postoperatively, leaving the mesh exposed.
- ▲ Leakage of gas at a trocar site or trocars that repeatedly fall out during a prolonged case can be quite frustrating. Replacing the leaking or loose trocar with a balloon-tipped trocar to reestablish a seal against the abdominal wall can save significant time and insufflation gas.
- ▲ For measuring large defects, an umbilical tape may be used internally. The tape is held at one of the needles and is stretched taut between the two points, marking the edge of the defect. The tape is brought out through the trocar and measured.
- ▲ One drawback to the laparoscopic repair of ventral hernias has been the inability to reapproximate the midline and reestablish a functional abdominal wall. Patient expectations should clearly be discussed preoperatively. In this instance, an open retrorectus mesh repair may be more beneficial. The ventral defect may be closed during a laparoscopic repair with transabdominal sutures. This technique is usually reserved for defects measuring less than 10 cm in width.
- ▲ Be cautious of the patient with a history of previous mesh infection! If the prosthetic was contaminated with methicillin-resistant *Staphylococcus aureus,* an open repair reinforced with a biologic or bioresorbable graft may be preferred. This approach may require a component separation to gain midline closure of the fascia.

Selected References

Carbonell AM, Harold KL, Mahmutovic AJ, et al: Local injection for the treatment of suture site pain after laparoscopic ventral hernia repair, *Am Surg* 69:688–691, 2003.
Cobb WS, Kercher KW, Heniford BT: Laparoscopic repair of incisional hernia, *Surg Clin N Am* 85(1):91–103, 2005.
Heniford BT, Park A, Ramshaw BJ, Voeller G: Laparoscopic repair of ventral hernias: nine years' experience with 850 consecutive hernias, *Ann Surg* 238:391–399, 2003.
Novitsky YW, Paton BL, Heniford BT: Laparoscopic ventral hernia repair. In Koltun W, editor: *Operative techniques in general surgery: techniques of laparoscopic hernia repair*, New York, 2006, Elsevier, Inc, Chapter 3, pp 4–9.
Rosen MJ: Polyester-based mesh for ventral hernia repair: is it safe? *Am J Surg* 197:353–359, 2009.
Stoppa RE: The treatment of complicated groin and incisional hernias, *World J Surg* 13:545–554, 1989.

CHAPTER 3

Laparoscopic Repair of Atypical Hernias: Suprapubic, Subxiphoid, and Lumbar

Benjamin K. Poulose, MD, MPH

1. Clinical Anatomy

▲ The laparoscopic repair of incisional hernias that occurs at the extremes of the abdomen either superiorly, inferiorly, or laterally can present many unique challenges to the surgeon. These hernias are often near major neurovascular or bony structures, making adequate overlap of mesh and fixation difficult. Typical locations for these types of hernias include the subxiphoid, suprapubic, or lumbar areas. These atypical hernias can often be approached and repaired laparoscopically with careful preoperative planning.

1. Suprapubic Hernia

▲ Correct and timely identification of the key structures in the lower anterior abdominal wall is critical for the safe laparoscopic repair of suprapubic hernias (Fig. 3-1). A careful preperitoneal dissection provides the needed landmarks for appropriate fixation to lessen the chance of postoperative recurrence.

2. Subxiphoid Hernia

▲ Identification of the costal margins and xiphoid process provide the laparoscopic bounds of transabdominal fixation for repair of subxiphoid hernias (Fig. 3-2). Generous overlap of the mesh over the diaphragm helps provide adequate coverage of the fascial defect in lieu of superior fixation.

Chapter 3 • Laparoscopic Repair of Atypical Hernias: Suprapubic, Subxiphoid, and Lumbar

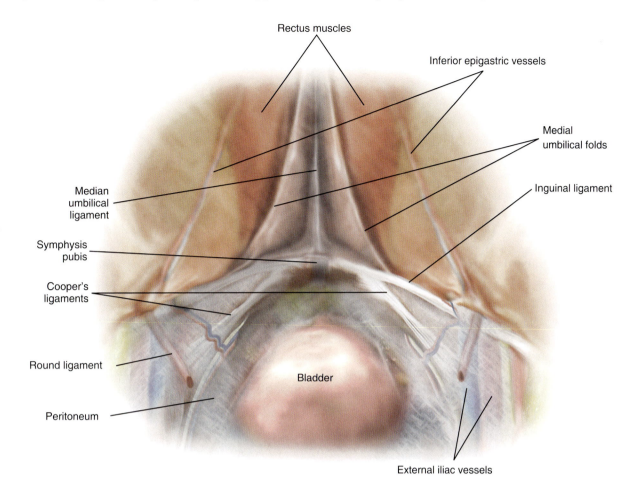

Figure 3-1.

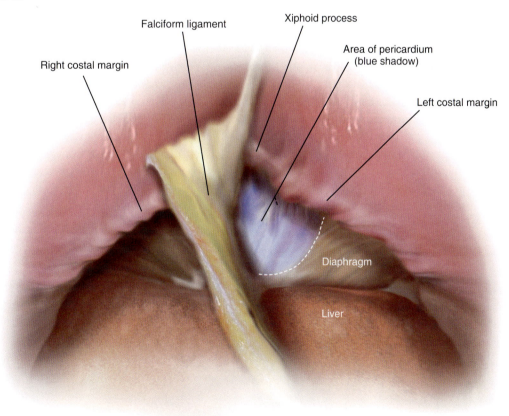

Figure 3-2.

3. Lumbar Hernia

▲ The lumbar triangle is defined superiorly and laterally by the latissimus dorsi muscle, medially by the external oblique muscle, and inferiorly by the iliac crest (Fig. 3-3). Weakness of the internal oblique and transversus abdominis musculature within the lumbar triangle leads to hernia formation (Fig. 3-4). An anterior abdominal approach can be used for laparoscopic repair, with proper patient positioning used to strategically expose the lumbar triangle.

2. Preoperative Considerations

1. Laparoscopic or Open Approach?

▲ The decision to proceed between a laparoscopic or open approach to atypical hernias rests on the surgeon's ability to estimate adequate coverage of the defect via laparoscopic approach and the candidacy of the patient for creation of a more physiologic repair via an open abdominal wall reconstruction. Relatively large fascial defects within 4 cm of the iliac crest are difficult to approach laparoscopically. Younger, active patients with sizable subxiphoid hernias may benefit from an open retrorectus or preperitoneal repair when dissection above the costal margins can be performed along with rectus medialization. Conversely, patients with smaller defects and those who may not tolerate an extensive abdominal wall reconstruction may benefit from a laparoscopic approach.

Chapter 3 • Laparoscopic Repair of Atypical Hernias: Suprapubic, Subxiphoid, and Lumbar

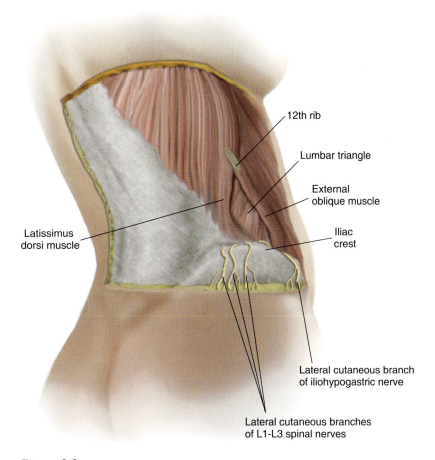

Figure 3-3.

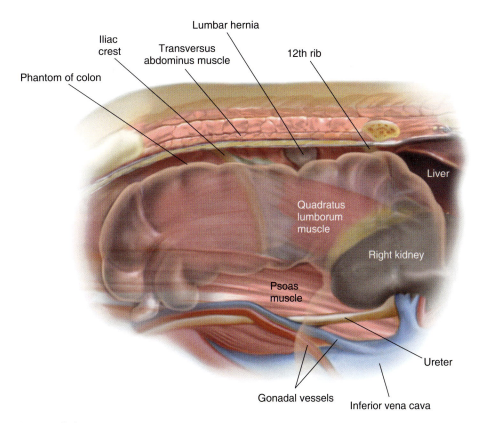

Figure 3-4.

2. Patient Positioning and Trocar Placement

▲ For laparoscopic suprapubic and subxiphoid hernia repairs, the patient is placed in the supine position, with arms tucked and carefully padded. Laparoscopic lumbar hernia repair often requires elevation of the ipsilateral side for posterior transabdominal fixation (Fig. 3-5). Usual trocar placement for laparoscopic ventral hernia repair should suffice for initial approach and lysis of adhesions (see Chapter 2, Fig. 2-3). These parts are placed more medially than usual on the contralateral side of the hernia defect. Access to the suprapubic region and myopectineal orifice is facilitated through three trocars at the level of the umbilicus; two are placed just lateral to the linea semilunaris, and one is placed at the umbilicus.

3. Special Considerations

▲ A three-way Foley catheter is placed before laparoscopic repair of suprapubic hernias to facilitate identification of the distended bladder during dissection.

Chapter 3 • Laparoscopic Repair of Atypical Hernias: Suprapubic, Subxiphoid, and Lumbar

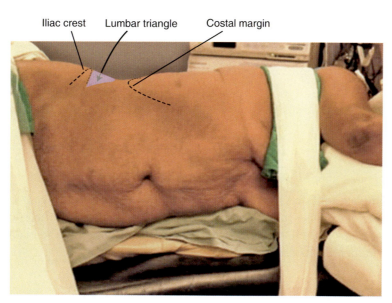

Figure 3-5.

3. Operative Steps

 1. Suprapubic

▲ After complete adhesiolysis and delineation of the hernia defect (Fig. 3-6), the relationship of the inferior extent of the hernia and the bladder is defined. The three-way Foley catheter is clamped and 300 mL of sterile normal saline is instilled into the bladder, distending it for ease in identification (Fig. 3-7).

Chapter 3 • Laparoscopic Repair of Atypical Hernias: Suprapubic, Subxiphoid, and Lumbar   49

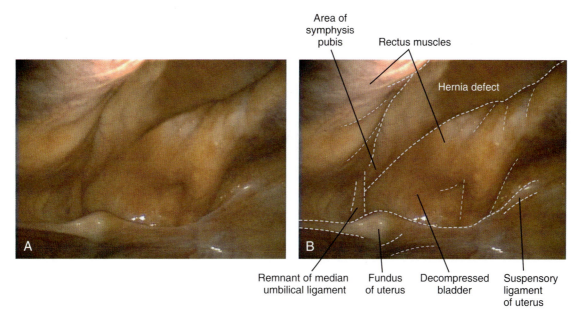

Figure 3-6.

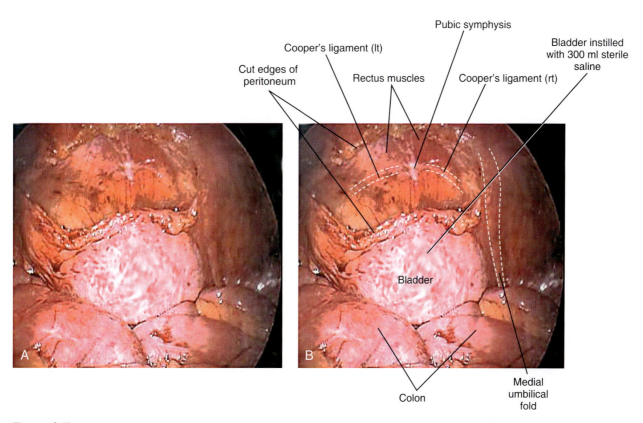

Figure 3-7.

▲ The inferior epigastric vessels are located on the opposite side of the operating surgeon and the preperitoneal space entered, mobilizing the flap medially. A preperitoneal tunnel is developed to identify Cooper's ligament. The preperitoneal space lateral to the inferior epigastric vessels is developed toward the iliopubic tract if needed. The peritoneum is then swept away from the inferior epigastric vessels, fully mobilizing the preperitoneal space on this side. A similar dissection is performed to expose the contralateral preperitoneal space. The bladder is then mobilized off the midline using electrosurgical current. The dissection is carried down to the pubis. Cooper's ligament is identified bilaterally, and the bladder is mobilized inferiorly into the space of Retzius. If the hernia abuts the pubis, it is important to mobilize the bladder sufficiently to allow several centimeters of mesh to be tucked under the pubis (Fig. 3-8).

Chapter 3 • Laparoscopic Repair of Atypical Hernias: Suprapubic, Subxiphoid, and Lumbar

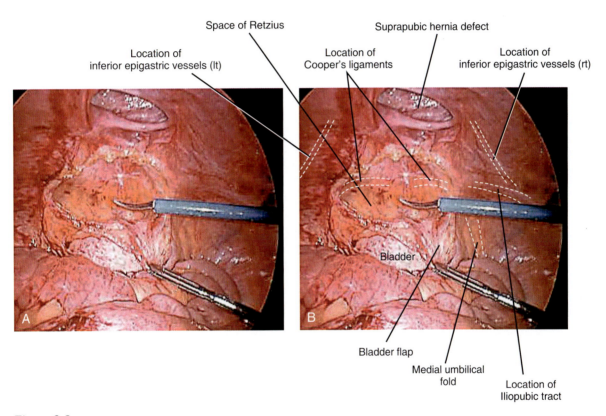

Figure 3-8.

▲ The mesh is fixated to Cooper's ligament bilaterally using tacks in addition to suprapubic transabdominal suture fixation (Figs. 3-9 and 3-10). If the defect is close to the pubis, the inferior transfascial suture is placed several centimeters off the edge of the mesh. In doing so, the surgeon is able to bring the suture adjacent to the pubic bone, and the mesh drapes several centimeters inferiorly for adequate overlap. When applying tacks to the lower abdominal wall, it is important to confirm bimanual palpation of the tip of the tacker externally. This ensures the tack is placed above the iliopubic tract and avoids major neurovascular injuries. If there is excess mesh below the iliopubic tract that cannot be secured with tacks, we occasionally apply fibrin sealant to secure the inferior edge of the mesh over the iliac vessels.

Chapter 3 • Laparoscopic Repair of Atypical Hernias: Suprapubic, Subxiphoid, and Lumbar

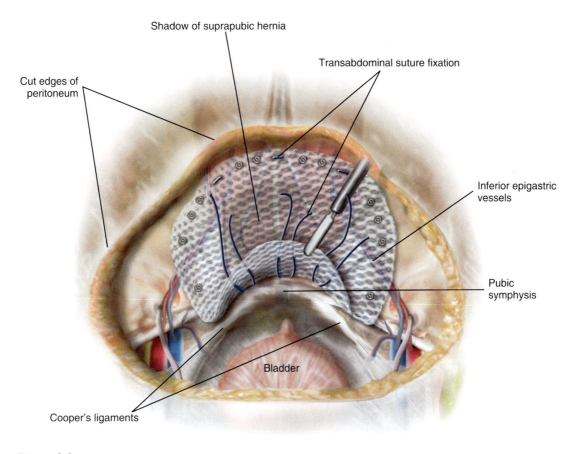

Figure 3-9.

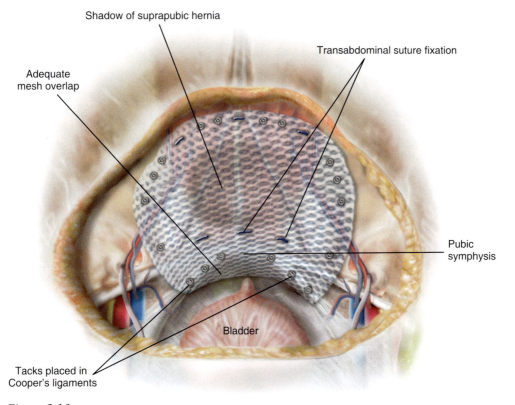

Figure 3-10.

2. Subxiphoid

- ▲ Space is created for cephalad overlap of the defect by dividing the falciform ligament toward the diaphragm. This often can be done with electrosurgical current; however, meticulous hemostasis should be confirmed at the conclusion of this step (Figs. 3-11 and 3-12).
- ▲ The mesh is fixated just below the costal margins bilaterally and allowed to drape generously over the diaphragm (Fig. 3-13). If the defect abuts the xiphoid process, adequate overlap can be challenging. We do not suture around ribs because of the risk of severe chronic pain, nor do we advocate placing tacks above the costal margin because of the risk of pericardial injury. In order to achieve adequate overlap, the cephalad suture can be placed several centimeters off the edge of the mesh (Fig. 3-14). The extra mesh is allowed to drape over the diaphragm. Typically this mesh doesn't require fixation because the liver will hold it in place; however, if the surgeon is concerned, applying fibrin sealant to the diaphragm can help secure the mesh.

 3. Lumbar

- ▲ The surgeon must be comfortable with retroperitoneal exposure. In order to gain adequate posterior coverage of the defect with the mesh, the colon must be mobilized medially. Careful identification of the ureter is paramount to safe fixation of the mesh. We prefer to clearly identify the psoas muscle. Once the psoas muscle is identified and the ureters delineated, the dissection stops and any major vascular structures are avoided (Figs. 3-15 and 3-16).

Chapter 3 • Laparoscopic Repair of Atypical Hernias: Suprapubic, Subxiphoid, and Lumbar   55

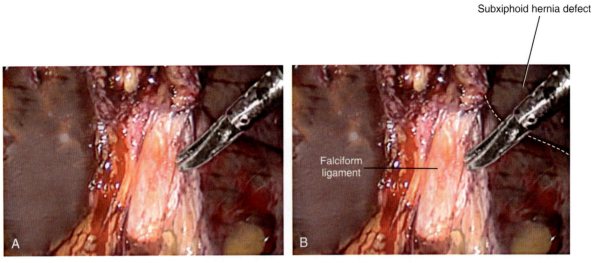

Figure 3-11.

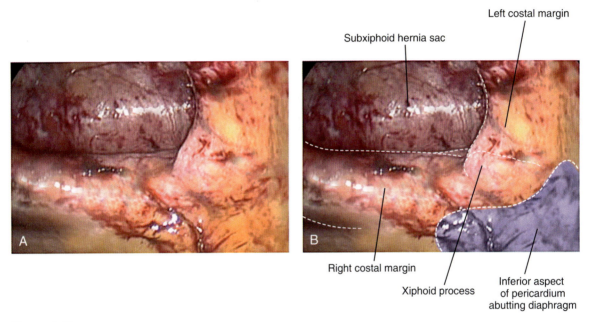

Figure 3-12.

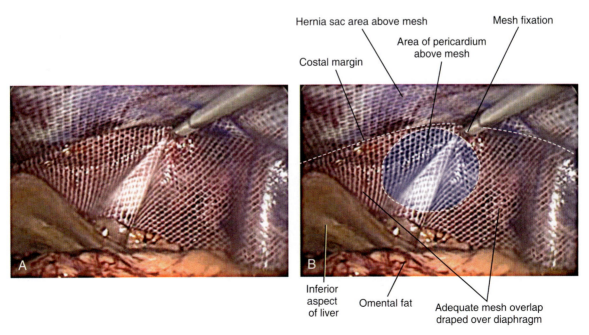

Figure 3-13.

56   Section II • Laparoscopic Repairs

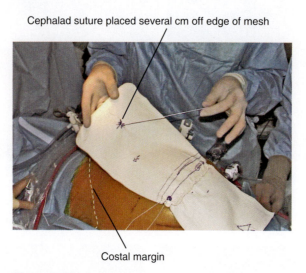

Figure 3-14.

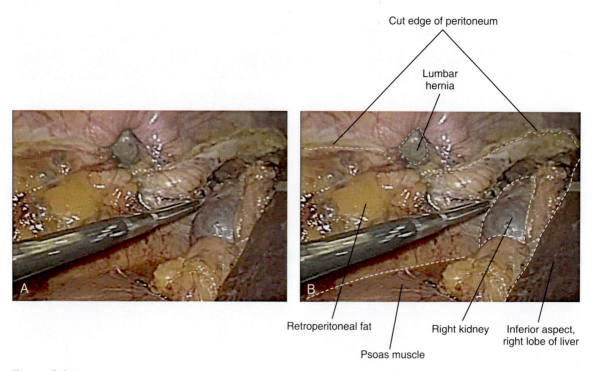

Figure 3-15.

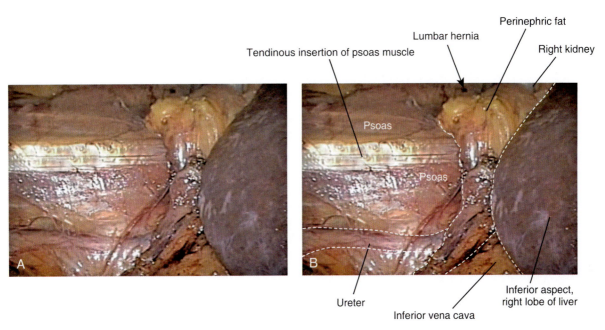

Figure 3-16.

▲ Space must be left for transabdominal fixation sutures to secure the mesh. Fixation to the iliac crest is usually not necessary if adequate inferior overlap is obtained (Fig. 3-17).

4. Postoperative Care

1. Immediate Postoperative Management

▲ In general, patients are allowed a clear liquid diet that is advanced as bowel function returns. Ambulation is begun on the night of operation with aggressive efforts at pulmonary toilet. An appropriately sized abdominal binder is employed to help minimize the formation of large seromas.

5. Pearls/Pitfalls

▲ Patients must understand the potential risks associated with these repairs. A complete discussion of the potential outcomes and management strategies for any neurovascular injury is paramount.

▲ The decision to mobilize the preperitoneal space in the laparoscopic repair of suprapubic hernias should be made preoperatively to ensure that adequate equipment and expertise are available for success. Unlike mobilization of the preperitoneal space during laparoscopic transabdominal preperitoneal inguinal hernia repair, this maneuver can be very difficult in the repair of suprapubic hernias. Often, this space has been entered multiple times because of lower abdominal or pelvic operations. This dissection can often be facilitated by developing the preperitoneal space on the medial aspect of the separated rectus muscles within the hernia sac.

▲ Atypical hernias often involve nearby bony structures in close proximity to the hernia defect (pubic bone, xiphoid process, iliac crest). When selecting the appropriately sized mesh, it is paramount to incorporate extra overlap beyond that included for transabdominal suture fixation. This allows additional overlap over difficult areas where fixation is impossible or ill-advised.

▲ One of the most common reasons for failure after repair of an atypical hernia is lack of mesh overlap. Regardless of the approach (laparoscopic or open), the surgeon should rely heavily on mesh overlap and not mesh fixation. Any mesh fixated to the edge of the defect will likely contract over time and eventually dissociate from any bony structure. Therefore, the true key to repairing an atypical hernia is the comfort in gaining appropriate lateral and inferior dissection planes to afford mesh overlap.

Selected References

Losanoff JE, Basson MD, Laker S, Weiner M, Webber JD, Gruber SA: Subxiphoid incisional hernias after median sternotomy, *Hernia* 11:473–479, 2007.

Varnell B, Bachman S, Quick J, Vitamvas M, Ramshaw B, Oleynikov D: Morbidity associated with laparoscopic repair of suprapubic hernias, *American Journal of Surgery* 196:983–987, 2008:discussion 987-988.

Yavuz N, Ersoy YE, Demirkesen O, Tortum OB, Erguney S: Laparoscopic incisional lumbar hernia repair, *Hernia* 13:281–286, 2009.

Chapter 3 • Laparoscopic Repair of Atypical Hernias: Suprapubic, Subxiphoid, and Lumbar

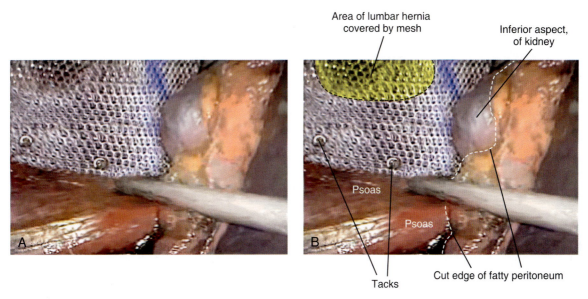

Figure 3-17.

CHAPTER 4

Laparoscopic Repair of Parastomal Hernias

Alan A. Saber, MD, FACS

1. Clinical Anatomy

1. Types of Parastomal Hernias

Parastomal hernia has been anatomically classified into four subtypes: (Fig. 4-1)
1. Subcutaneous: The hernia sac goes alongside the stoma into the subcutaneous tissue. This is the most common type of paracolostomy hernia.
2. Interstitial: The hernia sac is within the layers of the abdominal wall. This hernia is at a high risk for strangulation.
3. Peristomal: The bowel prolapses through a circumferential hernia sac enclosing the stoma.
4. Intrastomal: The hernia sac is between the intestinal wall and the everted intestinal layer.

2. Characteristics of the Facial Defect

▲ Most hernia defects are lateral to the rectus abdominis muscle, alongside the mesentery of the emerging bowel, and medially and cranially to the stoma loop.
▲ Commonly the parastomal hernia sac is very large with a relatively small fascial defect.

2. Preoperative Considerations

▲ The life expectancy of the patient and any predisposing factors, such as malignancy and obesity, should influence the decision to proceed with surgery.
▲ Accurate diagnosis and assessment of the anatomy of the hernia are essential. This is done with clinical examination, or more accurately, with a computed tomography (CT) scan.
▲ CT scan is useful to delineate parastomal defects, any associated incisional hernia, and the content of the hernia (Fig. 4-2).

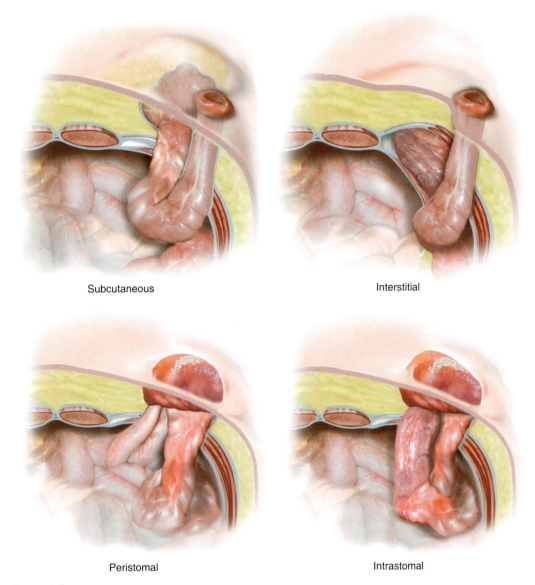

Figure 4-1.

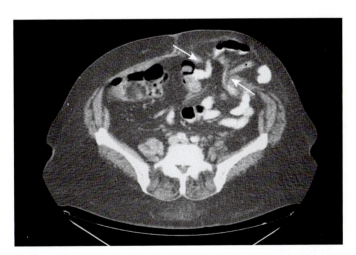

Figure 4-2.

- ▲ A preoperative bowel preparation may diminish the risk of infection if there is a colonic injury during laparoscopy.
- ▲ Intravenous prophylactic antibiotic therapy covering both skin and intestinal flora is initiated.
- ▲ A large Foley catheter may be inserted into the stoma to facilitate location of the bowel intraoperatively.
- ▲ Seal the skin and stoma from the operative field with adhesive plastic drapes after preparing the skin.

3. Operative Steps

There are two techniques for laparoscopic repairs of parastomal hernias: the keyhole and the Sugarbaker techniques. Keyhole technique may be associated with bowel herniation between the mesh hole and the stoma loop. We have developed a technique that closes the gap between the mesh and the stoma loop and facilitates intracorporeal mesh manipulations (Scroll technique) during keyhole repairs. The Sugarbaker technique avoids the risk of herniation through the keyhole, but it does create an acute angle as the bowel exits the mesh and can cause obstruction (see Fig. 4-11). Meticulous attention to the details of mesh fixation and placement can limit these complications.

 1. Laparoscopic Parastomal Hernia Repair Technique: The Scroll Technique

- ▲ *Operating Room Setup (Fig. 4-3)*

  - ▲ The patient is placed in the supine position with the arms extended laterally.
  - ▲ The surgeon and the assistant stand contralateral to the stoma site.
  - ▲ General anesthesia is administered.
  - ▲ The abdomen is prepared and draped, including the colostomy, in standard fashion; the stoma is covered with transparent adhesive drapes. Placement of a Foley catheter in the stoma is optional.

- ▲ *Trocar Placement (Fig. 4-4)*

  - ▲ For a left lower quadrant stoma, an initial 12-mm Hasson trocar is placed in the right upper quadrant away from the hernia defect.
  - ▲ Initial diagnostic laparoscopy usually reveals abdominal adhesions and the parastomal hernia.
  - ▲ Under direct vision, two 5-mm trocars are inserted into the right lower quadrant.
  - ▲ All the trocars are placed away from the hernia defect to facilitate surgical manipulation.

Chapter 4 • Laparoscopic Repair of Parastomal Hernias 63

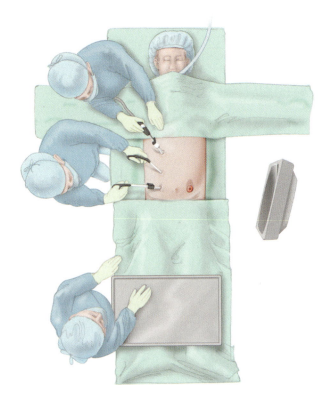

Figure 4-3.

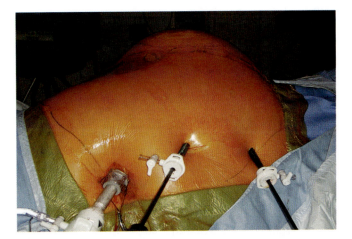

Figure 4-4.

▲ **Lysis of Adhesions**

  ▲ Lysis of adhesions is the most challenging part of this procedure; this is performed using sharp or blunt dissection as close as possible to the anterior abdominal wall.
  ▲ An energy source can be used only after ensuring no bowel is nearby to avoid lateral thermal injury.
  ▲ The hernia contents are reduced by a combination of external pressure and internal traction.
  ▲ One of the most challenging aspects of this type of laparoscopic repair is that one loop of bowel must remain on the abdominal wall. This can be difficult to differentiate with laparoscopic visualization. As mentioned, a Foley catheter, or occasionally, intraoperative endoscopy can guide the surgeon.
  ▲ The hernia margins are demarcated and measured, either extracorporeally or preferably intracorporeally, to determine the size of the mesh that would allow 5 cm of overlap circumferentially.

▲ **Mesh Choice and Preparation (Figs. 4-5 and 4-6)**

  ▲ We typically use ePTFE mesh (Dualmesh Plus, W.L. Gore). The lack of ingrowth on the peritoneal side is particularly advantageous when placing prosthetic mesh around the bowel.

▲ **Keyhole Technique**

  ▲ The mesh is fashioned by creating a 3 × 3 cm cruciate cut at the junction of two thirds and one third of the mesh (see Fig. 4-5).
  ▲ A split is made from the defect to the edge of the mesh.
  ▲ Long CV-0 nonabsorbable sutures are placed at each corner of the mesh and tied.
  ▲ The sutures are tied with the knot toward the rough surface of the mesh.
  ▲ The mesh is rolled tightly from each side to the middle like a scroll so that the rough surface of the mesh faces outward with sutures inside the rolled mesh. 2-0 Vicryl stay sutures are placed around the rolled mesh to keep it rolled tightly (Fig. 4-6).
  ▲ The rolled mesh is placed into the abdominal cavity through the 12-mm Hasson trocar; this will avoid mesh contamination from the skin.

Chapter 4 • Laparoscopic Repair of Parastomal Hernias 65

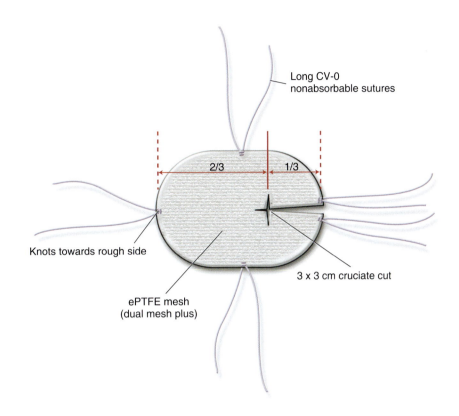

Figure 4-5.

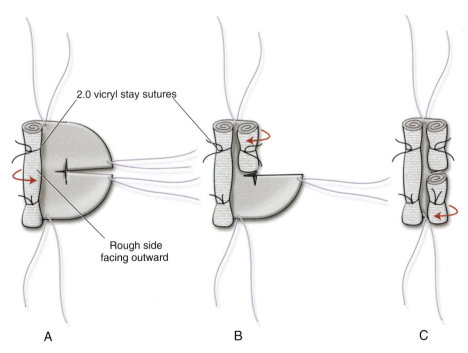

Figure 4-6.

▲ **Mesh Fixation**

- ▲ Once the mesh is inside the abdominal cavity, the two transfascial sutures at the sides of the mesh are pulled through the abdominal wall with the suture passer. This will bring the rolled mesh adherent to the abdominal wall, centering it over the defect with the mesh split toward the colostomy side (Fig. 4-7).
- ▲ Care must be taken that the rough surface faces the anterior abdominal wall and the smooth surface faces the viscera.
- ▲ The transabdominal sutures are tied. The Vicryl stay suture is cut, and the upper half of the mesh is unfolded (Fig. 4-8).
- ▲ By using a suture passer, the superior suture is pulled through the abdominal wall.
- ▲ Next, 5-mm hernia tacks are placed circumferentially, 1 cm from the edge of the mesh and 1 to 2 cm apart.

Chapter 4 • Laparoscopic Repair of Parastomal Hernias 67

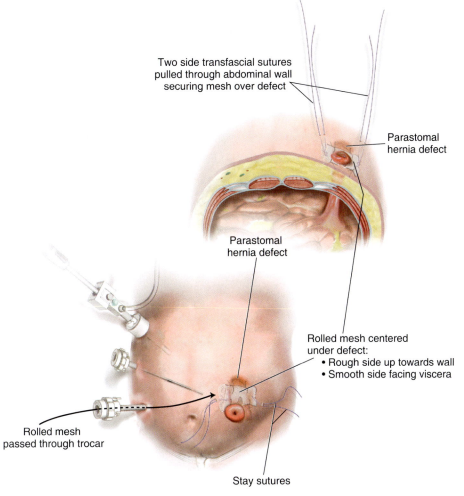

Figure 4-7.

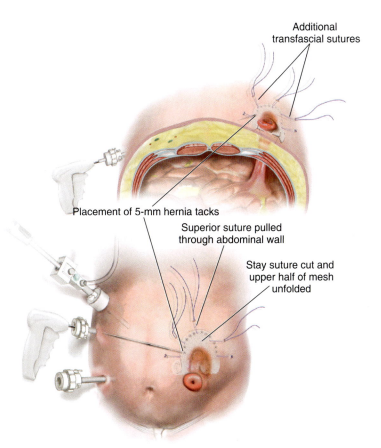

Figure 4-8.

- ▲ The same procedure is repeated on the other half of the mesh (Fig. 4-9), cutting the Vicryl stay suture and spreading each part of the lower portion of the mesh individually. The mesh portions are fixed using transabdominal sutures and 5-mm hernia tacks.
- ▲ After the mesh is secured properly to the abdominal wall, the gaps between the colostomy and the cruciate defect in the mesh are closed with interrupted 2-0 nonabsorbable sutures securing the mesh to the seromuscular layer of the colostomy loop.
- ▲ This will form a collar around the colostomy, eliminating potential spaces for future recurrence.
- ▲ Additional transfascial sutures are placed circumferentially at 5-cm intervals to augment long-term stability.
- ▲ At the completion of the procedure, the mesh covers the entire hernia defect with 5 cm of overlap while the mesh defect hosts the colostomy loop without restriction (Fig. 4-10).

Chapter 4 • Laparoscopic Repair of Parastomal Hernias 69

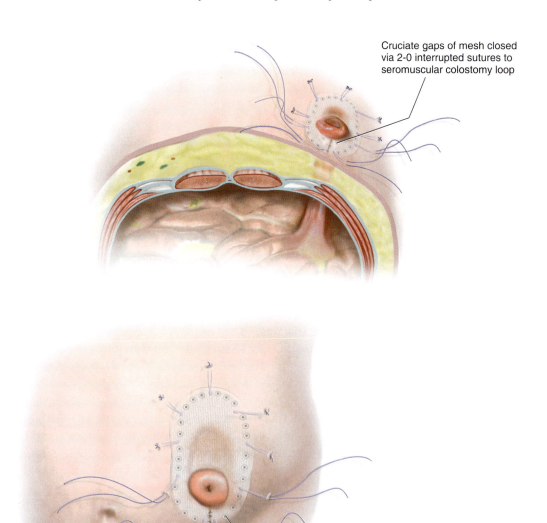

Figure 4-9.

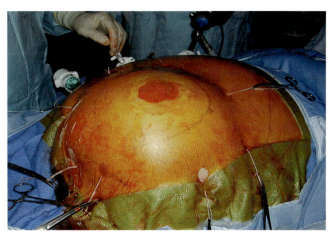

Figure 4-10.

2. Laparoscopic Sugarbaker Technique (Fig. 4-11)

- ▲ The laparoscopic Sugarbaker technique involves placing a flat sheet of mesh on the abdominal wall and lateralizing the stoma's loop of bowel. In order to perform this procedure, the bowel must have sufficient mobilization to allow it to be displaced laterally without excessive kinking. Occasionally, ileal conduit hernias cannot be lateralized because of the posterior fixation of the ureters.
- ▲ Once the defect is measured, an appropriately sized piece of mesh is designed to provide at least 5 cm of overlap.
- ▲ We typically suture the bowel to the lateral abdominal wall before bringing in the mesh. This allows the surgeon to see the angle of the bowel before being obscured by the prosthesis. Additionally it confirms that there is not too much tension on the bowel as it makes this angle and avoids the mesh acting as a sling on the bowel wall that is not secured to the abdominal wall.
- ▲ Placing the four cardinal transfascial sutures at each corner of the mesh aids in mesh positioning (see Fig. 4-11).
- ▲ The mesh is brought into the abdominal cavity through a trocar and unrolled.
- ▲ The inferior lateral suture is retrieved first, after 5 cm of overlap is measured. Given the typical lower lateral location of most stomas on the abdominal wall, it is important to retrieve this suture first, since you will often be limited by the major neurovascular structures of the pelvis.
- ▲ The superior lateral suture is subsequently retrieved. These sutures are then tightened on the abdominal wall. The surgeon can then see over the mesh and confirm that the bowel is not being too acutely angled as it exits the mesh.
- ▲ The remaining two sutures are then stretched out across the abdominal wall and secured.
- ▲ A tacking device is then used to secure the mesh to the anterior abdominal wall every 1 cm. When placing tacks next to the stoma site, great care must be used to avoid injuring or obstructing the lumen. There is no exact measurement to allow the surgeon to confirm appropriate mesh and bowel placement, and great care should be used. Because the mesh is placed during full insufflation, it is likely that as the abdomen is desufflated the mesh will loosen a bit.

4. Postoperative Care

- ▲ Use appropriate stoma care.
- ▲ Patients are allowed a liquid diet that is advanced as tolerated, although some degree of postoperative ileus may follow, depending on the operative trauma.
- ▲ There are no restrictions of activity.
- ▲ Abdominal binders aid in the management of postoperative pain and in the preventing of seromas.

Chapter 4 • Laparoscopic Repair of Parastomal Hernias

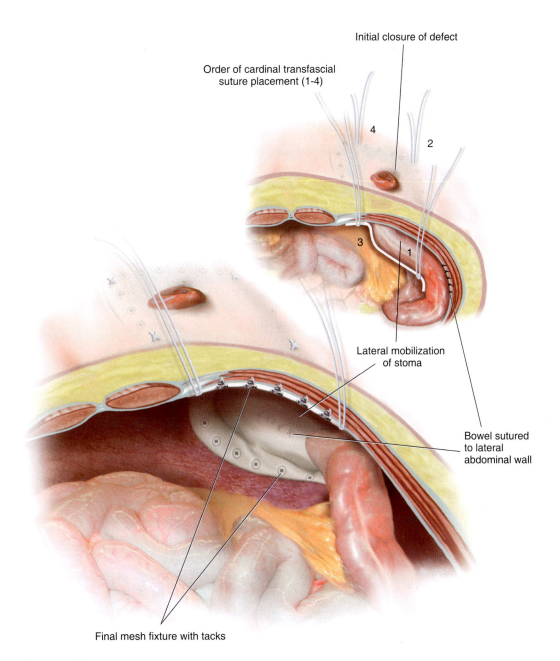

Figure 4-11.

5. Pearls/Pitfalls

- ▲ When dealing with parastomal hernias, we need to repair the hernia while maintaining the defect in the abdominal wall for the colostomy loop to pass without obstruction.
- ▲ Scroll technique facilitates intracorporeal mesh manipulation, maintains precise orientation of the mesh in relation to the hernia defect, and allows secure fixation of the mesh to the anterior abdominal wall.
- ▲ The rolled mesh is placed through the 12-mm Hasson trocar into the abdominal cavity; this will avoid mesh contamination from the skin.
- ▲ The fundamental components of a sound hernia repair of wide mesh overlap of the defect and transabdominal sutures are used.
- ▲ Full-thickness nonabsorbable sutures are crucial for long-term stability of the mesh to the abdominal wall while the 5-mm tacks close the gaps between the abdominal wall and the mesh, thereby preventing incarceration of a loop of bowel between the mesh and the abdominal wall.
- ▲ The laparoscopic approach visualizes the entire abdominal wall, thus detecting any impalpable hernia defect that also may be repaired at the same time.
- ▲ Large midline defects in addition to parastomal hernias can be very challenging to simultaneously repair, and occasionally, an open approach or the use of two meshes laparoscopically is warranted.
- ▲ Suture closure of the hernia defect and reinforcement with the mesh is an optional maneuver that adds security to the mesh repair. However, this may create a tension repair that may necessitate a concomitant component separation.
- ▲ These are challenging hernias to repair in a challenging patient population, and all techniques have a potential risk for complication and recurrence, mandating appropriate preoperative counseling.

Selected References

Berger D, Bientzle M: Laparoscopic repair of parastomal hernias: a single surgeon's experience in 66 patients, *Dis Colon Rectum* 50(10):1668–1673, 2007 Oct.

Craft RO, Huguet KL, McLemore EC, Harold KL: Laparoscopic parastomal hernia repair, *Hernia* 12(2):137–140, 2008 Apr.

Hansson BM, Bleichrodt RP, de Hingh IH: Laparoscopic parastomal hernia repair using a keyhole technique results in a high recurrence rate, *Surg Endosc* 23(7):1456–1459, 2009 Jul.

Muysoms EE, Hauters PJ, Van Nieuwenhove Y, Huten N, Claeys DA: Laparoscopic repair of parastomal hernias: a multi-centre retrospective review and shift in technique, *Acta Chir Belg* 108(4):400–404, 2008 Jul-Aug.

Muysoms F: Laparoscopic repair of parastomal hernias with a modified Sugarbaker technique, *Acta Chir Belg* 107(4):476–480, 2007 Jul-Aug.

Saber AA, Rao AJ, Rao CA, Elgamal MH: Simplified laparoscopic parastomal hernia repair: the scroll technique, *Am J Surg* 196(3):16–18, 2008 Sep.

SECTION III

Open Repairs

Open Retromuscular Ventral Hernia Repair

Yuri W. Novitsky, MD, FACS

1. Clinical Anatomy

- ▲ Retrorectus repair requires a thorough knowledge of the relative anatomy of the myofascial components of the abdominal wall.
- ▲ The rectus abdominis, a long, broad, strap-like muscle, is the principal vertical muscle of the anterior abdominal wall. Its origin is at the pubic symphysis and pubic crest. The muscle is inserted into the cartilages of the fifth, sixth, and seventh ribs. The rectus abdominis is three times as wide superiorly as it is inferiorly.
- ▲ The rectus abdominis is innervated by the thoracoabdominal nerves T7-T12. The main trunks of the intercostal nerves pass anteriorly from the intercostal spaces and run between the internal oblique and transversus abdominis muscles in a so-called neurovascular plane. The inferior intercostal, subcostal, and lumbar arteries accompany the nerves of this plane.
- ▲ In addition, the lateral cutaneous nerve branch of T12, as well as the ilioinguinal and iliohypogastric both enter the space between the internal oblique and transversus abdominis via the lateral border of the transversus muscle. These nerves, along with the ventral primary rami of the inferior six thoracoabdominal nerves (T7-11) innervate the anterolateral abdominal wall skin and musculature.
- ▲ The rectus sheath is the strong, incomplete fibrous compartment for the rectus abdominis muscle. It forms by the fusion and separation of the aponeurosis of the lateral abdominal muscles.
- ▲ At its lateral margin, the internal oblique aponeurosis splits into two layers, one passing anterior to the rectus muscle and the other passing posterior to it. The posterior layer joins with the aponeurosis of the transverse abdominis muscle to form the posterior wall of the rectus sheath. Muscle fibers of the transversus abdominis end in an aponeurosis, which contributes to the formation of the rectus sheath.
- ▲ The lateral abdominal wall consists of three flat muscles: external oblique, internal oblique, and transversus abdominis. The flat muscles cross each other similar to a three-ply corset that strengthens the abdominal wall and diminishes the risk of herniation between the muscle bundles. One important consideration for the retrorectus repair is the fact that in the upper third of the abdomen, the transversus abdominis extends medially beyond the overlying linea semilunaris as a primary muscular component not as fascia (Fig. 5-1).

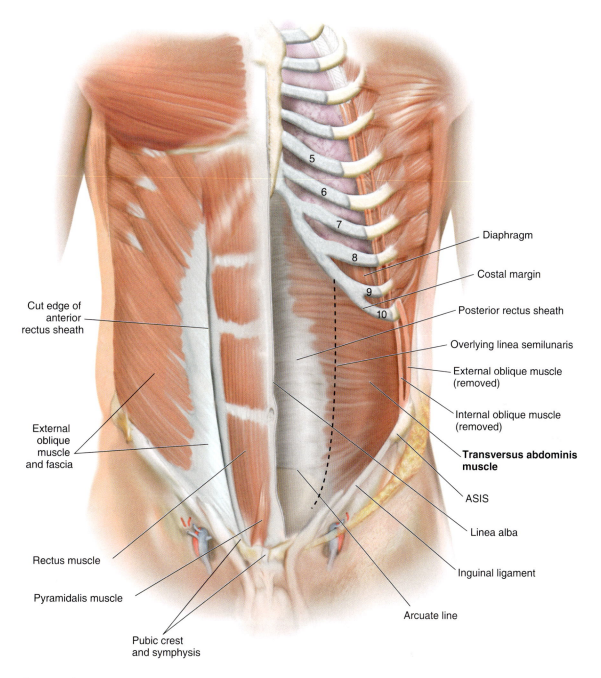

Figure 5-1.

2. Preoperative Considerations

▲ *Preoperative Imaging*

   ▲ I recommend routine abdominal/pelvic computed tomography (CT) imaging. CT delineates all abdominal wall defects, assessment of the integrity of the remaining abdominal wall musculature, allows for detection of previous synthetic meshes and/or occult infection, and facilitates perioperative planning. I also mandate a screening colonoscopy in appropriate patients before undertaking major abdominal wall reconstructions.

▲ *Preoperative Optimization*

   ▲ Nutritional evaluation and counseling for obese patients is paramount, and weight loss surgery should be considered.
   ▲ Smoking cessation is mandatory
   ▲ Cardiac and pulmonary status should be assessed and optimized.

▲ *Choosing the Type of Mesh*

- ▲ Use a large, synthetic mesh with or without an antiadhesive barrier. I prefer a large (30 × 30 cm) macroporous, reduced-weight polypropylene mesh.
- ▲ Composite synthetic mesh with an antiadhesive barrier may need to be used if visceral exposure through fenestrations in the posterior layer is possible/likely.
- ▲ Biologic or biodegradable mesh should be considered in all contaminated and potentially contaminated fields. Synthetic mesh should be avoided in patients with a previous history of mesh infection, especially methicillin-resistant *Staphyloccus aureus* (MRSA). In addition, biologic meshes should be considered in patients with multiple comorbidities (morbid obesity, diabetes, systemic steroids or other form of immunosuppression, etc) and resultant increased risks of wound/mesh infections.

3. Operative Steps

▲ *Planning Incision*

- ▲ A generous midline laparotomy is required.
- ▲ Elliptical incisions are used to incorporate previous scars, skin ulcerations, and/or defects. For most, and especially morbidly obese, patients with large midline hernias, I recommend excision of the umbilicus to minimize postoperative wound morbidity.
- ▲ Use an inverse "T" incision, if panniculectomy is contemplated.

▲ *Lysis of Adhesions, Removal of Old Mesh*

- ▲ Complete lysis of all visceral adhesions to the anterior abdominal and pelvic walls is performed. This is particularly important in cases where dissection lateral to the linea semilunaris is undertaken. Inter-loop adhesions are typically ignored.
- ▲ If possible, complete excision of all previously placed mesh is performed.

▲ *Incision of the Posterior Rectus Sheath (Rives-Stoppa-Wantz Technique)*

- ▲ To dissect the retromuscular space to the linea semilunaris, the posterior rectus sheath is incised sharply about 0.5 cm from its edge (Fig. 5-2, *A*). This typically is initiated at the level of the umbilicus. The retromuscular plane is then developed using a combination of blunt dissection and electrocautery. The lateral extent of this dissection is the linea semilunaris, confirmed by visualizing the junction between the posterior and anterior rectus sheaths (Fig. 5-2, *B*). Careful identification of the intercostal nerves and vessels is critical to maintaining an innervated functional abdominal wall (Fig. 5-2, *C*).

Chapter 5 • Open Retromuscular Ventral Hernia Repair 79

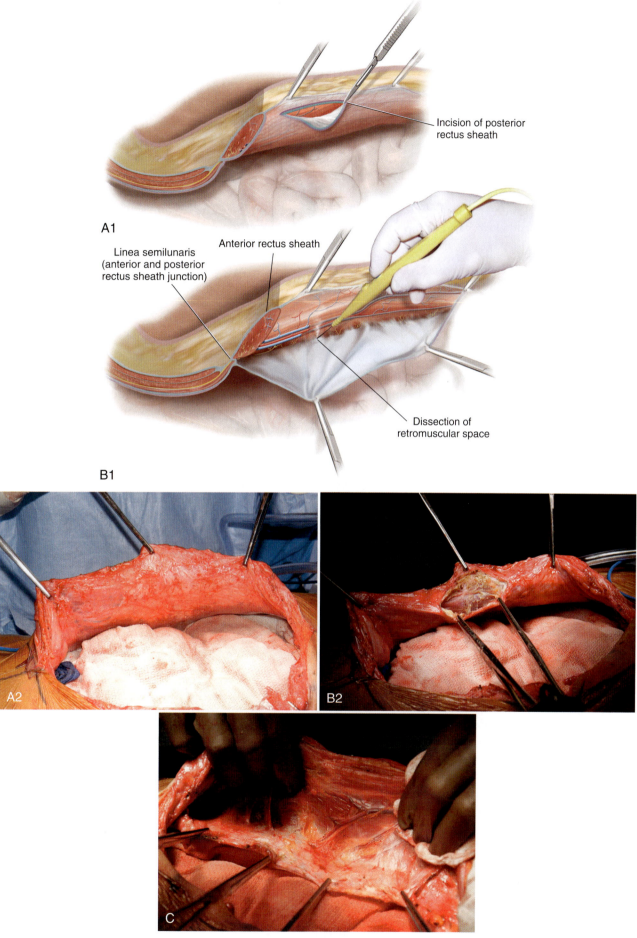

Figure 5-2.

▲ Exposure of Cooper's ligaments/pubis is shown in Figure 5-3. Inferiorly, the space or Retzius is entered to expose the pubis symphysis and both Cooper's ligaments. This dissection is blunt in what is typically a bloodless plane. Since this area is below the arcuate line, posterior layer includes peritoneum and transversalis fascia only. Because both of these layers are very thin, fenestrations are not uncommon and should be repaired. Care should be taken to identify and preserve inferior epigastric vessels that course along the deep surface of the rectus muscles. The urinary bladder may be filled with saline to facilitate its identification and dissection. This is particularly prudent in patients with a previous history of pelvic surgery.

▲ Exposure of the subxiphoid space is shown in Figure 5-4. The retromuscular plane can be extended cephalad to the costal margin and to the retroxiphoid/retrosternal areas.

▲ Lateralization of the Dissection Plane Beyond the Linea Semilunaris

▲ Traditional Rives-Stoppa-Wantz dissection is carried out to the lateral edge of the rectus sheath. However, such dissection is insufficient for some patients undergoing major abdominal wall reconstructions for three main reasons: (1) insufficient medial advancement of the posterior rectus sheath, (2) decreased potential for medialization of the rectus muscles, and (3) insufficient space for large prosthetic reinforcement.

▲ Three techniques for lateral extension of the retromuscular plane have been described. They are the preperitoneal, posterior component separation with intramuscular dissection, and the posterior component separation with transversus abdominis release (TAR). A description of each follows.

- Preperitoneal: The preperitoneal plane may be entered immediately at the medial border of the rectus sheath. Kocher clamps are placed on the edge of the posterior rectus fascia and peritoneum is incised. Alice clamps are then placed on the cut edge of the peritoneum and the plane is developed laterally using blunt dissection. Medial traction applied by the Alice clamps significantly facilitates the dissection. This technique has significant limitations, as it does not provide for any fascial release/advancement. In addition, peritoneal flap (especially its medial edge) is very tenuous in many patients and may tear easily. Such fenestrations should be repaired primarily or buttressed by underlying visceral fat and/or omentum. If complete exclusion of the peritoneal cavity is not possible, this plane should be bridged or buttressed with an absorbable, a biodegradable or a biologic mesh.
- The preperitoneal plane also can be entered from within the rectus sheath. Following a traditional retromuscular dissection (described above), the posterior rectus sheath is incised about 1 to 2 cm medial to the linea semilunaris. Once the plane is entered, the dissection is carried out as described above.
- Posterior component separation with intramuscular dissection (Fig. 5-5): Starting in the periumbilical area, the lateral edge of the posterior rectus sheath is incised, dividing the posterior aponeurotic sheath of the internal oblique muscle. This allows access to the plane between the internal oblique and transversus abdominis muscles. The dissection is carried out laterally using electrocautery. The main limitation of this technique is division of the neurovascular bundle to the abdominal musculature traversing this plane.

Chapter 5 • Open Retromuscular Ventral Hernia Repair 81

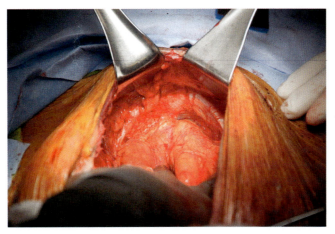

Figure 5-3.

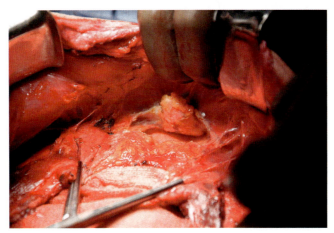

Figure 5-4.

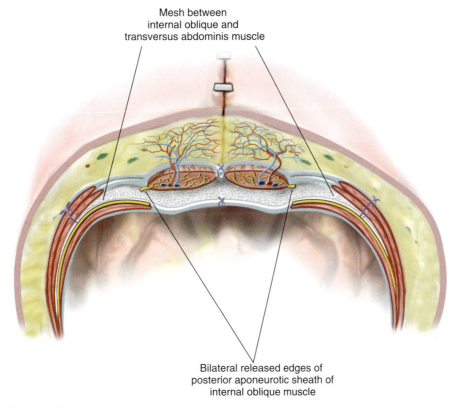

Figure 5-5.

- Posterior component separation with transversus abdominis release (TAR): Starting in the upper third of the abdomen, about 0.5 cm medial to the anterior/posterior rectus sheath junction (linea semilunaris), the posterior rectus sheath is incised to expose the underlying transversus abdominis muscle (Fig. 5-6, A and B). The muscle is then divided along its entire medial edge using electrocautery. The use of a right-angled dissector significantly facilitates this release and minimizes injury to the underlying transversalis fascia and peritoneum. Transection of the medial edge of the transversus abdominis muscle allows for entrance to the space between the transversalis fascia and the lateral

Chapter 5 • Open Retromuscular Ventral Hernia Repair   83

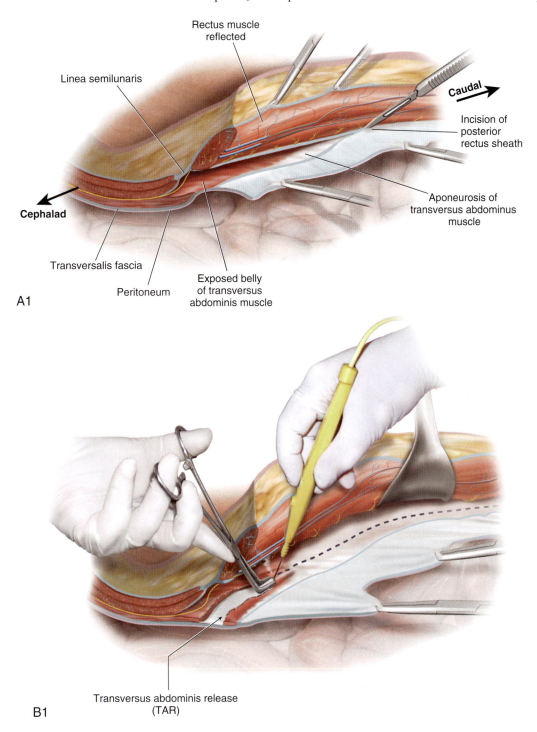

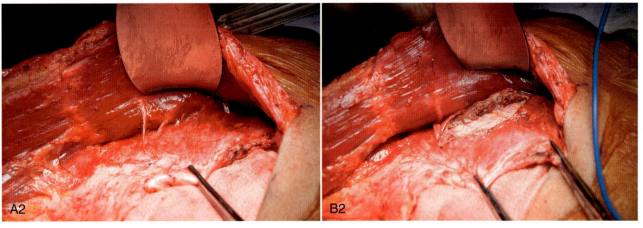

Figure 5-6.

edge of the divided transversus abdominis muscle (Fig. 5-7). The retromuscular space is bluntly developed further laterally to as far as the lateral border of the psoas muscle to allow for a reinforcement of a visceral sac with a large mesh (Fig. 5-8). Also, if needed, this dissection may be extended superiorly above the costal margin and inferiorly to expose both myopectineal orifices (Fig. 5-9).

▲ The key component to the release is the division of the entire medial edge of the transversus abdominis muscle. The main function of the transversus is to act as a "corset" around the abdomen. The synergistic action of the transversus and the posterior fibers of the internal oblique produce hoop tension through the thoracolumbar fascia. By dividing the transversus abdominis, I am able to release the circumferential muscle tension and not only provide for expansion of the abdominal cavity but also afford significant medial advancement of the posterior rectus fascia (Fig. 5-10).

Chapter 5 • Open Retromuscular Ventral Hernia Repair   85

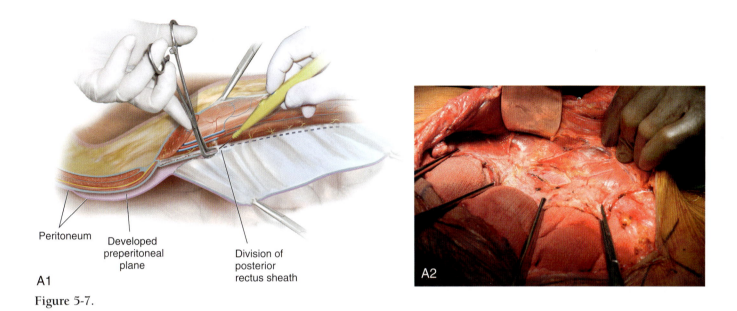

Peritoneum Developed preperitoneal plane Division of posterior rectus sheath

A1

Figure 5-7.

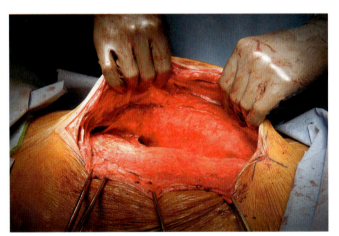

Figure 5-8.

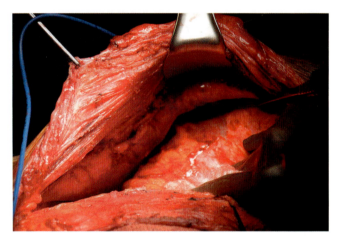

Figure 5-9.

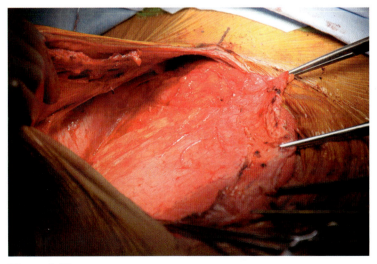

Figure 5-10.

▲ *Posterior Layer Reconstruction*

▲ Once release is performed on both sides, the posterior rectus sheaths are reapproximated in the midline with a running monofilament suture (Fig. 5-11, *A* and *B*). Interrupted figure-of-8 sutures may be used if there is significant tension or pulmonary plateau pressures increase by 5 mm Hg or more.
▲ Fenestrations in the posterior fascia and/or peritoneum laterally are closed primarily or buttressed with native tissue (i.e., omentum), absorbable, biodegradable, or biologic mesh.
▲ Hemostasis is ensured.
▲ Copious antibiotic-laden pulse lavage of the newly created extraperitoneal space is performed.

Chapter 5 • Open Retromuscular Ventral Hernia Repair 87

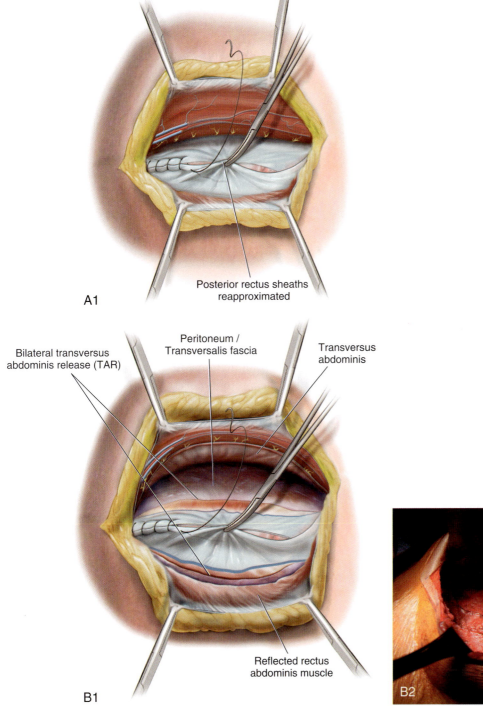

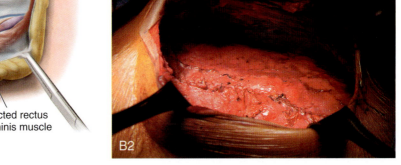

Figure 5-11.

▲ **Mesh Fixation**

- ▲ The mesh is placed as a sublay in the retromuscular space (Fig. 5-12).
- ▲ The inferior edge of the mesh is secured to both Cooper's ligament using 2 to 4 interrupted monofilament sutures. The mesh may be positioned to also reinforce both myopectineal orifices.
- ▲ Superiorly, the mesh could be placed in beyond the costal margin and in the retroxiphoid space. It is secured with interrupted sutures around the xiphoid process. Those sutures are placed 4 to 5 cm off the edge of the mesh to allow for large overlap, especially for subxiphoid defects. Similarly, even though the mesh edge may be significantly beyond the costal margin, fixation is performed below the margin to reduce the risks of lung injury.
- ▲ The mesh is then fixated circumferentially with full-thickness, transabdominal sutures using the Reverdin needle (Figs. 5-13 and 5-14, A and B).

Chapter 5 • Open Retromuscular Ventral Hernia Repair

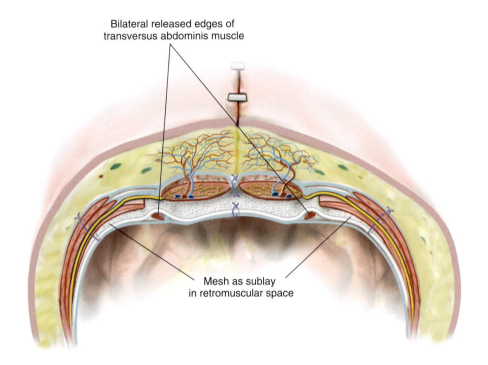

Figure 5-12.

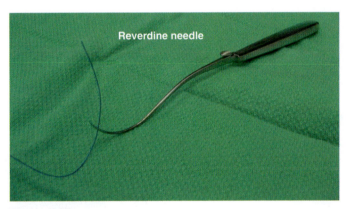

Figure 5-13.

90   Section III • Open Repairs

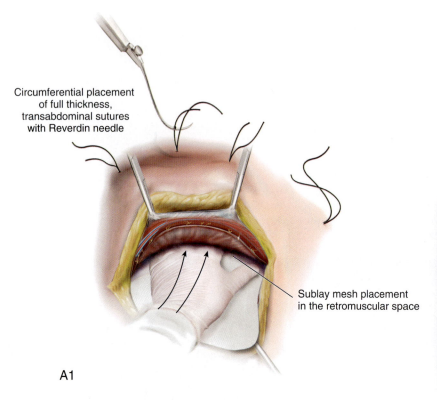
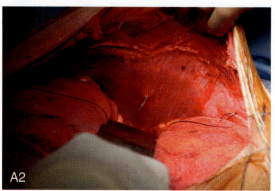
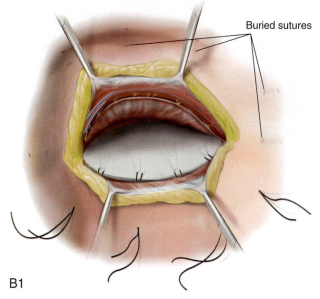
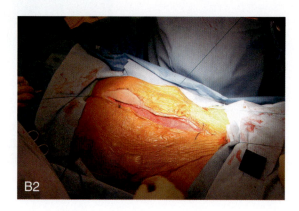

Figure 5-14.

- ▲ The mesh should be placed under appropriate "physiologic" tension. Laxity is of particular concern if biologic mesh is used because mesh "wrinkling" would lead to seromas, infections, and possible mesh degradation and/or weakening. The transfascial sutures should be placed under physiologic tension, so that when they are secured, they provide medialization of the rectus muscles. In doing so, the midline fascia is reapproximated while the mesh is taut, preventing wrinkling when closing the fascia. Alternatively, if the mesh is placed "tension free" and then the fascia is closed, the prosthetic will buckle.
- ▲ Drainage: Closed suction drains are placed ventral to the mesh. Subcutaneous drains are used selectively.

▲ Reconstruction of the Linea Alba

- ▲ The anterior rectus sheaths are then reapproximated in the midline to restore the linea alba. A running, slowly absorbable suture is used. Alternatively, interrupted figure-of-8 stitches can be used, especially when there is a potential predisposition to the abdominal compartment syndrome.
- ▲ In rare instances when the anterior rectus sheath cannot be reapproximated, external oblique fascia release (open or endoscopic) may be performed. However, it is important to not combine the anterior external oblique release with a transversus abdominus release. If both muscle layers are released, the lateral abdominal wall can become destabilized.

4. Postoperative Care

▲ General

- ▲ Intraoperative hemodynamics and airway pressures affect postoperative care. Overnight intensive care unit admission is recommended for patients undergoing major abdominal wall reconstructions. Long operative times and prolonged exposure of the abdominal cavity to room air lead to significant insensible losses and predispose to large fluid shifts. As a result, patients undergoing complex abdominal wall reconstructions often remain intubated overnight. In addition, those patients with poor pulmonary reserve and/or significant increase in plateau airway pressures are kept paralyzed for 24 to 48 hours postoperatively.

- ▲ The drains are kept in place until the output is <20 mL per day.
- ▲ When a biologic graft is used, the drains are left in place for at least 2 weeks, regardless of the output.
- ▲ Antibiotics are continued for up to 24 hours, unless otherwise indicated.
- ▲ Aggressive deep vein thrombosis prophylaxis is mandatory. I do not use systemic anticoagulation and/or caval filters, unless specifically indicated. Ambulation is avoided until the second postoperative day.
- ▲ Abdominal binders are used in the early postoperative period. Beyond the first week, their use is liberalized at the patient's discretion.

▲ Pain Management

- ▲ Epidural catheters are strongly recommended. Epidural catheters are maintained until patients are tolerating a diet and have full return of bowel function. In addition, scheduled (not prn) intravenous diazepam (Valium) is given for muscle relaxation and spasm prevention.

▲ Diet

- ▲ Routine nasogastric tube decompression is reserved for patients with intestinal resections, significant intestinal manipulations, and prolonged adhesiolysis. Diet advancement is very conservative in order to avoid early postoperative bloating, retching, and vomiting, which may lead to pulmonary complications, as well as disruption of the repair. As a result, diets are not advanced until return of bowel function occurs.

5. Outcomes

- ▲ Retromuscular (Rives-Stoppa-Wantz) repair has been shown to result in an effective repair of most ventral hernias. Recurrence rates of 3% to 6% at mid- to long-term follow-ups have been reported. In fact, in 2004, given its superior track record, this approach was proclaimed to be the gold standard for open ventral hernia repair by the American Hernia Society.

- ▲ The posterior component separation and retromuscular repair has the following advantages: (1) it is relatively easy to adopt, (2) it is applicable in a broad range of patients, (3) the creation of skin flaps is avoided, and (4) the risk of lateral laxity/bulging is low. An additional advantage is that sublay mesh placement allows for giant prosthetic reinforcement of the visceral sac and for proper mesh placement and sufficient mesh overlap for repair of hernias in difficult locations including the subxiphoid, suprapubic, flank, and parastomal areas.
- ▲ It may also be the best *space* for a biologic graft positioning to maximize the environment for graft integration and regeneration via superior blood supply.

6. Pearls and Pitfalls

1. Anatomy

- ▲ Neurovascular bundles supplying rectus muscles run in between transversus abdominis and internal oblique muscles and traverse posterior rectus sheath near the linea semilunaris, entering rectus muscle at its lateral edge. Care should be taken to identify and preserve these nerve bundles during the retrorectus dissection to prevent denervation of the rectus muscles
- ▲ The transversus abdominis muscle is the "corset" of the abdomen and is the muscle mostly responsible for intraabdominal pressure. It extends more medially than both internal and external obliques. These anatomic features allow for TAR in posterior component separation.

2. Preoperative Considerations

- ▲ Smoking cessation is mandatory. Abdominal wall reconstructions in smokers carry a high risk of wound morbidity and repair failures.
- ▲ Abdominal imaging (CT) should be performed routinely.
- ▲ Both synthetic and biologic meshes can be used in complex repairs even if component release has been performed. Mesh choices should be based on the multitude of patient factors and surgeon preferences and is more completely covered in Chapter 19.

3. Intraoperative Considerations

- ▲ Complete lysis of visceral adhesions to the abdominal wall is performed to facilitate fascial advancement and to avoid subsequent intestinal injuries during component release.
- ▲ Removal of ALL previous meshes is essential to allow optimum prosthetic integration and reduce postoperative infectious complications.

4. Technical Considerations

- ▲ In many patients, retromuscular dissection to the extent of the lateral edge of both rectus sheaths may be sufficient.
- ▲ Release of the posterior rectus sheath (posterior component separation) could be achieved with or without transversus abdominis muscle release. Posterior component separations should NOT be combined with any type of the anterior release. Traditional retrorectus dissection, on the other hand, could be an excellent adjunct to the anterior (external oblique) release to allow for sublay mesh placement.
- ▲ Fenestrations in the transversalis fascia should be repaired.
- ▲ If posterior rectus sheaths cannot be re-approximated, omentum, remnants of the hernia sac, or an absorbable mesh can be used to "bridge" the gap.
- ▲ Complete exclusion of the abdominal viscera is essential to both avoid intestinal herniations/strangulations through defects in the posterior layer of reconstruction and to avoid intestinal exposure to uncoated synthetic meshes.
- ▲ The mesh should be sized to provide significant reinforcement of the whole visceral sac. Typically, at least a 30 × 30 cm synthetic or a 20 × 20 cm biologic mesh is used.
- ▲ Mesh fixation is performed with a wide lateral overlap. Full-thickness transabdominal sutures are used to fixate the mesh and to provide physiologic tension across the entire abdominal wall. "Tension-free" repair of the abdominal wall is not adequate if preservation of the abdominal wall function is intended.

▲ Fixated biologic mesh should be taut without bucking/wrinkling.
▲ Follow pulmonary plateau pressures to minimize risks of postoperative abdominal hypertension and respiratory failures. In cases of significant (>5 mmHg) intraoperative plateau pressures elevation, fascial bridging, postoperative mechanical ventilation, and/or paralytics may be employed.

5. Postoperative Care

▲ Aggressive pain management, including epidural and intravenous antispasmodic agents, is mandatory.
▲ Advance diet slowly.
▲ Keep drains until output is <20 mL per day, especially when a biologic mesh used.

Selected References

Carbonell AM, Cobb WS, Chen SM: Posterior components separation during retromuscular hernia repair, *Hernia* 12(4):359–362, 2008.
Conze J, Prescher A, Klinge U, et al: Pitfalls in retromuscular mesh repair for incisional hernia: the importance of the "fatty triangle" *Hernia* 8(3):255–259, 2004.
Hammond DL, Ackerman L, Holdsworth R, Elzey B: Effects of spinal nerve ligation on immunohistochemically identified neurons in the L4 and L5 dorsal root ganglia of the rat, *J Comp Neurol* 475(4):575–589, 2004.
Iqbal CW, Pham TH, Joseph A, et al: Long-term outcome of 254 complex incisional hernia repairs using the modified Rives-Stoppa technique, *World J Surg* 31(12):2398–2404, 2007.
Novitsky YW, Porter JR, Rucho ZC, et al: Open preperitoneal retrofascial mesh repair for multiply recurrent ventral incisional hernias, *J Am Coll Surg* 203(3):283–289, 2006.
Rives J, Pire JC, Flament JB, et al: [Treatment of large eventrations. New therapeutic indications apropos of 322 cases], *Chirurgie* 111(3):215–225, 1985.
Rosen MJ, Fatima J, Sarr MG: Repair of abdominal wall hernias with restoration of abdominal wall function. *J Gastrointest Surg* 14(1):175–185.
Stoppa RE: The treatment of complicated groin and incisional hernias, *World J Surg* 13(5):545–554, 1989.
Wirhed R: *Athletic Ability & the Anatomy of Motion*, 1984, Wolfe Medical Publications Ltd.

CHAPTER 6

OPEN FLANK HERNIA REPAIR

Melissa S. Phillips, MD and Michael J. Rosen, MD, FACS

1. Clinical Anatomy

▲ Flank hernias can be divided broadly by etiology into those that are congenital in nature and those that are acquired, often after previous surgery or trauma. Congenital, or lumbar hernias, are less common than the acquired type and can be subclassified into superior triangle (Grynfeltt) or inferior triangle (Petit) defects. Acquired flank hernias can develop after previous operations such as iliac bone harvest, trauma, retroperitoneal aortic surgery, or nephrectomy. The anatomic proximity of flank hernias to bony prominences and major neurovascular structures presents a challenge in the durable repair of these hernias. Specifically, the proximity of these lesions with the iliac crest and twelfth rib can often limit the amount of tissue present for adequate mesh-tissue overlap.

2. Preoperative Considerations

▲ When considering surgical repair of flank hernias, it is important to perform a computed tomography (CT) scan of the abdomen and pelvis. First and foremost, this will distinguish a true hernia from a pseudohernia (e.g., abdominal wall laxity from denervation after division of the lower thoracic nerves). In addition, a CT scan is not only essential to understanding the patient's specific anatomy but also for delineating the presence of previous mesh repairs. It also will show the structure of remaining bone, because there may be alterations secondary to previous operations in this area. This information is important for planning the appropriate location for prosthetic deployment and any fixation or overlap issues that might arise.
▲ Preoperative counseling detailing the risks of nerve injury leading to numbness, weakness, or chronic pain, as well as the risks for vascular and intraabdominal injury is important.
▲ Given the large incision and extent of dissection, these patients may benefit from the placement of preoperative epidurals for postoperative pain management if no other contraindications exist. Routine preoperative antibiotics for skin flora should be administered.

3. Operative Steps

1. Patient Positioning

▲ The patient is positioned in the full lateral decubitus position on a beanbag as seen in Figure 6-1. A roll is placed in the axilla and the table is flexed to maximize the space between the lower border of the costal margin and the anterior superior iliac spine to optimize exposure. The beanbag is then engaged for support and padding. The patient should be secured to the table with padded tape to allow for full rotation of the bed during the operation.

2. Operative Steps

▲ The following anatomic landmarks are prepped into the sterile field: costal margin and pelvic brim including the anterior superior iliac spine, inguinal ligament, pubic tubercle, and umbilicus. The midline should be accessible as well if added exposure and mesh overlap are necessary. The incision should be made preferably 3 cm above the iliac crest. As many flank hernias are related to previous surgical interventions, the incision site will often be dictated by the site of the previous incision.

▲ Electrocautery is used to carry the dissection through the subcutaneous tissue including Camper and Scarpa fasciae to identify the musculature of the lateral abdominal wall. If the anatomic planes are intact, the external oblique, internal oblique, and transversus abdominis muscles will be divided. If the distinct muscle layers are obscured by the presence of the hernia or prior prosthetic, blunt dissection is used to identify the hernia sac and follow this down to the fascial edges, separating the hernia from the surrounding lateral abdominal wall musculature.

▲ If possible, an attempt is made to avoid entry into the peritoneum. In many circumstances, reduction of the hernia sac will lead to an inadvertent entry into the abdominal cavity. In this circumstance, the edges of the hernia sac are left attached to the surrounding peritoneum, and the defect in the peritoneum will be closed at the completion of the dissection. After division of the transversus abdominis muscle, the preperitoneal fat is encountered. This plane is easier to identify laterally than medially. Care is taken to confirm entry into the preperitoneal/retroperitoneal plane because this is the location to deploy the prosthetic and optimize overlap. A Kittner dissector is useful to bluntly extend the preperitoneal dissection in all directions. Often the hernia sac is attenuated and cannot be separated from the subcutaneous tissues safely. In these circumstances, we typically enter the abdominal cavity and perform a complete adhesiolysis. Subsequently, the preperitoneal space can be accessed at the border of the defect directly.

Chapter 6 • Open Flank Hernia Repair 99

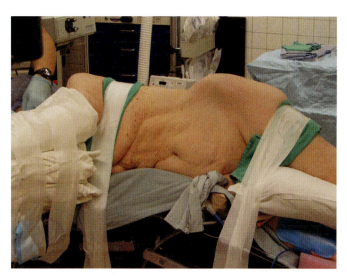

Figure 6-1.

▲ Establishing an area of overlap for mesh placement is essential in the repair of a flank hernia. Superiorly, the dissection and overlap one can achieve can be limited by the costal margin. However, the preperitoneal plane can be developed, separating the peritoneum off the diaphragm obtaining 8 to 10 cm of overlap underneath the ribs in the cephalad direction as illustrated in Figure 6-2 and Figure 6-3. Posteriorly, the psoas muscle and spine form an anatomic boundary. In this area, care is taken to identify and avoid injury to the ureter, gonadal vessels, and iliac vessels as shown in Figure 6-4 and Figure 6-5. Additionally, the genitofemoral, ilioinguinal, iliohypogastric, and lateral femoral cutaneous nerves are identified and avoided when securing the prosthetic. Medially, the peritoneum can be adhered densely to the posterior rectus sheath. We prefer to transition the dissection plane into the posterior rectus sheath just medial to the linea semilunaris (Fig. 6-6). This allows the dissection to be carried all the way to the linea alba. Inferiorly, the Cooper ligament and the pelvis are exposed by sweeping away the bladder. Care should be taken to avoid injuring the spermatic cord structures as they are often encountered at this point.

Chapter 6 • Open Flank Hernia Repair 101

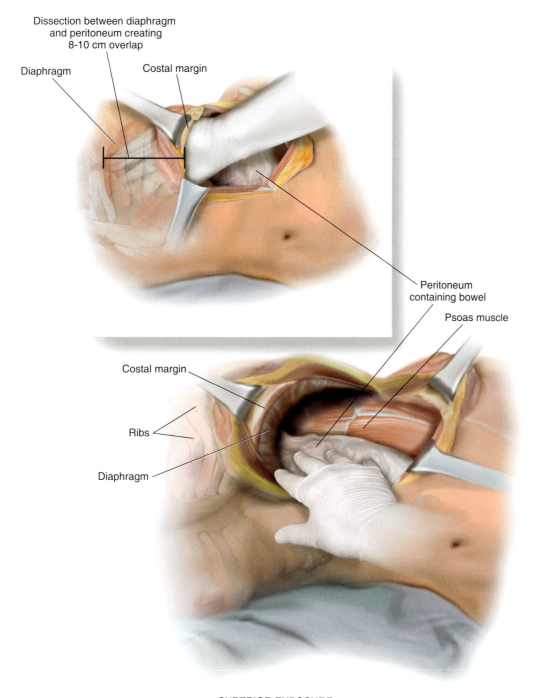

SUPERIOR EXPOSURE

Figure 6-2.

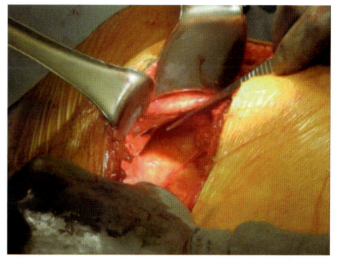

Figure 6-3.

102 Section III • Open Repairs

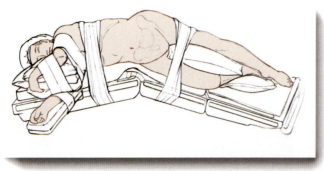

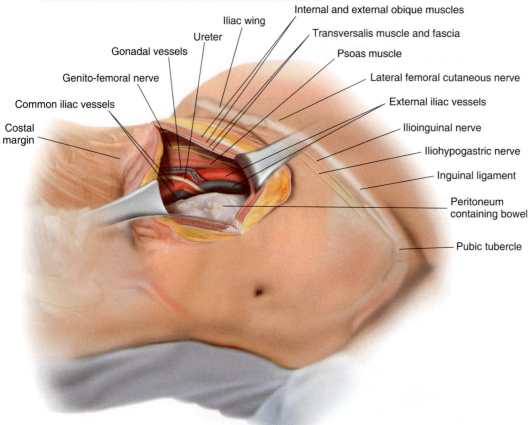

POSTERIOR EXPOSURE

Figure 6-4.

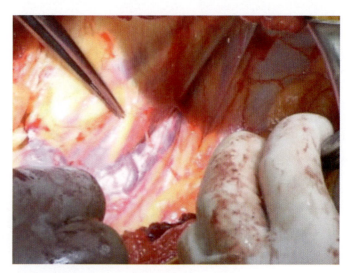

Figure 6-5.

Chapter 6 • Open Flank Hernia Repair 103

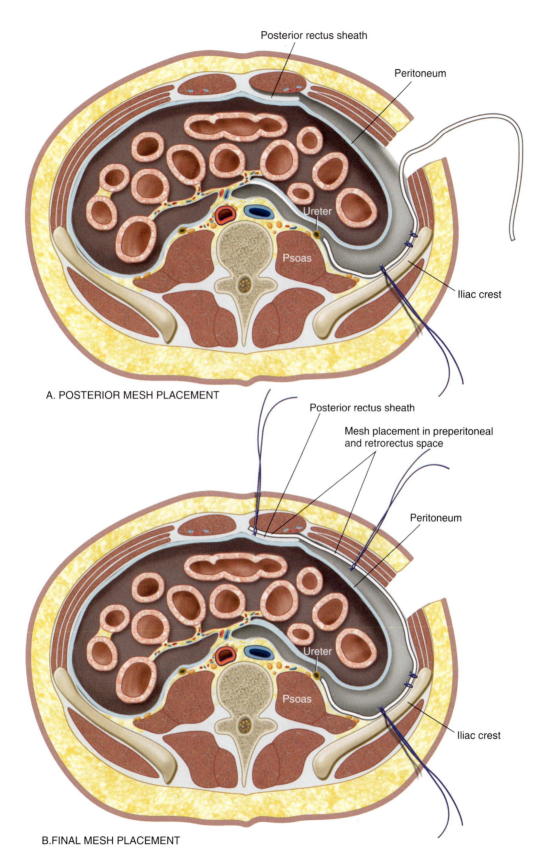

A. POSTERIOR MESH PLACEMENT

B. FINAL MESH PLACEMENT

Figure 6-6.

▲ If the peritoneum was entered during the hernia sac reduction or during the preperitoneal dissection, it is closed with a #2-0 absorbable braided suture. If this layer is not completely excluded, bowel can herniate through with a high strangulation risk or an internal hernia. The hernia sac may be used to provide additional coverage of the viscera in larger defects. If primary closure of this plane is not possible, the remaining defects may be buttressed using omentum or with a piece of vicryl mesh. An adequately sized piece of mesh (Fig. 6-7) is used to cover the entire retroperitoneal space from the Cooper ligament to the psoas muscle, under the costal margin, and to the midline. Since the mesh is placed extraperitoneally, an unprotected macroporous synthetic mesh is used.

▲ The mesh is placed into the preperitoneal space, folded in a "taco" configuration The mesh is initially fixed posteriorly (Fig. 6-8, A). The suture is placed off the edge of the mesh to allow the mesh to drape over the psoas muscle to the ureter. The sutures can now be passed with the Reverdin needle inferior to the lateral border of the psoas muscle to avoid major vascular injury. Inferiorly, the mesh is fixated to the iliac crest in the following fashion, illustrated in Figure 6-8, B and Figure 6-9. A surgical cordless drill is used to preplace the number of designated holes in the iliac crest. Mitek bone anchors (Mitek Surgical Products, Westwood, MA), which contain titanium anchors with double #2 braided polyester sutures, are placed into the tracts. Each arm of the bone anchor suture is passed through the mesh and tied, securing the mesh to the iliac crest. These sutures are not placed at the edge of the mesh. Instead the suture is placed 8 to 10 cm off the edge of the mesh. This allows the mesh to drape past the iliac crest for adequate overlap. A total of 8 to 10 fixation sutures are then placed The remaining transfascial sutures for mesh fixation are placed using a #1 polypropylene suture passed through the mesh and the needle removed. Once in place, the mesh is pulled to recreate normal physiologic tension. We recommend the circumferential fixation begin posteriorly, then medially, then inferiorly, and finally superiorly. After the inferior edge of the mesh is fixated, the flex in the table is removed and the patient is allowed to return to neutral position. It is important to return the anatomic position to allow appropriate tensioning of the mesh and avoid buckling. It is also critical to not overstretch the mesh excessively tight to limit lateral movements and stretching to the contralateral side. The cross sectional images in Figure 6-6 illustrate the location of mesh placement. At the completion of the mesh fixation, the boundaries of the fascial defect should be relatively reapproximated before closure, as seen in Figure 6-8, C and Figure 6-10. The fascia of the lateral abdominal wall is closed using a #1 absorbable monofilament suture in a figure of eight fashion.

Chapter 6 • Open Flank Hernia Repair   105

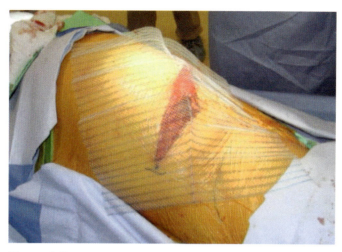

Figure 6-7.

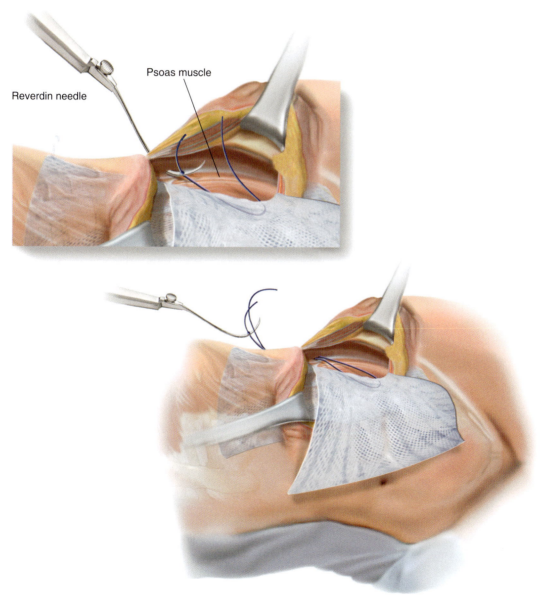

POSTERIOR TRANSFASCIAL SUTURE FIXATIONS

Figure 6-8.

106 Section III • Open Repairs

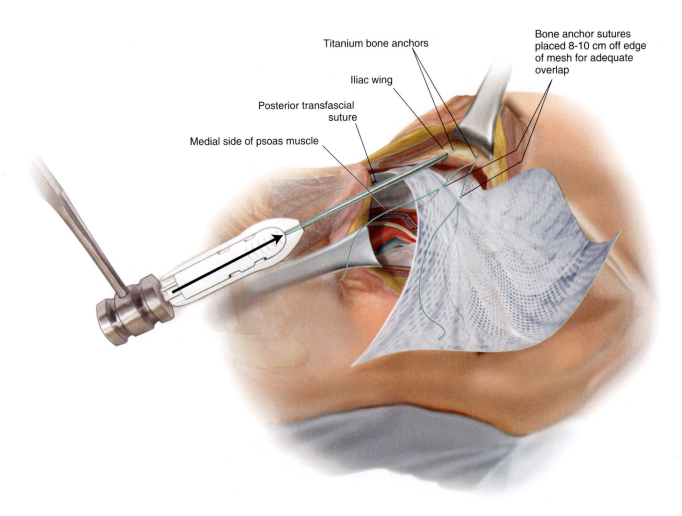

ILIAC BRIM BONE ANCHOR PLACEMENT

Figure 6-8—Cont'd

Chapter 6 • Open Flank Hernia Repair 107

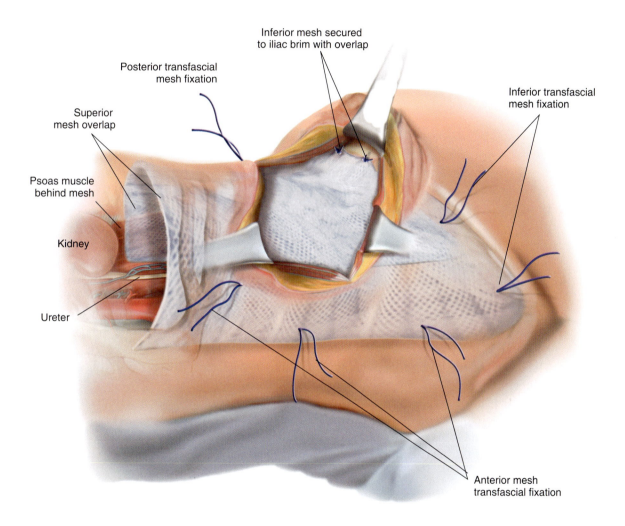

FINAL MESH PLACEMENT
(Taco shape)

Figure 6-8—Cont'd

4. Postoperative Care

▲ Abdominal distention should be avoided following this repair. If an extensive lysis of adhesions was required, oral intake should be delayed until there is evidence bowel function has returned. Patients should be kept in an abdominal binder following this operation for 6 weeks. Antibiotics are continued for 24 hours unless otherwise indicated. A drain is typically placed intraoperatively and removed within 3 days postoperatively.

5. Pearls and Pitfalls

▲ Knowledge of the anatomy is particularly important in this type of hernia because dissection is complex given the proximity to neurovascular and bony structures. Always obtain a preoperative CT scan to help delineate the anatomy, define overlap planes, and document previous mesh repairs.

▲ The most important technique to learn from this type of repair is that overlap may be superior to fixation. Reliance on transfascial or bony fixation as the backbone for a flank hernia repair implies that there is inadequate overlap. Dissection of the preperitoneal plane allows a 5- to 10-cm overlap that can overcome hernia defects and eliminate the need for excessive fixation.

▲ The described method for flank hernia repair may not be appropriate in a setting of contamination. Specifically, the patient and surgeon must consider the infectious risk of the procedure. If the risk is elevated beyond a clean case, the bony fixation described below may be contraindicated due to the risk for subsequent osteomyelitis.

▲ Appropriate mesh fixation to follow the contour of the abdominal wall can be technically challenging. Fixating laterally, medially, inferiorly, and finally superiorly can help minimize these issues.

Selected References

Carbonell AM, Kercher KW, Sigmon L, Matthews BD, Sing RF, Kneisl JS, Heniford BT: A novel technique of lumbar hernia repair using bone anchor fixation, *Hernia* 9(1):22, 2005.

Heniford BT, Iannitti DA, Gagner M: Laparoscopic inferior and superior lumbar hernia repair, *Arch Surg* 132:1141, 1997.

Stumpf M, Conze J, Prescher A, Junge K, Krones CJ, Klinge U, Schumpelick V: The lateral incisional hernia: anatomic considerations for a standardized retromuscular sublay repair, *Hernia* 13(3):293, 2009.

Yee JA, Harold KL, Cobb WS, Carbonell AM: "Bone anchor mesh fixation for complex laparoscopic ventral hernia repair." *Surgical Innovation* 15(4):292, 2008.

Chapter 6 • Open Flank Hernia Repair 109

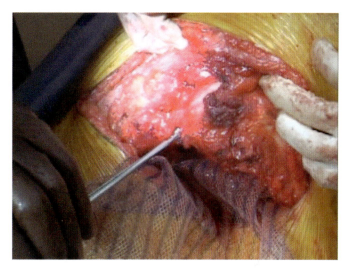

Figure 6-9.

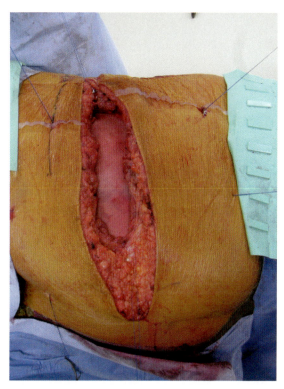

Figure 6-10.

CHAPTER 7

OPEN REPAIR OF PARASTOMAL HERNIAS

Harry L. Reynolds, Jr., MD, FACS, FASCRS

1. Introduction

▲ Multiple techniques of parastomal hernia repair have been described. This chapter outlines an open retrorectus biologic mesh placement technique that is suitable for simultaneous repair of large parastomal and midline hernias.

2. Clinical Anatomy

1. Dissection Planes

▲ Abdominal wall anatomy is discussed in detail in Chapter 1. It is essential to understand the anatomic layering of the abdominal wall for proper retrorectus/retroperitoneal mesh placement and anterior component separation.
▲ The linea semilunaris lies at the lateral aspect of the posterior rectus sheath. Rectus innervation is preserved and plane development is facilitated by entrance into the retroperitoneal space medial to the linea semilunaris. Dissection in the retroperitoneal space is below the transversus abdominis muscle and can be completed to the psoas. Mesh placement is in this retroperitoneal space.
▲ Anterior component separation involves division of the external oblique aponeurosis lateral to the rectus sheath. Access for this division can be achieved via subcutaneous flap or via laparoscopic techniques as described previously (see Chapters 8 and 11) (Fig. 7-1).

2. Ostomy Site Selection

▲ Ostomy sites are chosen with the assistance of an enterostomal therapist and are marked preoperatively. Patients should be examined while sitting and supine, and an appropriate location visible to the patient is found. Transrectus placement is typically preferred.

Chapter 7 • Open Repair of Parastomal Hernias 111

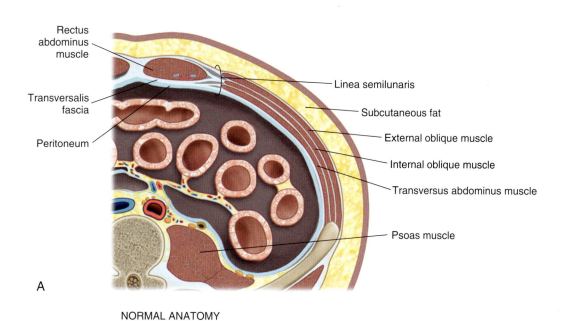

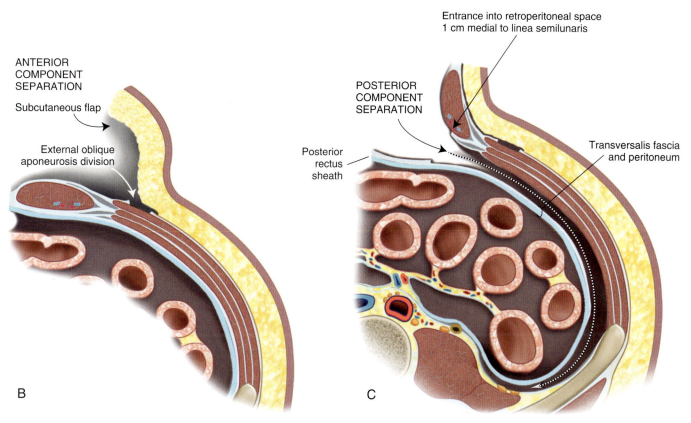

Figure 7-1.

Folds should be avoided to facilitate appliance adhesion. Thus, it is essential to examine the patient while he or she is sitting in order to visualize folds. Obese patients with a significant pannus should be sited in the upper abdomen. During complex abdominal wall reconstruction, excess skin and subcutaneous tissues are often resected, and therefore consideration must be given to the eventual placement of the stoma (Figs. 7-2 and 7-3).

3. Preoperative Considerations

1. Comorbidities

- ▲ Appropriate patient selection and optimization is essential. The procedure results in a significant physiologic insult. An extended operation with a long midline incision and prolonged adhesiolysis is typical. Significant fluid shifts should be expected. Those with extensive cardiac, pulmonary, or renal disease should be vetted carefully and optimized maximally. Risk of surgery may be prohibitive in some.
- ▲ Combined ventral and parastomal hernias are typical. With large hernias there may be significant loss of abdominal domain. Intraabdominal reduction results in increased abdominal compartment pressures with potential for pulmonary and renal compromise. The use of a large biologic mesh prosthesis partially mitigates this problem; however, perioperative intensive care including brief ventilator support is not unusual.
- ▲ Timing of the operation is important as well. An appropriate interval from previous surgeries should be allowed. This typically should be a minimum of 3 months. However, with a history of a significant inflammatory process or hostile abdomen on previous exploration, a longer interval (6 months to a year) may be appropriate. On exam before exploration, ideally, the abdominal skin overlying any midline hernia should be mobile and soft without significant adherence to underlying bowel loops.
- ▲ Those that present with infected prosthetic mesh with or without fistulas are particularly good candidates for this approach. The duration and complexity of operation can be expected to increase significantly in this situation.
- ▲ Preoperative imaging with abdominal pelvic computed tomography (CT) scans is routinely performed. These images provide important information as to the exact location of the stoma in the abdominal wall, the integrity of the rectus muscle and lateral abdominal wall musculature, and the size of the parastomal and midline hernias. In addition, the surgeon can be alerted to possible loss of abdominal domain and plan appropriately.

2. Two-Team Approach

- ▲ We have found a two-team approach particularly efficacious. One team focuses on adhesiolysis, intestinal mobilization, resection, and repair as appropriate. A second team proceeds with abdominal wall reconstruction. In our institution, we typically use a colorectal surgical team and a general surgical team. Although, one surgeon can certainly accomplish these procedures, fatigue of the operating team does become a factor with operative times averaging about 5 hours. A planned two-team approach helps facilitate procedure progression in these prolonged cases.

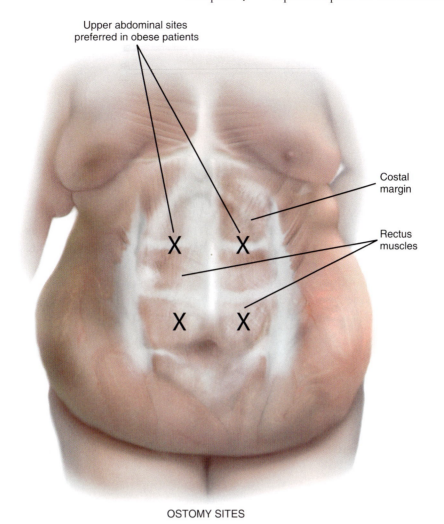

Figure 7-2.

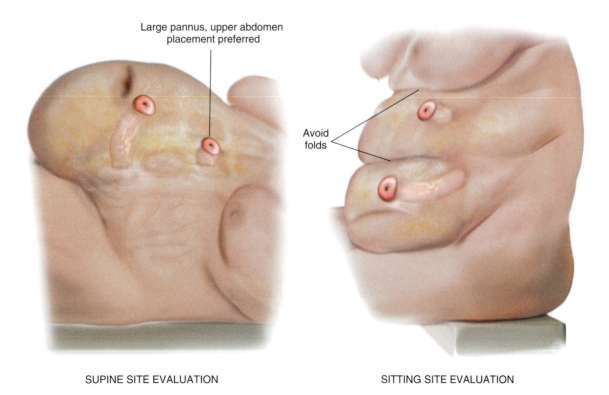

Figure 7-3.

3. Operative Options

- ▲ Multiple methods of parastomal hernia repair, both laparoscopic and open, have been described. The multiplicity of procedures belies the complex nature of the problem and the lack of a clear and simple, yet efficacious repair.
- ▲ Direct suture repair has been frequently described but has an unacceptably high recurrence rate. Mesh, either biologic or synthetic, placed in a subcutaneous overlay, or in a retrorectus underlay has been described with variable results. Stomal transposition with or without mesh use has been used also, and results have also been variable.
- ▲ Our preferred option, particularly for those with combined ventral and parastomal hernias, is component separation, stomal transposition, and retrorectus reinforcement with biologic mesh. This method is the focus of this chapter.

4. Operation Steps

1. Midline Laparotomy

- ▲ After preoperative bowel preparation, deep venous thrombosis prophylaxis, and intravenous antibiotics, the patient is approached through a midline laparotomy. Patients are placed in low lithotomy with Allen stirrups or Yellow Fin stirrups to allow easy access to the pelvis for adhesiolysis. The stoma is isolated and excluded with an impervious iodine impregnated sticky drape. Midline entry can be challenging in those with a previously placed mesh prostheses, which is commonly seen after previous attempts at repair. The previous scar is excised, fistulas are mobilized, and mesh is explanted. Particularly careful and tedious dissection is necessary to prevent enterotomy (Fig. 7-4).

2. Complete Adhesiolysis and Stomal Mobilization

- ▲ A complete adhesiolysis is undertaken to the root of the mesentery. It is essential to fully free the abdominal wall to allow complete mobility of the wall for reconstruction. The bowel proximal to the stoma is typically divided with a linear cutter intraabdominally, isolating the stoma to limit contamination. The mucocutaneous junction is then taken down, and the old stoma is excised. The intestinal segment used for the stoma is mobilized adequately to transpose it, preferably to the contralateral side. The ventral and parastomal hernia defect size is assessed, and a decision is made as to whether component separation will be necessary.

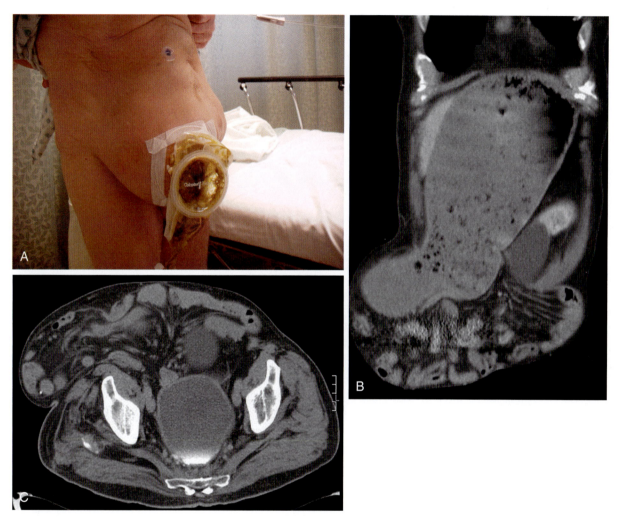

Figure 7-4.

3. Anterior Component Separation

▲ An open component separation technique is preferred for the old stoma site. This allows mobilization of a subcutaneous skin flap including the old stoma site. The skin flap is mobilized at least 2 cm lateral to the rectus sheath, and the external oblique aponeurosis is identified. The external oblique aponeurosis is opened from above the costal margin to the pelvis. In some cases, there may be enough redundant skin with this flap to allow complete resection of the skin and subcutaneous tissue containing the old stoma site after abdominal wall reconstruction. The fascial edges are assessed to see if closure will be feasible anteriorly. If deemed necessary to gain additional anterior abdominal wall mobilization, a contralateral anterior component separation is performed, either by lifting a flap or proceeding with an endoscopic technique, which we prefer for the side opposite the stoma. The endoscopic technique preserves the perforators to the abdominal wall skin and avoids a large skin flap around the new stoma, as described in Chapter 11 (Figs 7-5 and 7-6).

4. Retrorectus Mobilization

▲ The rectus sheath is now entered in the midline, and the muscle is mobilized anteriorly, allowing visualization of the posterior rectus sheath and the linea semilunaris laterally. This space can be difficult to access with a prior stoma. However, if one dissects above and below the old stoma site, the space can almost always be recreated. The parastomal hernia sac can be left in situ on the posterior rectus sheath if possible, although this is often difficult. Alternatively, the hole created in the posterior rectus sheath at the old stoma site can be reapproximated with sutures. One of the limits of the posterior rectus sheath is the lateral extent of mesh placement. For standard midline defects, this is often not a significant problem. For parastomal defects or when reinforcing new stomas, creating space for lateral overlap and fixation of the mesh can be difficult. Utilizing the preperitoneal dissection plane in the lateral abdominal wall, large sheets of mesh can be utilized to reinforce the old stoma site and the newly created stoma. To access this plane, the posterior rectus sheath is superficially opened approximately 1 cm medial to the linea semilunaris, and the retroperitoneal space is entered, posterior to the transversus abdominis muscle. By opening medial to the linea semilunaris, injury to the segmental intercostal nerves innervating the rectus is less likely. The dissection is continued laterally in the retroperitoneal space to the psoas muscles from the costal margin to the pelvis. This dissection is completed on the opposite side as well. It is more difficult on the side of the previous stoma, but with care, full mobilization can be accomplished, preserving the posterior sheath and the peritoneum laterally for closure over the bowel before mesh placement (Figs. 7-7 to 7-9).

Chapter 7 • Open Repair of Parastomal Hernias   117

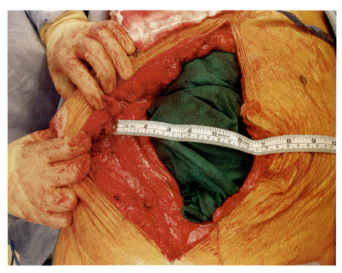

Figure 7-5.

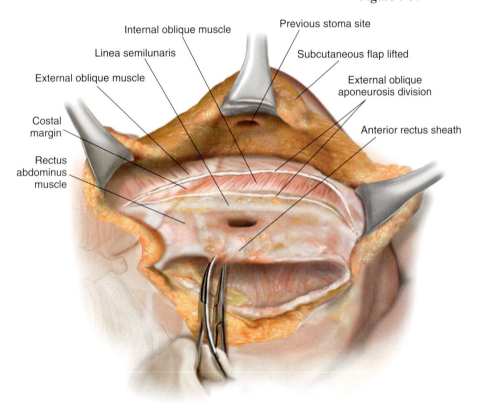

Figure 7-6.

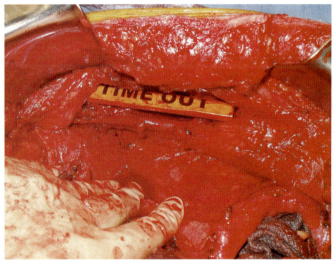

Figure 7-7.

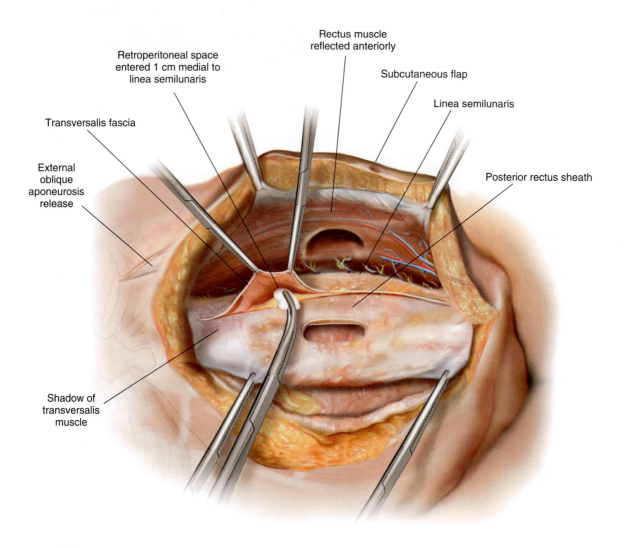

Figure 7-8.

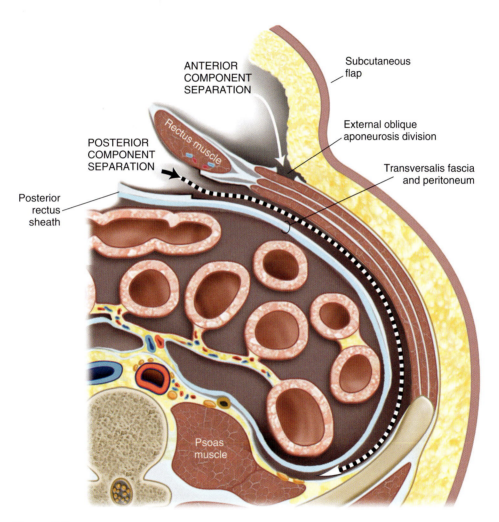

Figure 7-9.

5. Stoma Site Transposition and Posterior Sheath Closure

▲ The previous stoma site in the posterior sheath is closed with a long-term absorbable suture, and the stoma is brought through the posterior sheath on the *contralateral* side at a site corresponding to the point marked on the skin preoperatively by the enterostomal therapist. In order to establish the appropriate track for the new stoma, it is important to bring all layers of the component separated abdominal wall together in the midline simulating the recreated linea alba. Skin, anterior sheath, rectus muscle, and posterior sheath must all be aligned as the new ostomy aperture is created to ensure that there is no angulation through any layer that could potentially obstruct the stoma. We typically create a circular defect in the skin, sized appropriately for the intestinal diameter. The defect in the rectus sheath and the rectus muscle is created longitudinally and is typically at least two finger breadths in size, again sized appropriately for intestinal diameter. The intestinal segment for the stoma is then brought through the posterior sheath only at this time. The posterior sheath is closed in the midline, completely covering all intestine, except the segment brought up for the new stoma.
▲ Alternatively, one can choose to wait to create the rectus muscle, anterior sheath, and skin apertures until after mesh placement and fixation to help ensure no excessive angulation (Figs. 7-10 and 7-11).

Chapter 7 • Open Repair of Parastomal Hernias   121

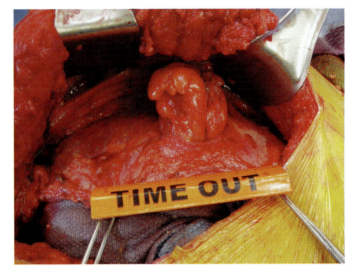

Figure 7-10.

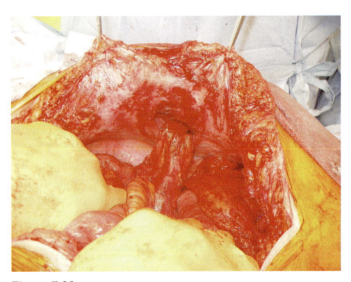

Figure 7-11.

6. Reapproximation of Previous Stoma Site in Anterior Sheath and Retrorectus Placement of Biologic Mesh

▲ The previous stoma site is closed in the anterior sheath with long-term absorbable suture. Typically, a 20 × 20 cm sheet of biologic mesh is used and positioned in a diamond shaped configuration in the retrorectus and retroperitoneal spaces. The mesh is secured cephalad and caudad initially with two #1 polypropylene sutures brought through the abdominal wall through skin stab incisions with the Reverdin needle. The mesh is then secured laterally on the side opposite the new stoma, initially with three heavy polypropylene sutures brought transabdominally through the skin stab incisions in the same manner with the Reverdin needle. Keyholes are made in the mesh for passage of the stoma, and the stoma is pulled through; the mesh is resecured with a polypropylene suture laterally to keep the soft biologic mesh just adjacent to the stoma. More recently we have been making a cruciate incision in the mesh and pulling the stoma through instead of using keyholes. A small gap of about one finger breadth is allowed adjacent to the stoma to prevent constriction at the mesh level. Again, importantly the hole in the mesh must be made to align with the hole previously made in the posterior sheath. If the rectus muscle, anterior sheath, and skin apertures are not already created, the rectus, anterior fascia, and skin are now pulled toward the midline, so one can determine where a properly aligned aperture can be made for the new stoma site through the remaining abdominal wall. This aperture should be made while simulating the linea alba, reapproximated in the midline. An appropriately sized circle of skin is excised, and a longitudinal, muscle-splitting incision is made in the anterior rectus sheath and rectus muscle. The ostomy is then pulled up through the mesh only. The mesh is then secured in the retrorectus and retroperitoneal spaces to the abdominal wall via three skin stab incisions just as it was on the opposite side (Figs. 7-12 to 7-16).

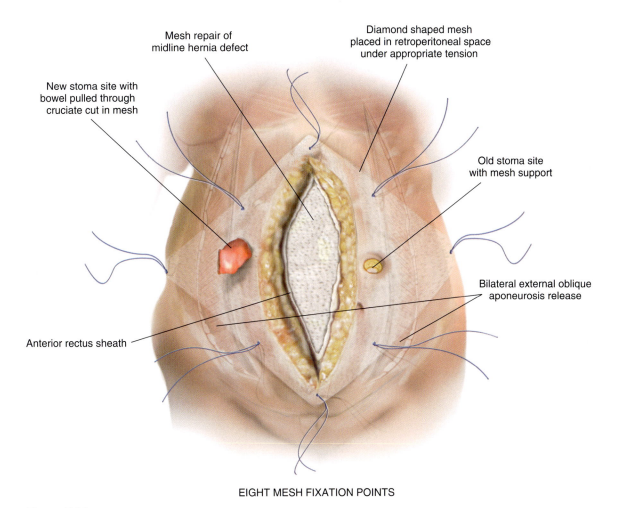

Figure 7-12.

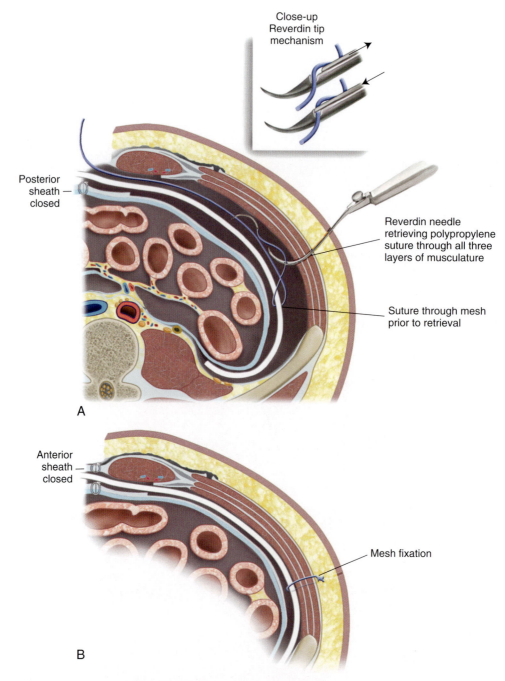

Figure 7-13.

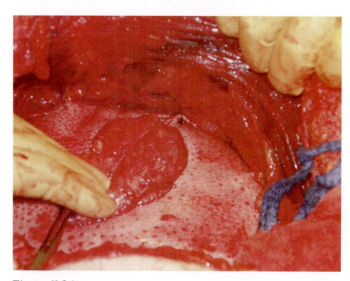

Figure 7-14.

Chapter 7 • Open Repair of Parastomal Hernias 125

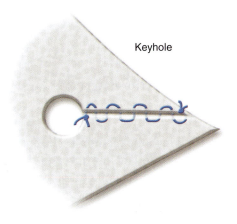

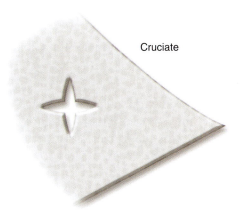

OPTIONS FOR STOMA APERTURES IN MESH

Figure 7-15.

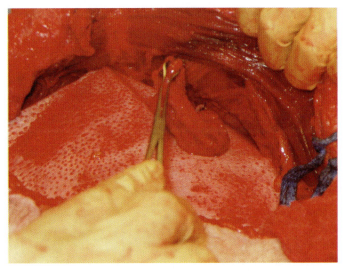

Figure 7-16.

7. Reapproximation of Midline Anterior Fascia over Mesh, Pull Through of Stoma

▲ The stoma is now pulled through the rectus muscle, anterior sheath, and skin. Two 10-mm flat closed suction drains are brought out through the inferior abdominal wall through stab incisions just above the mesh. The midline fascia is closed with a heavy #1 long-term absorbable suture over the biologic mesh (Fig. 7-17).

8. Resection of Redundant Skin and Old Stoma, Skin Closure

▲ Redundant skin is excised, sometimes allowing excision of the old stoma site. A 10-mm flat drain is placed under the skin flap if there is significant dead space. The midline skin is then closed with staples as is the former ostomy site. The ostomy is matured after all wounds are closed.

5. Postoperative Care

▲ Patients with larger hernias and any loss of abdominal domain are typically observed in the intensive care unit immediately postoperatively. Careful monitoring of pulmonary and fluid status is essential in these patients. Drains are typically maintained for 2 weeks, then discontinued. Antibiotics are stopped at 24 hours, and they are not continued for the duration of the drains unless signs of superficial infections are present.

▲ Early respiratory difficulties and renal difficulties related to loss of domain and resuscitation can be seen. In an early series of 12 patients, we had one early postoperative death, but the cause was unclear because the family refused postmortem examination. Thirty-three percent had significant perioperative complications, including one transient renal failure requiring hemodialysis, one who acutely thrombosed an aortobifemoral graft, and one wound infection requiring local care. We have not had to explant any mesh. No symptomatic recurrences were noted in our 11 patients at 1 year. CT follow-up was obtained in all, and two small recurrences were noted radiographically only.

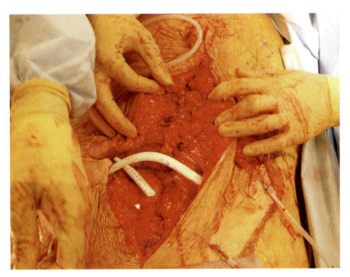

Figure 7-17.

6. Pearls and Pitfalls

▲ Careful selection of patients for this extensive surgical repair is essential. Thorough preoperative evaluation and optimization of cardiac, pulmonary, and nutritional status is essential. Counseling of patients on the complexity of the planned operation and expected perioperative course must be complete so that realistic expectations can be maintained. In patients with excessive comorbidities, this operation may be inappropriate

▲ Knowledge of abdominal wall anatomy and careful attention to planes of dissection are critical to success, allowing for adequate mobilization of the preperitoneal space for wide tension-free mesh reinforcement of the abdominal wall. If you are going to access the lateral abdominal wall via incision of the posterior rectus sheath, great care should be taken to avoid injuring the transversus abdominis muscle and internal oblique, particularly if you are going to add an anterior component separation with external oblique release because this can destabilize the lateral abdominal wall. In most circumstances we find that a posterior release is sufficient and the anterior external oblique release is not necessary.

▲ Kinking of the stoma through the layers of the abdominal wall must be avoided. A careful, sequential creation of aligned stoma apertures is important to ensure a straight, non-obstructing path. Reapproximation of the abdominal layers to simulate linea alba at the midline as the stoma apertures are created is essential to create this aligned path.

▲ A biologic mesh is most suited for this repair in order to avoid erosion into the stoma and to avoid infection in these potentially contaminated cases. We have typically used a non–cross-linked porcine dermis mesh, noting its 20 × 20 cm available size, softness, and easy handling. The biologic meshes are expensive, but with the infection and erosion risk, we feel they should be chosen over polypropylene or other synthetic mesh types. The availability of large sizes in these porcine meshes makes them ideal for good overlap of the component separation repair. Importantly, the mesh is placed in a diamond configuration to assist with appropriate, wide underlayment. With our increasing experience with biologic mesh, we have become more comfortable allowing the biologic graft to touch the bowel at the new stoma site. The aperture for allowing the bowel to traverse the abdominal wall is a common point for recurrence. The use of a biologic graft likely reduces the risk of erosion and permits a more physiologic aperture.

Selected References

Rosen MJ, Reynolds HL, Champagne B, Delaney CP: A novel approach for the simultaneous repair of large midline incisional and parastomal hernia with biological mash and retrorectus reconstruction, *Am J Surg* 199(3):416–420, 2010 Mar.

The Ventral Hernia Working Group: Breuing K, Butler CE, Ferzoco S, Franz M, Hultman CS, Kilbridge JF, Rosen M, Silverman RP, Vargo D. Incisional ventral hernias: Review of the literature and regarding the grading and technique of repair, *Surgery*. 2010 Mar 19. [Epub ahead of print].

SECTION IV

Component Separation

CHAPTER 8

OPEN COMPONENT SEPARATION

Ronald P. Silverman, MD, FACS

1. Surgical Anatomy

A clear understanding of the anatomy of the abdominal wall is critical when performing a component separation operation. The two vertically oriented rectus abdominis muscles, with their overlying anterior rectus sheaths should normally lie side by side in the midline. In between the rectus muscles is the tendinous linea alba, which functionally is actually the tendinous insertion of the fascial extensions of the six lateral abdominal wall muscles (bilateral external oblique, internal oblique, and transverses abdominis). A midline incisional hernia is caused by a disruption of the linea alba, which in turn leads to unopposed contraction of the lateral abdominal wall muscles. It is this constant unopposed pull from the lateral muscles in combination with intraperitoneal pressure that leads to the gradual increase in size of these hernias and ultimately loss of abdominal domain. The position of the arcuate line is also important to understand. The arcuate line lies approximately three fourths of the way from the pubis to the umbilicus, or to use a bony anatomic landmark, approximately 2 cm cephalad to a line drawn between the two anterior superior iliac spines. Below this line there is no posterior rectus sheath (Cunningham, 2004). There is also a small triangular muscle called the pyrimidalis that overlies the most inferior portion of the rectus muscles just as they attach onto the pubis. This muscle is not relevant clinically.

The main blood supply to the rectus abdominis muscles is from the superior and inferior epigastric arteries, with the inferior epigastric being more dominant. The entire muscle can easily survive however on either blood vessel. There are additional vascular contributions from the intercostal arterial branches that come in laterally in a segmental fashion. The blood supply to the lateral musculature comes from intercostal branches that travel deep to the internal oblique muscle in the so-called neurovascular plane. In this plane are also the nerves to the abdominal wall that are branches of the lower six thoracic and the first lumbar segmental nerves.

2. Preoperative Considerations

The preoperative evaluation should include a complete medical history that includes any operative reports from previous operations. In cases where there have been previous hernia repairs, it is important to know what type of mesh repairs have been done, including the specific brand of mesh and the plane in which the mesh was placed and whether or not a component separation has been previously attempted. It should be noted in the history whether or not there were wound complications or infections after any of the previous operations.

Certain comorbidities are associated with higher rates of complications, and if any of these comorbidities can be managed before the surgery, every effort should be made to do so. Examples include losing weight, controlling diabetes, quitting smoking, maximizing nutritional status, maximizing a patient's cardio/pulmonary health, and taking appropriate prophylactic measures for thromboembolic disease.

It should be noted that in many circumstances, although patients can be quite miserable, incisional hernia repairs can be categorized as elective surgery. Those patients with hernia defects with a very wide base are at a low risk for bowel strangulation and obstruction. In patients like this, with non–life-threatening hernias, where the extent of their comorbidities carry an unacceptably high mortality risk, surgery should be avoided. One particular comorbidity, that of being super-obese (body mass index [BMI] >45), in addition to other general morbidities, carries a very high risk of hernia recurrence, reported to be as high as 50% (Vargo, 2008). In these patients, the risk-to-benefit scale is certainly tilted toward risk, and a serious effort at weight loss should be attempted before opting for elective surgery.

3. Operative Steps

The first step in performing a component separation is lysis of adhesions from the bowel to the undersurface of the abdominal wall. This allows for a good underlay of any mesh that may be used but also helps to untether the abdominal wall musculature and allow it to advance toward the midline. The next step is identification of the healthy fascial edges. This is performed by undermining the skin and subcutaneous fat until healthy rectus abdominis anterior fascia is identified. It is important to do this very carefully and avoid getting underneath the anterior rectus fascia. It is also important not to confuse dense scar tissue from healthy fascia, which is a common mistake that leads to recurrence over time as that dense scar tissue slowly remodels and ultimately gives way. In the case of skin graft or secondarily healed scar on top of bowel there are two options. One option is to remove the skin graft or scar completely with sharp dissection. This can sometimes be difficult and may lead to enterotomies. If it becomes clear that this technique is too risky, then another option is to leave the skin graft or scar on the bowel and simply de-epithelialize it. This is done with a number 10 scalpel blade by tangentially shaving off the epidermis, leaving what is left of the dermis or the scar tissue behind. At the periphery, the normal skin and subcutaneous fat can be undermined in the usual fashion until healthy fascia is identified.

Once the fascia is identified, undermining should continue until the lateral edge of the rectus abdominis is identified. This often can be visualized; however, a better way to find it is to pinch the abdominal wall musculature by placing the hand and fingers intraperitoneally with the thumb above the fascia and feeling for the thickening of the edge of the rectus muscle while the hand is slid medially. Some descriptions of open component separation describe continuing to undermine the skin all the way to the anterior axillary line. In my opinion this is not necessary and only leads to more risk for wound complications. I believe the undermining of the skin should end just at the point of where the external oblique fascia is divided.

A small nick in the external oblique fascia should then be made just 1 cm lateral to the lateral aspect of the rectus abdominis muscle. If the surgeon notices that there are still vertically oriented muscle fibers under the fascia, then the nick has been made too medial and another nick should be made a centimeter or so more laterally. Once the incision in the external oblique fascia is made, it is important to carry this incision all the way to just below the hernia defect (stopping short of the inguinal ligament) and all the way up over the costal margin superiorly. Generally, when going over the costal margin, the surgeon is dividing not only the fascial aponeurosis, but the actual muscle fibers of the external oblique muscle itself. It is important to completely transect these external oblique muscle fibers high up at the level of the costal margin. This allows for a much easier closure in the epigastric area. Figure 8-1 shows the division of the external oblique fascia just lateral to the lateral edge of the rectus abdominis muscle. Figure 8-2 is an intraoperative photograph showing the division of the external oblique fascia. In this photo, the rectus abdominis muscles have already been sutured together.

Once the external fascia is divided on both sides, the surgeon should assess the tension on the closure and whether or not the fascia will actually come together in the midline. A few additional maneuvers can then be attempted if there is still more advancement required to get a closure without undue tension. The next maneuver is to actually undermine the external oblique fascia/muscle all the way to the anterior axillary line. One must be careful to stop short of the blood vessels supplying the external oblique. If this is not enough, the last maneuver is to enter the medial edge of the rectus sheath and lift the muscle off of the posterior rectus sheath. This last step is only minimally effective in most cases, adding perhaps 1 to 2 cm of advancement on each side, with the exception of those cases where the rectus abdominis muscles have become tubularized.

In those cases where the rectus muscles will come together in the midline, I then proceed with performing a running closure with a #1 size loop suture made of monofilament slowly resorbable material (polydioxanone). In those situations where the fascial edges do not come together (which occurs less than 15% of the time in my practice), then a fascial bridge must be performed with some sort of mesh placed as an underlay. In this circumstance, the mesh must be placed in the intraperitoneal position, underneath the fascia and all the way to approximately the lateral edge of the rectus abdominis. Synthetic mesh should be avoided in circumstances where there is bacterial contamination or infection and also in those patients where comorbidities put the patient at an unacceptably high risk for developing a surgical site infection or wound breakdown. For those patients where synthetic mesh is undesirable, a biologic material should be used. It is important to note that there is a large and at times overwhelming variety of synthetic and biologic materials available to surgeons today, many of which have little in the way of data to support their use. Surgeons should obviously base their decision for material selection on the best available data at the time of use.

Chapter 8 • Open Component Separation   135

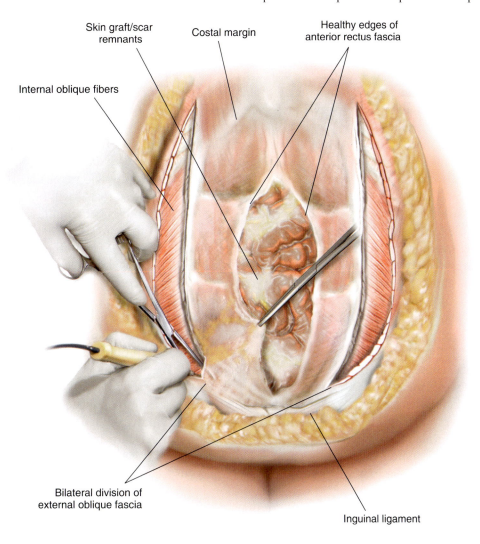

Figure 8-1.

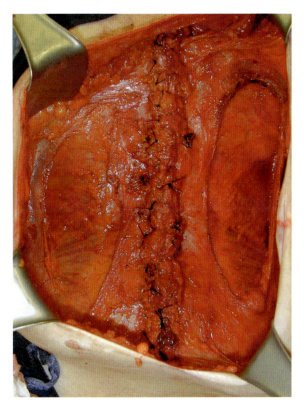

Figure 8-2.

When the muscles do reach together in the midline, and are able to be closed primarily, a reinforcing material (synthetic or biologic as discussed in the previous paragraph) should be placed either as an underlay or as an overlay to reduce the risk for recurrence. It is my preference to place the material as an overlay. I prefer the overlay because it allows me to reinforce not only the midline repair, but the lateral areas of the abdominal wall where the external oblique has been divided. I run the material along the cut lateral free edge of the external oblique fascia. I then pull the material taught across the midline and suture it with another running suture to the cut lateral edge of the opposite external oblique fascia under physiologic tension. It is important that this be under some tension and not completely loose so that it will off-load some of the tension on the midline repair. This added layer reinforces not only the midline but also the two lateral areas where the external oblique has been cut. Furthermore, by placing the material under some tension it re-medializes the two external oblique muscles that otherwise retract laterally and become useless. By effectively reinserting the two external muscles across the midline to one another it allows these muscles to continue to act as functional muscle units. It is important to quilt the material down to the anterior abdominal wall (Figs. 8-3, 8-4, and 8-5). This is done with size 0 polydioxanone suture. These quilting sutures must be placed only over the top of the rectus abdominis muscles because they are placed in a blind fashion. The needle is placed through the onlay material, then placed in a skiving fashion through the anterior rectus fascia and then brought back up through the implant material. This is safe as long as the rectus muscle is present. Laterally, the abdominal wall may be too thin to safely place these sutures without risk of entering the peritoneal space. The quilting sutures are important to place because they further offload tension from the midline by further distributing the tension and they prevent seroma formation between the implant material and the fascia, allowing vascular ingrowth into the material more readily. Our group has recently reported a 7% recurrence rate with a mean follow-up of 1 year in 60 consecutive patients using this technique (Stromberg, 2010).

One of the negatives of performing the open component separation technique is the risk of wound complications; however, several techniques can be used to minimize wound breakdown. Already mentioned is limiting the undermining of the skin and fat to only just lateral to the rectus abdominis muscle. Additional maneuvers include excision of any redundant skin and fat. Sometimes this requires a formal panniculectomy, and sometimes it is simply a matter of removing a few centimeters of skin and fat from each side of the incision. Next, for the remaining skin flaps, it is important to remove any sub-Scarpa fat. This is particularly important in patients with thick subcutaneous layers. This deeper fat is generally ischemic, and leaving it puts the patient at risk for fat necrosis and therefore at risk for seromas and wound infections. Next is the suturing down the skin flaps to the abdominal wall. These quilting sutures reduce dead space and help reduce the risk for seromas. Perhaps most important is the liberal use of drains. I put at least two but up to four 19-French round fluted drains. I never remove them during the patient's hospitalization and never sooner than 1 week after the procedure. After 1 week, I like to see <30 mL/drain/24-hour period for at least 2 days in a row before pulling out the drain. Typically, drains are removed in the 2- to 4-week range, but sometimes the drains are left in as long as 6 weeks.

A final maneuver that has helped with wound breakdown in my practice is the use of negative pressure therapy over the top of my closed incision. I perform an intradermal or subcuticular closure with resorbable sutures and then place a nonadherent porous dressing over the top of the suture line. On top of that I place the foam and the adhesive layer and place the dressing on negative 125 mm Hg suction. This dressing draws away any drainage from the suture line, but more importantly, it draws blood flow to the wound edges and reduces edema while mechanically pulling together the skin edges and stabilizing the suture line. This dressing is left in place for the patient's entire hospitalization (up to 8 days). This has remarkably improved outcomes in even the most challenging large panniculectomy incisions.

Chapter 8 • Open Component Separation 137

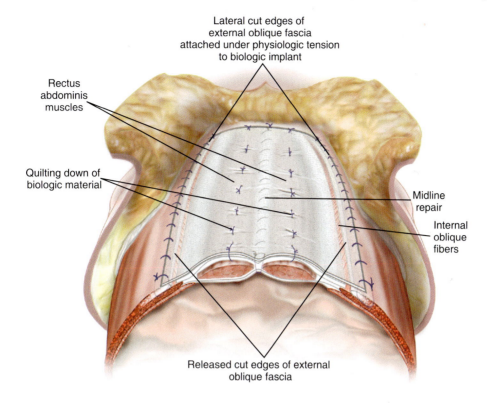

Figure 8-3.

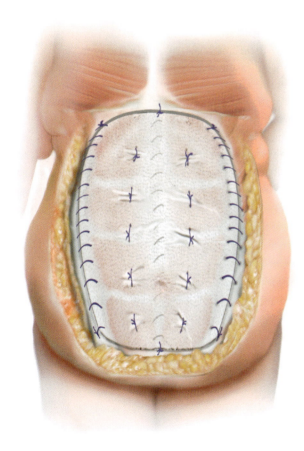

Figure 8-4.

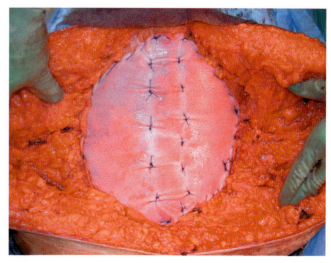

Figure 8-5.

4. Postoperative Considerations

Postoperatively, I do not tend to use abdominal binders until after the drains are removed. I am concerned that a binder being placed two tightly may interfere with skin perfusion, may irritate the suture line as well as the drain exit sites. Once the drains are removed, I have the patient wear the binder at all times (except when showering) for a period of 6 weeks. After this I tell the patients to continue to wear the binder whenever they are doing anything even moderately strenuous for the rest of their lives.

Patients are instructed to not lift anything heavier than their shoes for 6 weeks post operatively. After that, I explain to patients that they always have a risk of recurrence and so they should alter their lifestyles if they want to help reduce that risk. I recommend that they avoid heavy lifting if at all possible, even if that means changing occupations. They can resume moderate aerobic type exercise such as walking or bicycling, however they should never perform sit-ups or weight lifting.

5. Pearls and Pitfalls

One major pitfall is failure to identify the healthy medial edge of good fascia. Scar tissue, although it may seem strong at the time, will ultimately fail and lead to recurrence. Excessive undermining of the skin and fat also is a pitfall than can lead to ischemic skin edges and fat and wound complications. Finally closing the fascia under too much tension is another key pitfall. It is tempting to force together the fascial edges when they are very close but in time this will often lead to a recurrence. It is better to leave the edges apart and use an underlay technique to bridge the gap then to truly force together the fascial edges. Unfortunately the question of how tight is too tight is only answerable at this time with surgical judgment that comes from experience. One pearl that has given me additional fascial advancement when needed is the maneuver of undermining the external oblique fascia laterally, all the way to the anterior axillary line. Keep in mind that the fascia stays attached to the overlying fat to avoid devascularization of the fat. Also, a considerable amount of medial advancement of the fascia in the epigastric area can be achieved by carrying the division of the external oblique fascia over the costal margin. Finally, many of the potential negatives of the open component separation technique, such as wound problems and seromas, can be mitigated by proper management of the skin flaps. A summary of this management includes minimizing skin undermining to just lateral to the rectus muscles, excision of redundant skin and fat before closure, removal of sub-Scarpa fat from the remaining skin flaps, liberal use of drains, quilting down the Scarpa fascia to the abdominal wall, and the use of negative pressure therapy on top of the closed incision. With these techniques, the wound complications and seroma problems have become minimal in my practice.

Disclosure Statement

Dr. Silverman is the Chief Medical Officer and Sr. Vice President of KCI Corporation, of which LifeCell Corporation is a division. Elsevier does not endorse any products or services of KCI Corporation.

Selected References

Cunningham SC, Rosson GD, Lee RH, Williams JZ, Justman C, Slezak S, Goldberg NH, Silverman RP: Localization of the arcuate line from surface anatomic landmarks: a cadaveric study, *Annals of Plastic Surgery* 53(2), August 2004.

Stromberg J, Hamidi R, Silverman RP, Singh D: *Abdominal wall reconstruction with component separation and porcine acellular dermal matrix onlay*, May 23-26, 2010, 2010 Plastic Surgery Research Council.

Vargo DJ: *long term follow up of human acellular dermal matrix in 100 patients with complex abdominal wall reconstruction*. Hernia Update 2008, March 12-16, 2008, American Hernia Society, P 262.

CHAPTER 9

Periumbilical Perforator Sparing Components Separation

George DeNoto III, MD, FACS and Ron Israeli, MD, FACS

1. Clinical Anatomy

1. Rationale for Sparing the Periumbilical Perforators

- ▲ Components separation for ventral hernia repair requires release of the external oblique muscle lateral to the linea semilunaris and separation of the avascular plane deep to the external oblique. This allows midline advancement of the rectus abdominis in continuity with the internal oblique and transversus abdominis muscles. As originally described, components separation requires wide undermining of the skin and subcutaneous layer to adequately expose the external oblique muscles for subsequent division. Consequently, perfusion of the undermined skin flaps can be compromised, which increases the risk of skin flap necrosis, infection, and dehiscence. In addition, extensive elevation of abdominal skin flaps creates a large wound surface predisposing to postoperative hematomas and seromas.
- ▲ To address this major shortcoming of conventional components separation, a modified technique of elevating partial subcutaneous flaps with preservation of the periumbilical perforating vessels arising from the inferior epigastric vessels can be performed. The rationale for using the technique of periumbilical perforator sparing (PUPS) components separation is to maximize skin blood supply. The preservation of blood flow to the midline abdominal wall should minimize complications, especially skin flap ischemia and infection. In addition, by avoiding wide undermining, subcutaneous dead space is minimized, which may reduce the incidence of seromas or hematomas. Furthermore, preservation of blood supply to the abdominal wall in ventral hernia repair allows expanded applications for patients with obesity, diabetes mellitus, a recent smoking history, and for those with stomas as well as those who require concomitant panniculectomy.

2. Innervation and Blood Supply to the Abdominal Wall Muscles

- ▲ In performing all techniques of components separation abdominal wall reconstruction, it is important to understand the musculofascial anatomy, innervation, and blood supply of the anterior abdominal wall. The anterior and posterior releases in components separation allow preservation of the blood supply and innervation of the abdominal wall muscles.
- ▲ The intercostal neurovascular bundles that contribute to the external oblique, internal oblique, transversus, and rectus muscles are preserved because they run deep to the internal oblique. They are therefore preserved during all techniques of components separation.
- ▲ In addition, the deep inferior epigastric vessels and the superior epigastric vessels, which run in a longitudinal orientation deep to and within the substance of both rectus muscles, are also preserved regardless of which components separation technique is performed. Preservation of these vessels maintains the blood supply to the abdominal wall muscles.
- ▲ On the other hand, blood supply to the overlying skin relies on branches of these vessels, as well as on a number of additional vessels, which are preserved to varying degrees, depending on the technique of components separation performed.

3. Blood Supply to the Abdominal Wall Skin

- ▲ The blood supply to the abdominal wall skin is based on direct cutaneous vessels in addition to numerous branches of deep vessels that are known as musculocutaneous perforators. Whenever abdominal wall skin is undermined, as in components separation, defining the source of vascularity to the remaining skin in critical.
- ▲ The three Huger zones of abdominal wall vascular anatomy can help guide the surgeon in planning a safe abdominal wall operation. Huger zone I, the central abdominal wall, is supplied by the deep inferior epigastric and superior epigastric vessels. Zone II, the lower abdominal wall, is supplied by the superficial inferior epigastric, superficial external pudendal, and superficial circumflex iliac arteries. Zone III, the lateral abdominal wall, is supplied by the intercostal, subcostal, and lumbar arteries. Skin flap elevation during conventional components separation abdominal wall reconstruction results in complete division of the cutaneous blood supply of Huger zone I, supplied by the deep epigastric vessels. The PUPS components separation approach preserves the vessels of Huger zone I, which allows improved perfusion to minimize any potential vascular related complications.
- ▲ The concept of vascular territories called angiosomes further elucidates our understanding of the blood supply to the abdominal wall skin. From a clinical perspective, preservation of the primary angiosome to an anatomic territory of skin maximizes blood flow to that territory. The primary central anterior abdominal wall angiosome is supplied by multiple cutaneous perforator branches of the deep epigastric artery system. Microdissection analysis of the vascular anatomy of the anterior abdominal wall skin and subcutaneous tissue has confirmed that perforator branches of the deep inferior epigastric vessels provide the main blood supply to this region. More specifically, the periumbilical region, mostly just inferior and lateral to the umbilicus is the region with the highest concentration of these perforator vessel branches (Fig. 9-1). The PUPS components separation technique focuses on maintaining this rich vascular network, thereby maximizing blood supply without compromising the degree of muscle flap advancement possible.

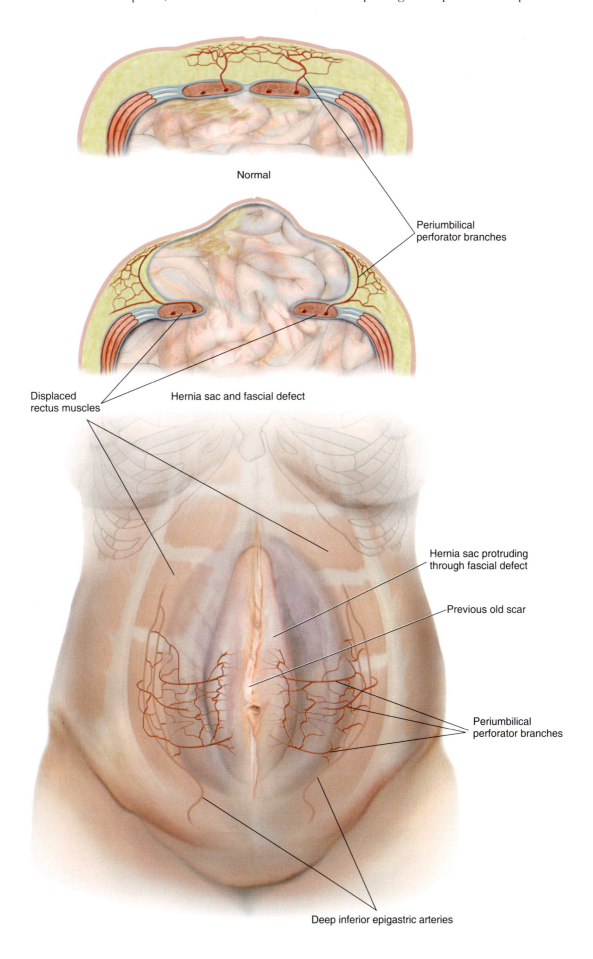

Figure 9-1.

2. Preoperative Considerations

1. Optimization of Comorbidities

- ▲ The primary goal in the management of the ventral hernia patient is to repair the hernia while minimizing the incidence of postoperative complications, including recurrence. As with any surgical procedure, preoperative patient optimization is vital to reducing the risk of postoperative complications. This includes smoking cessation, control of diabetes mellitus, weight loss, maximization of nutritional status, establishing an exercise routine, preoperative *Staphylococcus aureus* screening, and optimization of pulmonary and cardiac status.

2. Defining the Defect and Patient Anatomy

- ▲ *Preoperative Physical Examination*

  - ▲ A focused preoperative physical examination is very important in planning the operative approach in abdominal wall reconstruction and helps identify the appropriate candidate for PUPS components separation. Components separation procedures are useful for midline and paramedian hernias in which the fascia cannot be approximated without flap release and advancement. In general, components separation can allow fascial approximation for most midline defects smaller than 20 cm at the waistline.
  - ▲ The size of the defect and loss of domain can be estimated by physical examination. The combination of a large hernia sac and a large hernia defect are the typical findings on exam that may predict the need for a components separation. A large sac with a small defect frequently does not require a components separation procedure to obtain fascial closure, whereas a large defect with a small sac may. However, there is no exact size of defect that predicts the need for a components separation procedure because abdominal wall compliance varies from patient to patient.
  - ▲ Preoperative surgical scars and the position of any stomas, if they are present, should be noted. This can help in surgical planning of a PUPS procedure.

- ▲ *Preoperative Abdominal CT Scan*

  - ▲ Preoperative imaging studies also are useful in planning the operative procedure. A preoperative computed tomography (CT) scan provides an accurate measurement of the size of the ventral hernia defect and can demonstrate the size and contents of the hernia sac (Fig. 9-2). This information can help predict the need for a components separation procedure. A CT scan also may reveal the presence of any other hernia defects or other pathology otherwise not appreciated on physical examination. Other hernia defects potentially identified on a CT scan can then be addressed at the time of abdominal wall reconstruction.

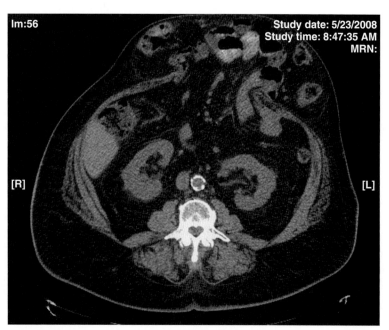

Figure 9-2.

▲ In patients who have had a prior wide subcutaneous flap procedure or other abdominal surgery where the periumbilical perforator blood supply to the abdominal wall may have been divided, a CT angiogram can be performed. CT angiography can identify the remaining blood supply to the central abdominal wall in order to help operative planning. The location of intact perforators can be identified preoperatively and thereby preserved during PUPS components separation.

3. Choosing the Type of Components Separation

▲ The technique of PUPS can be performed in essentially any patient thought to be a candidate for components separation.
▲ In all cases, the choice is made between two categories of components separation procedures: those that preserve the periumbilical perforators and those that do not. While this choice can be made preoperatively, the final selection of procedure may rely on findings at the time of surgery.
▲ The conventional components separation (as described in Chapter 8) requires significant skin undermining and division of the periumbilical perforators and should be performed only if extensive subcutaneous skin flap elevation is necessary (i.e., as done during removal of an infected onlay synthetic mesh). Otherwise a periumbilical perforator sparing technique, performed open or laparoscopic should be attempted in all cases requiring components separation.
▲ Procedures that preserve the periumbilical perforators include the open PUPS components separation and the laparoscopic components separation procedures.

- ▲ If dissection and removal of the hernia sac results in partial subcutaneous flap creation then one should continue that dissection around the periumbilical perforators and perform an open PUPS components separation. If there is no skin flap creation during removal of the hernia sac then a laparoscopic components separation can be performed (as described in Chapter 11).
- ▲ One of the limitations of the laparoscopic components separation technique is that it may not always provide the same degree of fascial release as compared to conventional components separation. In our experience, the extent of fascial release provided by open PUPS components separation is equivalent to the degree of release possible with the conventional open approach.

4. Choosing the Type of Mesh

- ▲ Mesh placement is strongly advised once the PUPS components separation procedure is completed in order to minimize post operative hernia recurrence.
- ▲ In the patient with multiple comorbidities, who is at higher risk for developing a postoperative surgical site infection, the implantation of a biologic matrix to reinforce fascial closure after components separation may be more appropriate than a synthetic mesh. Similarly, if the patient has a clean-contaminated or contaminated wound, then a biologic matrix should be implanted. A patient with minimal or no comorbidities and a clean operative wound class can have a synthetic mesh implanted for fascial reinforcement. If the wound is too contaminated or dirty, then mesh implantation should be avoided and a staged repair with mesh implantation at a later date should be considered.

3. Operative Steps

1. Hernia on Physical Exam (Fig. 9-3 and Fig. 9-4, A)

▲ The patient is examined and the hernia defects and surgical scars are noted.

2. Preoperative Markings (Fig. 9-4)

▲ Before surgery, the patient's abdominal wall is marked. The hernia defect is outlined, and the locations of the periumbilical perforators are marked in reference to the rectus abdominis muscles (Fig. 9-4, B). The perforators are usually located within a 6 cm radius of the umbilicus but can be more laterally positioned in the presence of a large hernia sac.
▲ The planned subcutaneous tunnels along each costal margin and each inguinal region are drawn on the abdomen.
▲ All old incision lines are identified and marked. The planned skin incisions are marked, including any planned excisions of old scar and excess skin (Fig. 9-4 C).
▲ The planned transection of the external oblique aponeurosis will be within the connecting tunnels on each side. Panniculectomy incisions can be marked if planned to occur simultaneous with the PUPS components separation.

3. Patient Positioning

▲ Whenever possible, an epidural catheter is placed. The patient is then positioned on the operating room table supine with the arms abducted. Following induction of anesthesia, an orogastric tube and Foley catheter are placed.

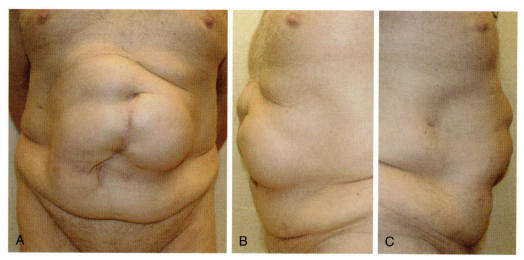

Figure 9-3.

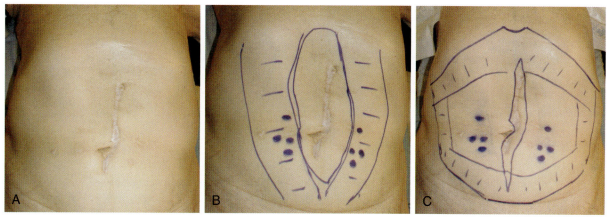

Figure 9-4.

4. Exposure

▲ The old scar and subcutaneous tissue posterior to the scar is excised. This is performed usually en bloc with the ventral hernia sac (Fig. 9-5, A). Care is taken during dissection of the ventral hernia sac not to undermine too widely from the sac in order to avoid injury to the periumbilical perforators. Once the dissection is completed to the edge of the fascial defect, the hernia sac is opened and excised (Fig. 9-5, B).

5. Adhesiolysis

▲ Any adhesions to the hernia sac and posterior abdominal wall must be fully lysed. If the patient has a history of adhesive small bowel obstruction, then all intraabdominal adhesions are lysed and consideration is given to placement of an antiadhesion material. Any concommitant intraabdominal procedure is performed at this time if necessary.

6. Assessment of Fascial Approximation and Tension

▲ Assessment of fascial approximation is performed by placement of two or three Kocher clamps on each medial fascial edge (Fig. 9-5, C). If the fasciae can be easily approximated with minimal or physiologic tension then a components separation is not required. If the fascial edges do not approximate easily, then a components separation should be performed.

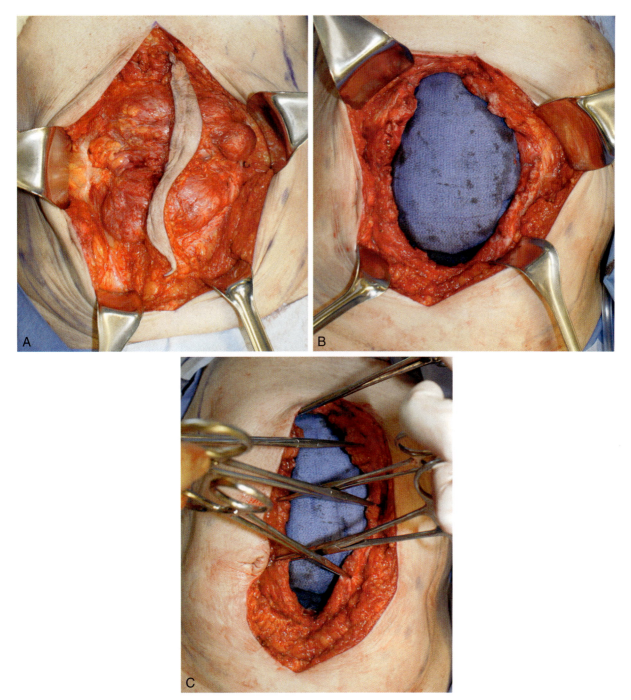

Figure 9-5.

7. Creation of Subcutaneous Tunnels

- ▲ The PUPS components separation is now begun with creation of subcutaneous tunnels that will allow exposure of the anterior aspect of the external oblique fascia bilaterally (Fig. 9-6 and Fig. 9-7).
- ▲ At the epigastric and suprapubic levels, using fiber optic lighted retraction, the skin and subcutaneous tissues are dissected off the anterior rectus sheath extending just lateral to the linea semilunaris. The epigastric tunnel typically exposes the costal margin and extends inferiorly from the xiphoid to a level 2 to 4 cm superior to the umbilicus (Fig. 9-8, A). The suprapubic tunnel typically exposes the inguinal ligament and extends superiorly from the pubic tubercle to a level 6 to 8 cm inferior to the umbilicus (Fig. 9-8, B).
- ▲ The intact subcutaneous tissue between the epigastric and suprapubic tunnels remains attached to the underlying anterior rectus sheath, thus preserving the periumbilical perforators of the deep inferior epigastric vessels.

Chapter 9 • Periumbilical Perforator Sparing Components Separation 151

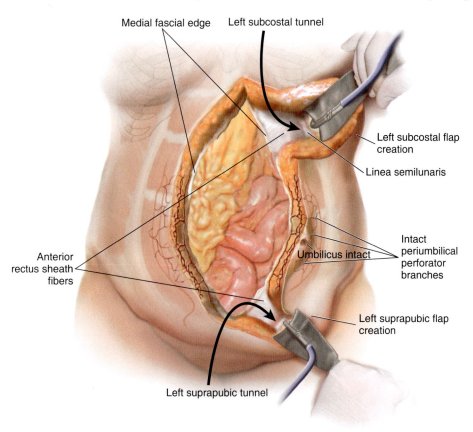

Figure 9-6.

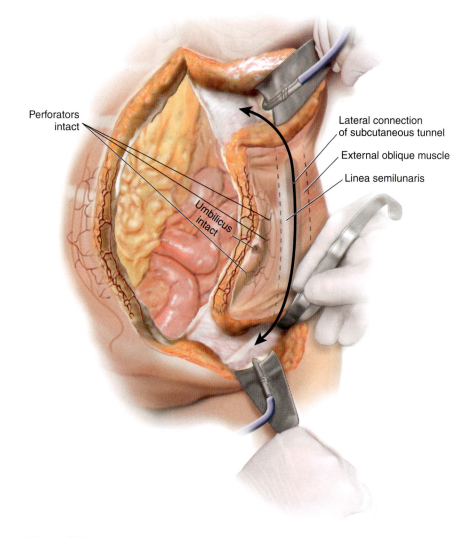

Figure 9-7.

8. Connecting the Subcutaneous Tunnels

▲ The epigastric and suprapubic subcutaneous tunnels can be connected before or during the division of the external oblique muscle.
▲ Using a deep fiber optic lighted retractor or a headlight and deep Deaver retractor, these tunnels are connected from the top down and from the bottom up using cautery dissection. In this way, they can be joined together lateral to the linea semilunaris while avoiding injury to the periumbilical perforators (Fig. 9-8, C).

9. Division of the Aponeurosis of the External Oblique Muscle

▲ Exposure for division of the external oblique muscle fascia is through the epigastric and suprapubic tunnels. The rectus abdominis can be manually retracted medially and the aponeurosis of the external oblique muscle is divided with cautery in a longitudinal orientation approximately 2 cm lateral to the linea semilunaris (Fig. 9-8, C) (Fig. 9-9). Note that at this distance from the linea semilunaris, the external oblique is comprised of thin fascia inferiorly and thicker muscle superiorly.
▲ The external oblique division can continue superiorly approximately 5 to 6 cm over the costal margin onto the thoracic ribcage and can extend inferiorly to the external inguinal ring if necessary (Fig. 9-9). Fiber optic lighted retraction allows maintenance of an optical cavity lateral to the linea semilunaris such that the periumbilical perforators are preserved during fascial incision.
▲ Once the external oblique muscle is completely divided, it is then separated from the underlying internal oblique muscle in an avascular plane laterally toward the flank (Fig. 9-8, D).
▲ Using the PUPS approach, the longitudinal division of the external oblique muscle and its separation from the internal oblique muscle allows medial advancement of the rectus abdominis in continuity with the internal oblique and transversus abdominis muscles towards the midline.

Chapter 9 • Periumbilical Perforator Sparing Components Separation 153

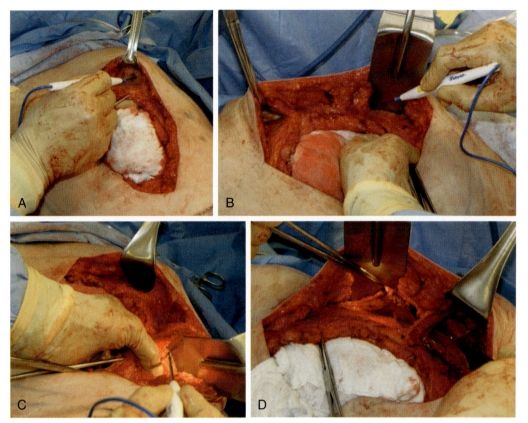

Figure 9-8.

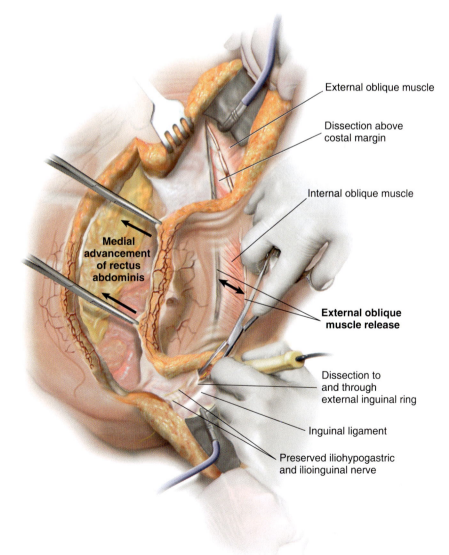

Figure 9-9.

10. Reassessment of Fascial Approximation

▲ Once the external oblique PUPS components separation release has been performed bilaterally, midline fascial approximation is reattempted. If successful, then mesh implantation can be performed. If unsuccessful, a posterior rectus release can be performed to increase the amount of rectus abdominis muscle advancement medially.

11. Division of Posterior Rectus Fascia

▲ If the posterior release is needed, the medial rectus abdominis edge can be retracted anteriorly and laterally with Kocher clamps, and the posterior rectus sheath can be incised longitudinally with cautery approximately 2 cm from the midline. From superior to inferior, this release can extend from under the costal margin to the arcuate line of Douglas where the posterior rectus sheath terminates (Figs. 9-10 and 9-11). Division of the posterior rectus sheath in this fashion typically yields another 1 to 2 cm of release per side. Fascial approximation at the midline is again assessed.

Chapter 9 • Periumbilical Perforator Sparing Components Separation   155

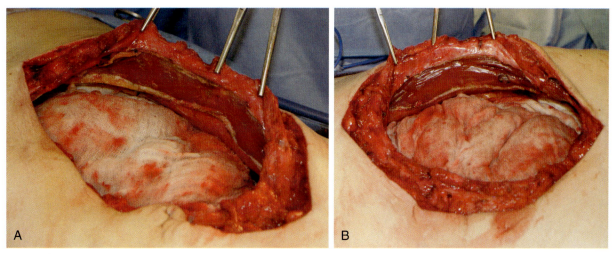

Figure 9-10.

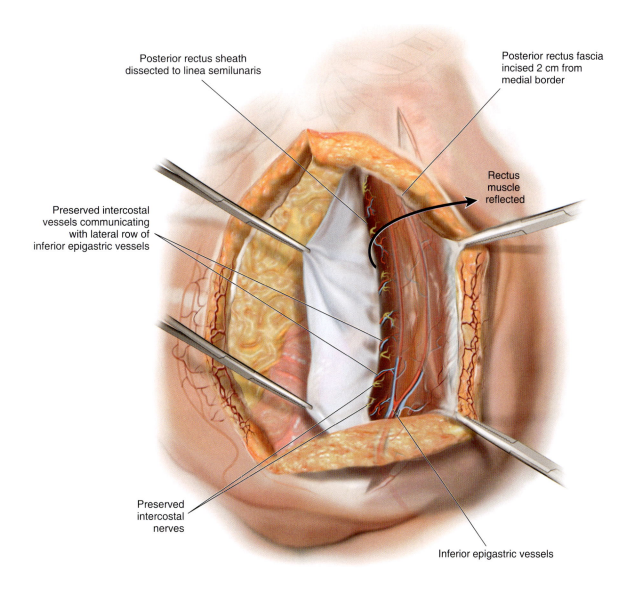

Figure 9-11.

12. Mesh Placement

▲ Once the PUPS components separation has been completed, mesh placement is performed. The mesh is typically placed as an underlay in a retro-rectus or intraperitoneal location, whether a synthetic mesh or a biologic matrix is chosen, because the periumbilical perforators have been preserved (Fig. 9-12).

▲ In placing the mesh as an underlay, the subcutaneous tunnels are used for placement of horizontal mattress transfascial sutures laterally to secure the mesh, thereby avoiding the periumbilical perforator vessels. The lateral sutures can be passed through the laterally displaced cut edge of the external oblique if the mesh underlay is wide enough. Otherwise, sutures can be placed through the medial cut edge of the external oblique at the linea semilunaris just lateral to the perforators (as noted in Fig 9-13 and 9-14). However, placement of sutures through the internal oblique and transversus abdominis muscles in the lateral subcutaneous tunnel can be performed to secure the underlay mesh as well. The mesh can be sutured with permanent or long-lasting absorbable sutures.

▲ Before fascial closure, a drain should be placed anterior to the mesh to minimize the incidence of subfascial fluid accumulation (see Figs. 9-12 and 9-13, A). This fluid could otherwise be a source of postoperative discomfort or infection, and it can be a barrier preventing apposition of the mesh to the rectus muscle, thereby preventing early fibroblast and vascular ingrowth and incorporation.

▲ A "double lay" mesh placement, combining both an underlay and onlay mesh, can be performed in cases of biologic matrix implantation in an attempt to minimize the chance of hernia recurrence (Fig. 9-14). A 4- to 6-cm wide segment of mesh is cut from the lateral side of the original piece. The underlay component is sutured in with at least a 5- to 7-cm underlayment; a drain is placed anterior to the underlay mesh, and the fascia is closed primarily over the drain. The onlay mesh piece is "pie-crusted" before implantation to avoid seroma entrapment between the anterior rectus sheath and the onlay mesh. The onlay portion of the double lay matrix may need to be "hour-glassed" at the level of the periumbilical perforators in order to preserve them. The onlay mesh can be sutured along its perimeter with a running long-lasting absorbable or permanent suture.

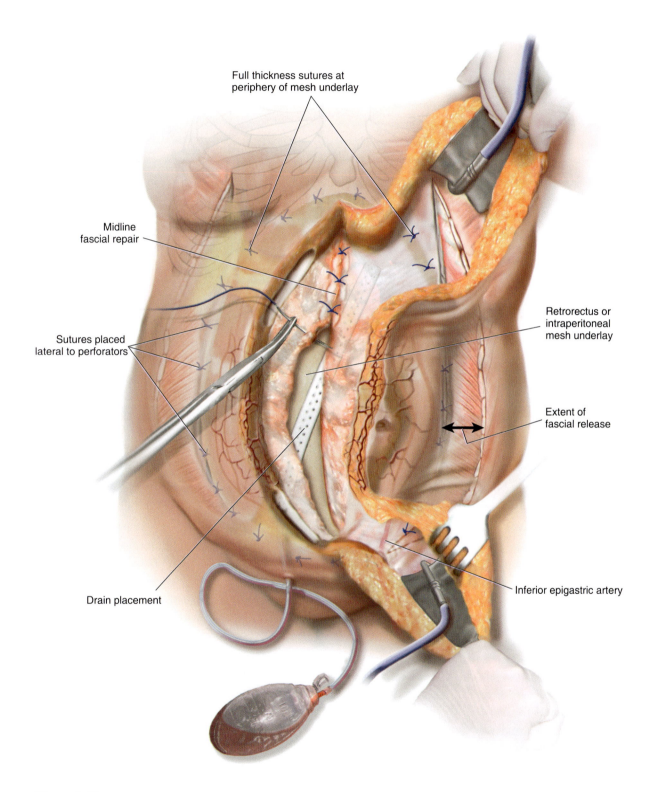

Figure 9-12.

158 Section IV • Component Separation

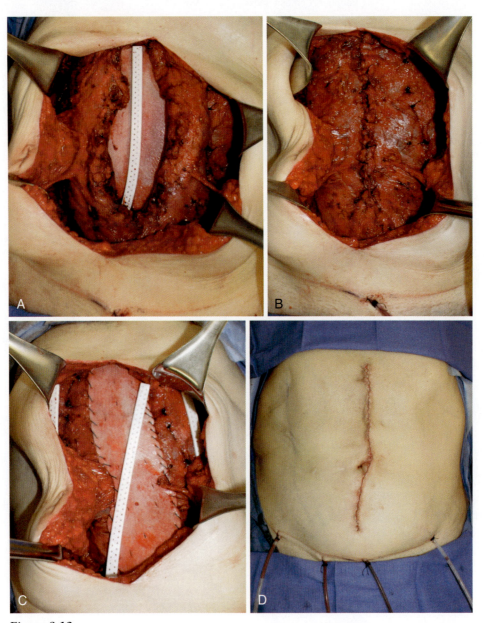

Figure 9-13.

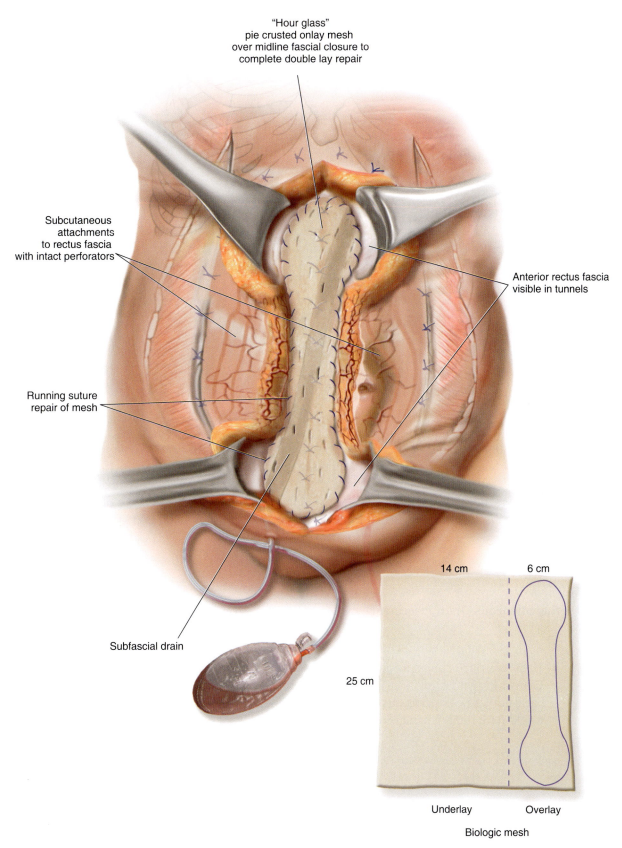

Figure 9-14.

13. Midline Fascial Closure

▲ Midline fascial closure is performed following completion of the underlay mesh placement (see Fig. 9-13, B). If the fasciae approximate with some tension, an interrupted figure of eight closure is used. This can be performed from the top down and from the bottom up until the point of maximal tension is closed. If the fascial edges approximate easily, a running closure can be performed.
▲ A long-lasting absorbable suture or a permanent suture can be used for fascial closure.

14. Onlay Mesh Placement

▲ A wide onlay mesh is not the primary mesh placement position in PUPS components separation because its placement would require division of the periumbilical perforators with creation of large subcutaneous flaps.
▲ In the setting of PUPS components separation, a narrow onlay mesh can be placed as part of a double lay technique when using a biologic matrix as described previously.

15. Subcutaneous Drain Placement

▲ There are three subcutaneous compartments following a PUPS components separation. There is a right lateral, a left lateral, and a central abdominal subcutaneous compartment. Each of these compartments should have a subcutaneous drain. Therefore, each patient would have three subcutaneous drains and one subfascial drain (Fig. 9-15).

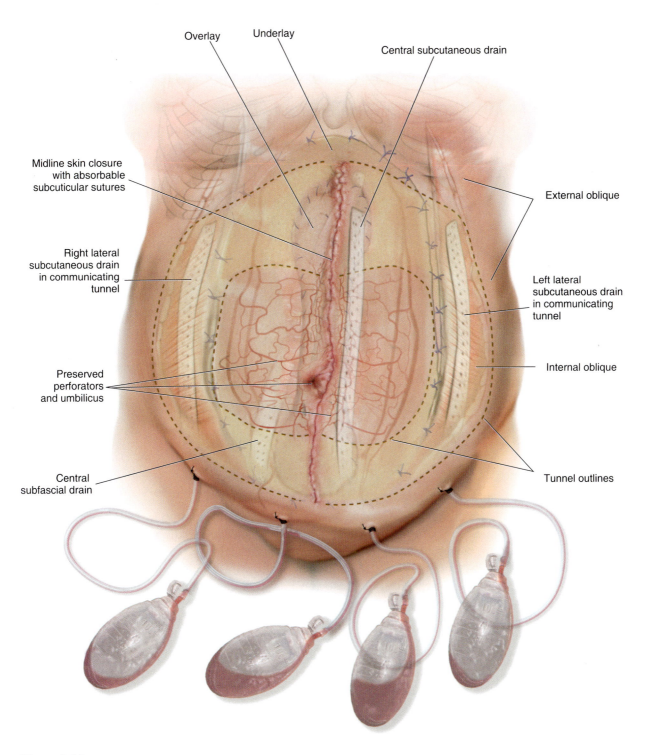

Figure 9-15.

16. Skin Closure

- ▲ The subcutaneous tunnels are closed with absorbable quilting sutures between the deep subcutaneous tissue and the anterior rectus abdominis fascia. This is done to reduce dead space and minimize the risk of seroma formation.
- ▲ Midline abdominal wall closure includes the placement of interrupted absorbable sutures for approximation of Scarpa fascia, as well as a deep dermal repair. The skin closure can be performed with staples or with absorbable subcuticular sutures covered by a liquid epidermal bonding agent (Fig. 9-13, D and Fig. 9-16).

17. Abdominal Binder

- ▲ An abdominal binder is used postoperatively to support the abdominal wall. Patients can be instructed to wear the binder for the first 1 to 3 months following surgery and during strenuous activities thereafter.
- ▲ If there is any concern about viability of the abdominal wall skin flaps, an abdominal binder should not be placed.

4. Postoperative Care

- ▲ Perioperative antibiotics are given as one dose preoperatively and up to 24 hours postoperatively unless the patient has a documented active infection. If the patient has an active infection, antibiotics are given until the infection is cleared.
- ▲ Most of the patients who require abdominal wall reconstruction are at higher risk for development of deep venous thrombosis (DVT) or pulmonary emboli. Therefore a dose of subcutaneous heparin is given before induction of anesthesia and is continued postoperatively until the patient is freely ambulating. Compression stockings also are used for DVT prophylaxis until the patient is ambulatory.
- ▲ Postoperative pain control is achieved with the epidural catheter. If an epidural catheter cannot be used, then an intravenous patient controlled analgesia system is used for postoperative pain management.
- ▲ The patient can be advanced to a regular diet once there is return of bowel function.
- ▲ The subfascial drain usually stops draining in the first week postoperatively and is removed before discharge from the hospital. The other drains are left in place until the output is less than 20 to 30 mL per day for 2 consecutive days. If a double lay placement of the mesh was performed, it is not uncommon for the central compartment subcutaneous drain to stay in for 3 to 6 weeks postoperatively.

Chapter 9 • Periumbilical Perforator Sparing Components Separation

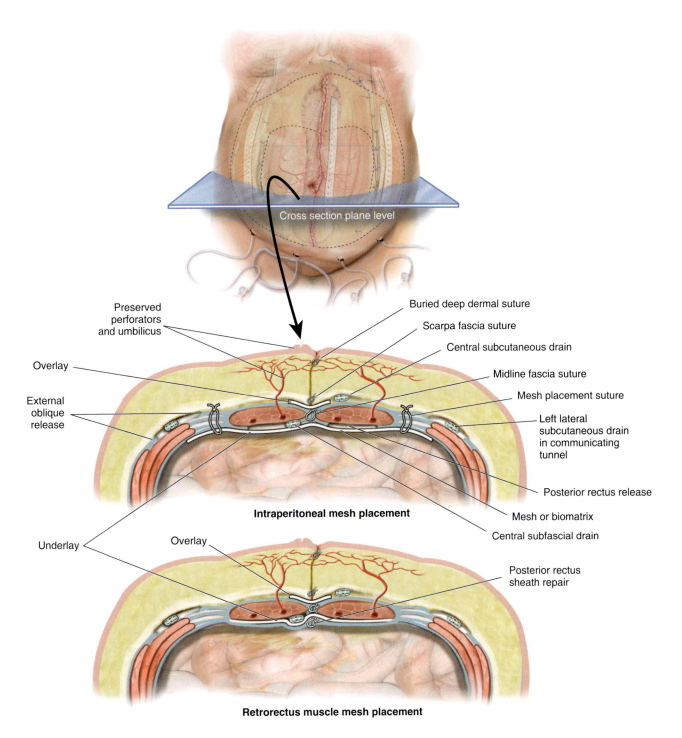

Figure 9-16.

5. Pearls/Pitfalls

1. Managing the Reoperative Patient

▲ *Patients with Previous Ventral Hernia Repair*

- ▲ Many patients who require a components separation operation have already undergone prior ventral hernia repair. Skin flaps may have been created and the periumbilical perforators may have already been divided.
- ▲ In such patients, a CT angiogram can be useful in establishing the presence or absence of periumbilical perforators and thereby determining if a PUPS procedure is warranted. The CT angiogram also may identify collateral blood flow to the abdominal wall such as prominent superficial inferior epigastric vessels, which should then be preserved to ensure vascular supply to the skin.

▲ *Prior Surgical Scars*

- ▲ During the preoperative evaluation, it is critical to note all healed surgical scars, including old laparoscopic trocar site scars. This is because release of the external oblique muscle during components separation across a healed fascial incision may leave weakened or attenuated internal oblique and transversus abdominis muscle fasciae. This will result in a significant risk for the development of a lateral postoperative hernia at that site.
- ▲ While these areas of fascial scar are best avoided, a components separation on that ipsilateral side can still be performed up to but not through the scar, leaving a margin of several centimeters.

▲ *Management of Stomas and Stoma Sites*

- ▲ Stomas, when properly constructed, pass through the rectus abdominis muscle and are not a contraindication for PUPS components separation. A stoma that passes through the rectus abdominis muscle does not interfere with division of the external oblique muscle fascia. When completing a PUPS components separation procedure, the entire area of subcutaneous tissue surrounding the stoma, or surrounding the site of a stoma reversal, is preserved, and the external oblique muscle can be easily divided laterally while still preserving the periumbilical perforators (Figs. 9-17 and 9-18). This allows PUPS components separation to be safely accomplished simultaneously with a stoma reversal operation. The site of the old stoma remains completely separate from any area of skin undermining.
- ▲ If a stoma is not properly located, passing lateral to the rectus abdominis and through the obliques, then the components release on that side should be avoided or should stop several centimeters from the stoma leaving the fascia surrounding the stoma intact.

Chapter 9 • Periumbilical Perforator Sparing Components Separation 165

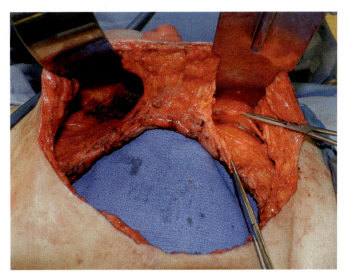

Figure 9-17.

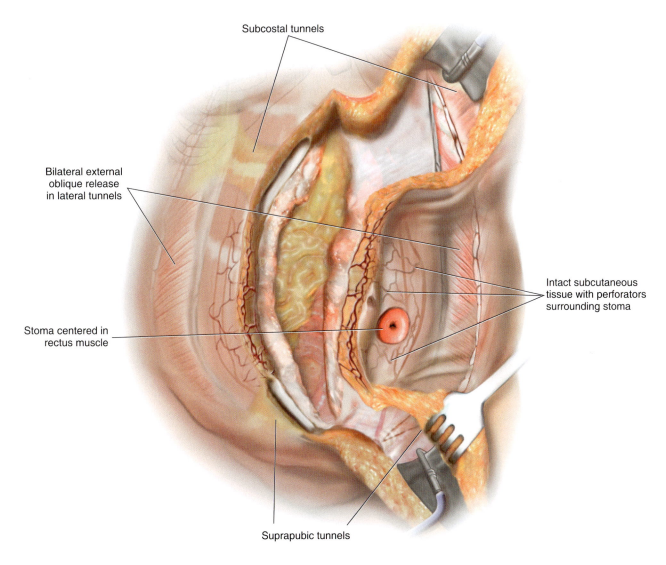

Figure 9-18.

2. Proper Identification of the External Oblique Fascia

▲ If the rectus abdominis muscle is wide or displaced laterally, identification of the external oblique fascia lateral to the linea semilunaris may require added attention. Confirmation of proper identification of the external oblique fascia can be done with gentle cautery. If cautery stimulation causes the underlying muscle to twitch in a longitudinal orientation, consistent with the rectus abdominis muscle contracting, a more lateral exposure is required. When cautery stimulation reveals muscle twitching in an oblique orientation, identification of the external oblique fascia is confirmed.

▲ Once the external oblique fascia is incised longitudinally, the cut fascial edge can be elevated to identify the underlying internal oblique with its muscle fibers directed inferolaterally and the underside of the external oblique muscle with its fibers directed superolaterally. If longitudinally oriented muscle fibers are seen after fascial division (rectus abdominis muscle), the exposure is likely medial to the linea semilunaris. In this case, the anterior fascia should be repaired and dissection should extend more laterally.

3. Maximizing Midline Fascial Advancement

▲ Midline flap advancement can sometimes be limited by the ribs at the epigastric region. In order to maximize advancement at this level, the longitudinal external oblique muscle release incision can extend superiorly 5 to 6 cm over the ribs.

▲ Even further release at this level can be gained by incising the anterior rectus fascia transversely, extending medially from the superior limit of the external oblique incision.

▲ If needed, the posterior rectus release can add a few additional centimeters of advancement.

▲ In cases in which fascial reapproximation was not possible despite an external oblique and posterior rectus release. The medial side of the cut posterior rectus sheath can be flipped medially to help achieve midline fascial closure. The integrity of this closure can be suboptimal; therefore, a double lay mesh placement is ideal in providing additional fascial support in this setting.

4. Determining Appropriate Tension During Mesh Suturing

▲ Mesh needs to be sutured maintaining physiologic tension, especially with biologics, to avoid laxity. In general, the mesh should be taut, so that an imaginary sterile quarter could bounce on the mesh.

5. Panniculectomy

▲ Patients with obesity or with a history of massive weight loss may benefit from simultaneous panniculectomy in the setting of ventral incisional hernia repair (Fig. 9-19, A).

Chapter 9 • Periumbilical Perforator Sparing Components Separation 167

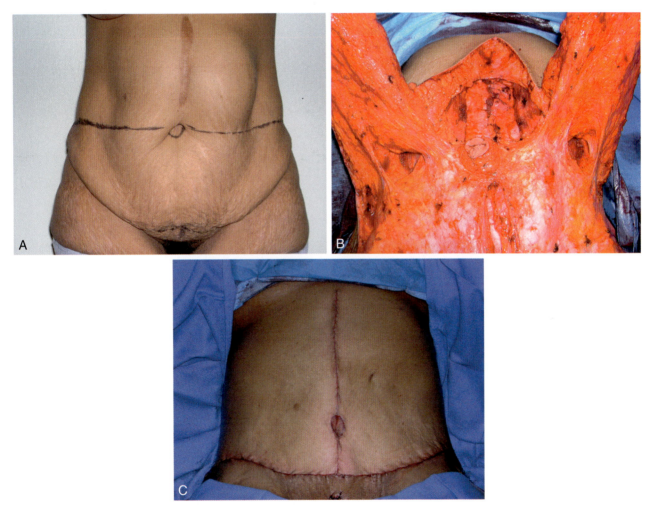

Figure 9-19.

- ▲ The transverse excision of infraumbilical skin and subcutaneous tissue in a panniculectomy results in division of the superficial inferior epigastric blood vessels. As such, when doing a components separation procedure simultaneously with a panniculectomy, preservation of the periumbilical perforator blood supply to the upper abdominal wall skin is critical in order to avoid skin ischemia and wound healing problems.
- ▲ The PUPS approach to components separation allows safe simultaneous panniculectomy. The hernia defect is approached through the previous midline incision. The external oblique fascial incision lateral to the linea semilunaris can then be approached through a longitudinal subcutaneous tunnel created following the panniculectomy (Figs. 9-19, B and 9-20). With fiber optic lighted retraction, dissection with incision of the external obliques can extend several centimeters superior to the costal margin through this approach.
- ▲ The upper abdominal medial subcutaneous attachments maintain the periumbilical perforator blood supply to the remaining skin, which is closed vertically and transversely (Fig. 9-19, C).

6. Management of Wound Complications

▲ *Infection*

- ▲ Cellulitis is treated with appropriate antibiotics. Infected collections need to be drained, in some cases, with the assistance of an interventional radiologist.

▲ *Wound Ischemia or Dehiscence*

- ▲ Skin necrosis should be addressed early with debridement, and the subcutaneous tissue should then be treated with wet-to-dry dressings or a vacuum-assisted closure device.

▲ *Seromas and Hematomas*

- ▲ Symptomatic or possibly infected seromas are percutaneously drained. Symptomatic or infected hematomas often require operative drainage.

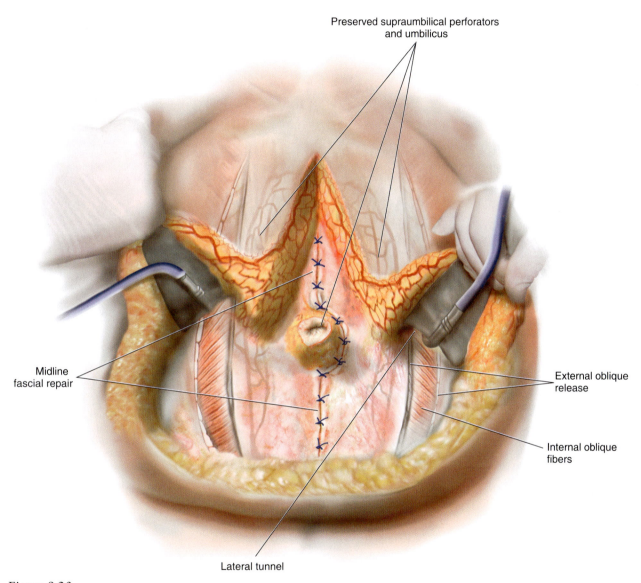

Figure 9-20.

Selected References

Agnew SP, Small W Jr, Wang E, Smith LJ, Hadad I, Dumanian GA: Prospective measurements of intra-abdominal volume and pulmonary function after repair of massive ventral hernias with the components separation technique, *Ann Surg* 25(5):981–988, 2010.

Ceydeli A, Rucinski J, Wise L: Finding the best abdominal closure: An evidence based review of the literature, *Curr Surg* 62:220–225, 2005.

Dunne JR, Malone DL, Tracy JK, Napolitano LM: Abdominal wall hernias: risk factors for infection and resource utilization, *J Surg Res* 111:78–84, 2003.

El-Mrakby HH, Milner RH: The vascular anatomy of the lower anterior abdominal wall: a microdissection study on the deep inferior epigastric vessels and the perforator branches, *Plast Reconstr Surg* 109(2):539–543, 2002:discussion 544-7.

Finan KR, Vick CC, Kiefe CL, Neumayer L, Hawn MT: Predictors of wound infection in ventral hernia repair, *Am J Surg* 190:676–681, 2005.

Huger WE Jr: The anatomical rationale for abdominal lipectomy, *Am Surg* 45:612, 1979.

Ramirez OM, Ruas E, Dellon L: Component separation method for closure of abdominal wall defects: an anatomic and clinical study, *Plast Reconstr Surg* 86:519–526, 1990.

Kolker AR, Brown DJ, Redstone JS, Scarpinato VM, Wallack MK: Multilayer reconstruction of abdominal wall defects with acellular dermal allograft and component separation, *Ann Plast Surg* 55:36–42, 2005.

Reid RR, Dumanian GA: Panniculectomy and the Separation-of-Parts Hernia Repair: A Solution for the Large Infraumbilical Hernia in the Obese Patient, *Plast Reconstr Surg* 116:1006–1012, 2005.

Rosen MJ, Williams C, Jin J, McGee MF, Schomisch S, Marks J, Ponsky J: Laparoscopic versus open-component separation: a comparative analysis in a porcine model, *Am J of Surg* 194(3):385–389, 2007.

Saulis AS, Dumanian GA: Periumbilical rectus abdominis perforator preservation significantly reduces superficial wound complications in 'separation of parts' hernia repairs, *Plast Reconstr Surg* 109:2275–2280, 2002.

Shestak KC, Edington HJ, Johnson RR: The separation of anatomic components technique for the reconstruction of massive midline abdominal wall defects: anatomy, surgical technique, applications, and limitations revisited, *Plast Reconstr Surg* 105:731–738, 2000.

Taylor GI, Palmer JH: The vascular territories (angiosomes) of the body: experimental study and clinical applications, *Br J Plast Surg* 40:113, 1987.

The Ventral Hernia Working Group, Breuing K, Bulter CE, Ferzoco S, Franz M, Hultman CS, Kilbridge JF, Rosen M, Silverman RP, Vargo D: Incisional ventral hernias: Review of the literature and recommendations regarding the grading and technique of repair, *Surgery*, 2010:epub.

CHAPTER 10

Modified Minimally Invasive Component Separation

Charles E. Butler, MD

1. Clinical Anatomy

- ▲ One of the goals of minimally invasive component separation (MICS) is to avoid dissecting the subcutaneous tissue overlying the anterior rectus sheath and the vessels that penetrate the rectus abdominis muscle, thereby minimizing subcutaneous dead space and improving vascularity to the overlying skin. The inferior epigastric vessels penetrate the inferior lateral aspect of the rectus abdominis muscle and travel through the muscle, branching off into myocutaneous perforating vessels that provide vascular supply to the overlying abdominal skin and subcutaneous tissue.
- ▲ The external oblique, internal oblique, and transversalis muscles insert laterally into the rectus abdominis complex at the semilunar line. In MICS, the aponeurosis of the external oblique muscle is released without disrupting much of the subcutaneous tissue attachments to the anterior rectus sheath and the rectus abdominis perforating vessels within the anterior rectus sheath. The transversalis and internal oblique musculature remains attached to the rectus complex and vascularized and innervated by the intercostal neurovascular bundles. The plane between the external and internal oblique muscle aponeuroses is relatively avascular and easily dissected to facilitate medialization of the rectus complex for the closure of moderate or large defects. Cranially, toward the costal margin, interdigitations between the external and internal oblique muscles require electrocautery dissection.

2. Preoperative Considerations

Surgeons must consider the risks of surgery and anesthesia, including cardiopulmonary comorbidities and other general health issues.
- ▲ Each patient's risk for perioperative wound complications, infection, and hernia recurrence must be considered.
- ▲ Realistic expectations of the potential outcomes must be clearly defined and discussed with each patient; topics should include the anticipated surgical outcome, possible complications, risk of recurrence, length of hospital stay, need for drainage catheters, and commitment to restrictions on activity.

▲ Patients should be encouraged to cease tobacco use for at least 2 weeks before surgery. Many patients benefit from participating in nutrition and exercise programs to achieve safe weight loss before MICS for hernia repair.

1. Pain Control

▲ Preoperative placement of an epidural catheter for anesthesia is highly recommended for patients undergoing MICS. When oral diet is initiated, patients transition to oral narcotic and non-narcotic analgesics before discharge from the hospital.

2. Musculofascial Considerations

▲ The surgeon must consider the size and location of the defect, particularly in difficult hernia repairs in the epigastric or low suprapubic area where the possibility of medializing musculofascial tissue is limited by a lack of tissue laxity. Previous surgeries and previously placed mesh materials that have failed also must be considered. Violation of the rectus complex with stomas, stomal site hernias, port site hernias, and/or indwelling catheters also must be considered but generally are not contraindications to MICS.

▲ The surgeon should ascertain whether the rectus abdominis myocutaneous perforators have been elevated and ligated during previous surgeries (usually from undermining the skin flap laterally over the anterior rectus sheath). The most important musculofascial consideration is semilunar line violation. Previous musculofascial incisions and/or trauma that transected the semilunar line complicate MICS or render this procedure contraindicated on the ipsilateral side. Transverse and oblique incisions that cross the semilunar line from the oblique muscles to the rectus muscle complex are relative contraindications to performing ipsilateral MICS. Subcostal incisions, transplant incisions, and in some patients, long appendectomy scars traversing the semilunar line, may limit the extent of or preclude component separation.

3. Intraperitoneal (Visceral) Considerations

▲ Previous surgeries and/or intraperitoneal infections may increase intestinal and visceral adhesions, thereby complicating laparotomy and adhesion lysis before MICS.

▲ If macroporous synthetic mesh is being considered for defect repair, the availability, quality, and surface area of the greater omentum should be evaluated intraoperatively for its potential use as a barrier between the mesh and intraperitoneal viscera.

4. Skin Considerations

- ▲ The patient should be evaluated for sufficient availability and laxity of good-quality skin to ensure reliable cutaneous closure over the musculofascial repair. Sufficient closure must be achieved to reduce the risk of skin dehiscence after surgery.
- ▲ The vast majority of patients have redundant, attenuated, poor-quality skin in the midline that is associated with the hernia sac. Most or all of this skin is usually resected to allow the more lateral, adequate-quality skin to be medialized and serve as the primary closure without tension.
- ▲ If the umbilicus is involved in the hernia, is considerably thin, or is ulcerated, it is generally resected along with the central skin.
- ▲ Previous scars on the abdominal wall also must be considered because they can limit the vascularity available to the central skin and reduce the skin's potential for medialization.

5. Defect Considerations

- ▲ Potential bacterial contamination, including infected mesh, contamination of the surgical field, inadvertent enterotomy, existing ostomy, and/or active open-wound infection, must be considered before MICS. To reduce the risk of infection, the surgeon should aggressively debride devitalized tissue, give perioperative therapeutic antibiotics, employ pulsatile lavage, reduce subcutaneous dead space, and drain subcutaneous space with closed-suction drainage catheters.
- ▲ The quality of the existing musculofascia and overlying skin should be assessed before MICS. Previous infections, incisions, or irradiation may limit the musculofascia's wound-healing capability and potential for medialization.
- ▲ The thickness, tensile strength, and overall quality of the tissues surrounding the defect should be evaluated. Systemic immunosuppression, multiple comorbidities, and intercostal denervation from previous surgeries can significantly reduce the quality of the musculofascia.

3. Operative Steps

- ▲ After making a midline incision for laparotomy, the surgeon performs adhesion lysis to mobilize all the adhesions from the dorsal aspect of the abdominal wall. The surgeon incises the musculofascia exactly at the midline of the abdomen without violating the rectus complex. The surgeon then incises the midline defect superiorly and inferiorly to combine all areas of midline herniation into a single defect. In patients who have had previous surgeries, the surgeon should palpate intraperitoneally any areas of unopened midline incisions to identify sites possibly subject to future herniation. At this time, any planned or unplanned intraperitoneal or intrapelvic surgeries should be performed before MICS.
- ▲ The surgeon dissects preperitoneal fat from the posterior sheath of the rectus abdominis muscle complex to facilitate the direct placement of implantable surgical mesh to the posterior rectus sheath. The majority of the preperitoneal fat pad is generally located in the central portion of the abdominal wall near the linea alba and is more extensive, thicker, and wider near the costal margin and the pubis than in the central, periumbilical area. Dissecting the preperitoneal fat pad flap at least 5 cm in the most cranial and caudal aspects

of the defect facilitates mesh implantation. Patients with numerous previous surgeries and patients with a very thin body habitus may not have a well-defined preperitoneal fat layer. After adhesion lysis and preperitoneal flap dissection has been completed, the surgeon should place a moist, radiopaque-tagged towel or sponge on the intraperitoneal viscera to help protect it from inadvertent trauma and dissection.

▲ Surgeons may choose to place mesh in the retrorectus rather than the preperitoneal plane, particularly if macroporous, synthetic mesh will be used. This minimizes mesh exposure directly to abdominal viscera. The retrorectus plane is developed by incising the posterior rectus sheath just lateral to the linea alba and dissecting between the rectus abdominis muscle and posterior rectus sheath. Below the arcuate line, where there is no posterior rectus sheath, the preperitoneal fat pad can be elevated in continuity. After MICS is completed and before insetting mesh to the semilunar lines, the posterior sheath and preperitoneal fat pad from each side are closed in the midline, thereby separating the intraperitoneal contents from the mesh.

▲ To facilitate suture placement for insetting implantable surgical mesh and fascial closure, the surgeon dissects the subcutaneous tissue from the anterior rectus sheath approximately 2 to 4 cm circumferentially. The dissection should extend laterally to the medial row of the rectus abdominis myofascial perforators, which is preserved.

▲ Depending on the length of the defect and body habitus of the patient, the surgeon accesses the semilunar line through one or two narrow tunnel incisions between the anterior rectus fascia and subcutaneous tissue. The hernia sac, which typically extends laterally towards the semilunar line, is often used to initiate tunnel access. Generally, a single tunnel incision is used in the supraumbilical area centered between the umbilicus and the costal margin. A narrow Deaver retractor is used to elevate the subcutaneous tissue, and electrocautery is used to dissect an approximately 4-cm-wide tunnel laterally to approximately 2 cm lateral to the semilunar line (Fig. 10-1). These lateral access tunnels allow creation of vertically oriented subcutaneous lateral tunnels over the anticipated external oblique aponeurosis release sites (depicted in Fig. 10-1) later in the procedure.

▲ It is imperative to identify the semilunar line to ensure that the appropriate plane is entered for the component separation release. Palpation is used to identify the edge of the rectus muscle, lateral edge of the rectus sheath, and transition of oblique musculature to aponeurosis, which serve as landmarks (Fig. 10-2). The presence of a fat pad between the internal and external oblique aponeuroses is a good indication of being in the correct plane. The optimal location of the release of the external oblique muscle is through its aponeurosis medial to the muscle body and lateral to its insertion into the rectus sheath complex, that is, generally 1.5 cm lateral to the lateral edge of the rectus complex. The area is marked with a pen and incised with a scalpel or electrocautery for 1 cm in the craniocaudal direction (see Fig. 10-2). In the event that the incision enters the rectus sheath (revealing the rectus abdominis muscle), the incision is closed and a new incision is made more laterally.

Chapter 10 • Modified Minimally Invasive Component Separation

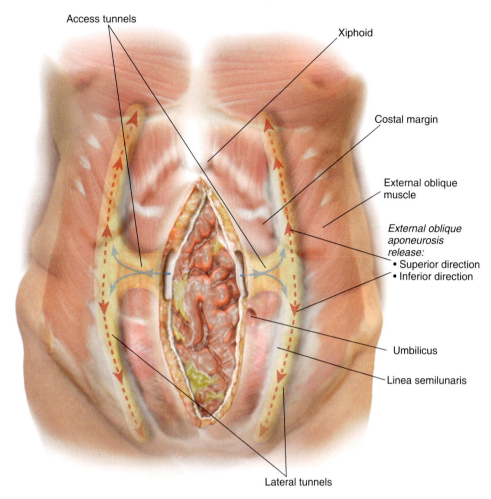

Figure 10-1.

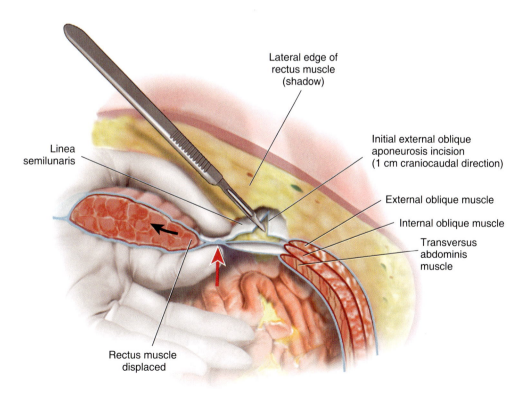

Figure 10-2.

▲ Blunt dissection between the internal and external oblique aponeuroses and muscle is performed through the 1-cm vertical incision in the external oblique aponeurosis. The surgeon uses a blunt-tip, metal Yankauer suction handle (not connected to suction) to start the dissection between the internal and external oblique aponeuroses inferiorly and superiorly to the initial external oblique aponeurosis incision (Fig. 10-3). This should slide easily just lateral to the rectus complex superiorly over the costal margin (shown) and inferiorly toward the pubis (not shown). This sweeping blunt dissection provides separation between the internal and external oblique aponeuroses for a safe separation of the external oblique aponeurosis in a minimally invasive fashion without inadvertent injury to the underlying internal oblique structure muscular aponeurosis. The surgeon then inserts the suction handle inferiorly between the internal and external oblique aponeuroses and positions the handle against the rectus abdominis muscle complex and uses the suction handle as a palpable guide to create vertical, 3-cm-wide, subcutaneous tunnels (Fig. 10-4, A). Using a narrow Deaver retractor and electrocautery, dissection over the external oblique aponeurosis release site is performed inferiorly and superiorly (see Fig. 10-4). The external oblique aponeurosis is then freed anteriorly and posteriorly and can be easily transected without injuring the overlying subcutaneous tissue or underlying oblique muscle or aponeurosis.

▲ The external oblique aponeurosis incision can be performed inferiorly and superiorly to the initial external oblique aponeurosis incision through the initial lateral tunnel incision. The blunt tip suction handle is again used as a guide to avoid inadvertently entering the rectus complex medially (Fig. 10-4, B). The surgeon uses scissors to release the inferior half of the external oblique aponeurosis, which extends towards the pubis. The same technique is applied superiorly to fully release the aponeurosis of the external abdominal oblique muscle; however, electrocautery becomes necessary as more muscle and less aponeurosis are present at and above the costal margin. The release is continued cranially to 8-12 cm cranial to the costal margin. Electrocautery for hemostasis and dissection is often required for the considerable interdigitation between the external oblique muscular aponeurosis and the underlying musculature at and above the costal margin. After the external oblique aponeurosis is completely released, the internal oblique muscle should be clearly visible.

▲ Sharp and electrocautery dissection between the internal and external oblique muscles should be completed through the initial lateral tunnel incision. Narrow Deaver retractors and a headlight or lighted retractor are helpful in performing this maneuver. The lateral extent of the dissection between the internal and external oblique muscles continues laterally to the anterior axillary line to facilitate maximal medialization of the rectus complex. The surgeon must avoid injuring the underlying internal oblique muscle and aponeurosis, which can cause potential weakness or herniation.

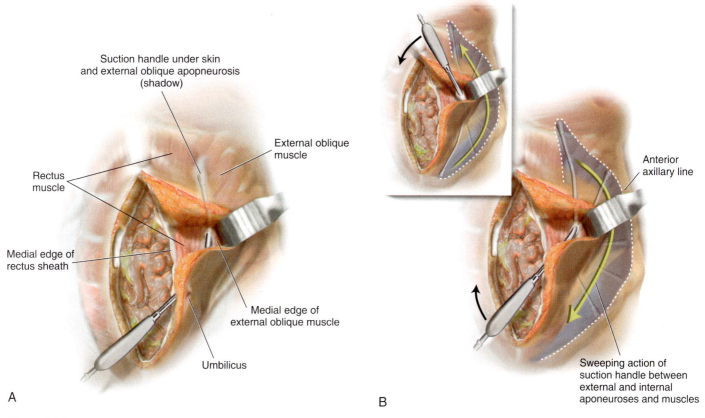

Figure 10-3.

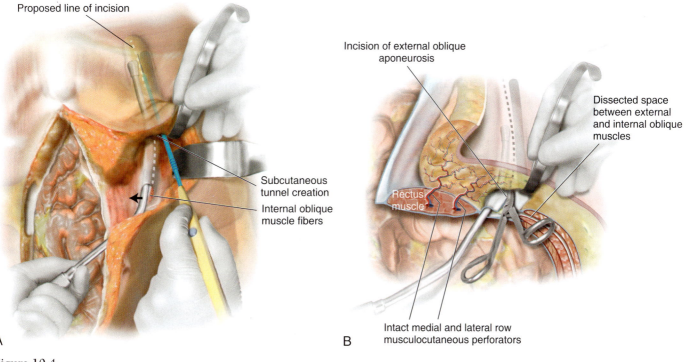

Figure 10-4.

- After the minimally invasive release on one side is complete, a medialization of the rectus complex and overlying attached soft tissue should be visible. If additional access to the semilunar line is required, the surgeon can perform a second tunnel incision 10 to 15 cm inferior to the initial tunnel incision. The entire procedure is then performed identically on the contralateral side.
- To determine whether primary fascial midline closure is possible, the surgeon places Kocher clamps on the fascial edge and retracts the fascial edges toward the midline. Inlay mesh is used to reinforce the primary fascial closure. If primary fascial closure is not possible in all or some areas of the defect, an inlay-bridging mesh is required.
- The defect's condition and the surgeon's preferences determine the type of implantable surgical mesh to be used. To avoid the consequences of adhesions, macroporous synthetic mesh should not be placed directly onto the intraperitoneal viscera. Instead, for simple defects, composite antiadhesive barrier mesh may be used. For complex defects, particularly defects with bacterial contamination, defects in which mesh may be placed directly over viscera, defects with a high risk of skin dehiscence with subsequent mesh exposure, and/or defects in patients at an increased risk for perioperative wound healing complications, bioprosthetic mesh is generally used. The procedure has been described by the author, Charles Butler, as the MICSIB (Minimally Invasive Component Separation with Inlay Bioprosthetic Mesh) technique when minimally invasive component separation is used with an inlay bioprosthetic mesh. The mesh is inset with at least 4-5 cms of overlap with the musculofascial edges to ensure a reliable repair. The surgeon cuts the mesh, orients it into the defect, and marks the midline of the mesh with a marker. The surgeon then resects any devitalized, attenuated, or severely scarred midline tissue. The surgeon marks the anticipated suture line on the mesh and the musculofascia to ensure that once the inset sutures have been placed and tied, the fascial edges meet at the midline without tension over the reinforcing mesh inlay if primary fascial closure is possible (reinforced repair). If bridging mesh is required, the surgeon marks the area of bridging and the anticipated positions of central suture lines where the true musculofascial edges are inset to the mesh.
- The surgeon then performs a circumferential, interrupted #1 polypropylene suture inlay inset through the full thickness of the musculofascia, through the mesh, and then back out through the musculofascia. In Figure 10-5 the separation of the internal and external oblique muscles laterally and the completed external oblique aponeurosis release are shown with the discontinued external oblique aponeurosis on both sides. The rectus complex on both sides is now able to be medialized toward the midline. Bioprosthetic mesh is being inset with interrupted monofilament sutures. Suture knots are oriented ventral to the musculofascia. The distance between the entry and exit of a suture through the fascia should be at least 1.5 cm to avoid suture pull-through and sutures should be placed at approximately 2-cm intervals on the musculofascia during the inset. The most superior suture is placed first, often through or around the xiphoid process, and the remainder of the costal margin inset is performed with all sutures placed on hemostats and left untied. Next, the most inferior suture is placed to provide midline orientation and establish the appropriate physiologic tension of the inlay mesh. The remaining sutures are then placed in the appropriate positions to enable primary fascial closure (reinforced repair) or placement of bridging mesh (bridged repair) as previously determined. The surgeon must identify the inferior epigastric vessels as they penetrate the rectus muscles to avoid inadvertently occluding them with a suture and thereby compromising the vascularity of the rectus complex and overlying skin.

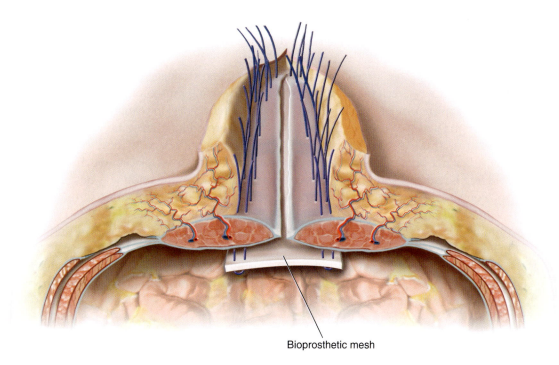

Figure 10-5.

- Once all inset sutures are placed and tagged with hemostats, the surgeon applies tension to them to confirm that the physiologic tension of the inset mesh will be appropriate and ensure that primary fascial closure is possible. The inset sutures are then individually tied under tension with the adjacent sutures above and below the placed on tension to facilitate an appropriate inset tension of the suture being tied. The surgeon should carefully visually inspect the intraperitoneal space and manually palpate each suture to ensure that any inclusion of intraperitoneal viscera within the suture loops has not occurred. After tying the inset sutures, the surgeon places a closed-suction drainage catheter to remove fluid from the space between the inset mesh and the overlying musculofascial closure.
- When complete primary fascial closure is planned, the surgeon reapproximates the fascial edges in the midline with either a running or interrupted long-term monofilament resorbable suture (Fig. 10-6). The vascularity of the rectus muscle is then assessed to ensure that it has not become congested or devascularized after inset placement. In areas where bridging is required and primary fascial reapproximation at the midline is not possible, the surgeon should use resorbable sutures to carefully tack the fascial edges to the surface of the mesh without injuring the underlying intraperitoneal structures (Fig. 10-7). To protect from inadvertent injury to intraperitoneal sutures while placing these central sutures, it is helpful to have left several peripheral inset sutures untied and placed on hemostats. A wide malleable retractor (not shown in Fig. 10-7) can be inserted through this area and placed just under the bioprosthetic mesh to protect the bowel during central inset suture placement. The few untied inset sutures are then tied.
- The surgeon then carefully measures the amount of skin redundancy for a vertically oriented central skin and subcutaneous tissue resection, which is performed to minimize dead space and to remove central, less vascularized tissue.
- Large-bore, round, channeled, closed-suction drainage catheters are placed with the drains exiting the suprapubic area. One drain is placed laterally in each MICS donor site, and depending on the volume of subcutaneous space, two to five drains are placed centrally in the subcutaneous space.

Chapter 10 • Modified Minimally Invasive Component Separation 181

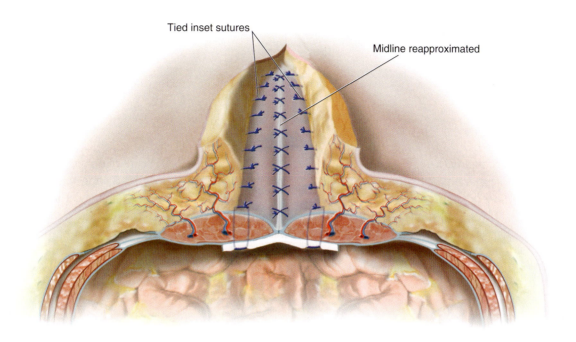

Figure 10-6.

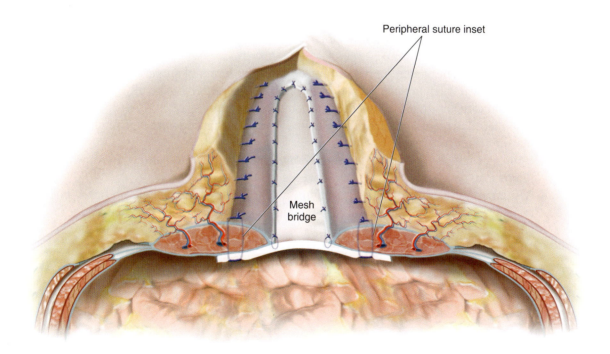

Figure 10-7.

- Generally, 3 to 5 interrupted 3-0 resorbable sutures are placed in a vertical line between drainage catheter channels to quilt the elevated skin flaps from Scarpa fascia to the musculofascial repair to eliminate dead space and reduce shear. Figure 10-8 shows a completed closure in three-dimensional cross section, indicating location of drainage catheters inset sutures, and quilting sutures. This technique has minimized the need for extensive skin flap elevation and preserved the rectus perforator vascularity to the overlying skin.
- The skin is then meticulously closed in a layered fashion including closure of the Scarpa fascia with resorbable sutures and closure of the dermis with interrupted resorbable sutures and a running resorbable subcuticular suture.

4. Postoperative Care

- Patients are generally hospitalized for 3 to 6 days after MICS, depending on the complexity of the reconstruction and whether other intraabdominal procedures were performed.
- Patients are encouraged to walk either the day of surgery or the following morning. Depending on a patient's risk factors, an anticoagulant may be prescribed to prevent venous thromboembolism.
- Perioperative antibiotics are discontinued within 24 hours of surgery unless indicated to treat an existing contamination and/or infection. Pain control is generally managed with an epidural catheter until the patient can tolerate oral narcotics.
- Oral diet is advanced gradually as tolerated, generally starting with sips of clear fluid the morning after surgery.
- Drains are removed when the output volume is less than 25 mL per day. In some patients, drains may be left in place for up to 3 weeks.
- Assuming no perioperative complications, activity restrictions include no heavy physical maneuvering for 8 weeks, followed by a transition to unrestricted normal activity by 12 weeks.

Chapter 10 • Modified Minimally Invasive Component Separation

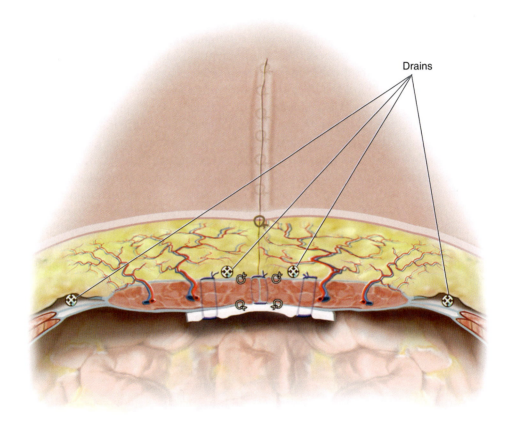

Figure 10-8.

5. Pearls/Pitfalls

▲ Surgeons must actively manage patients' expectations before patients undergo MICS. Patients must understand that MICS is a complex procedure, that indwelling drainage catheters will be present after surgery, that the umbilicus may be resected, that they may experience pain after surgery, that they must restrict their activity after surgery, and that complications can occur.

▲ Meticulous attention to detail during tissue dissection, component separation release, and mesh inset is critical to the success of MICS. The appropriate physiologic tension of the mesh inset must be achieved to reduce the risk of bulge and/or early hernia recurrence (tear) owing to insets that are too loose or too tight, respectively.

▲ Eliminating dead space reduces the risk of potentially chronic and/or infected subcutaneous and retrorectus fluid collections. To help reduce the risk of fluid collection, the surgeon should place drainage catheters and use quilting sutures.

▲ The vascularity of the rectus abdominis muscle must be confirmed during and after mesh inset. If venous congestion or arterial insufficiency of the muscle is suspected, the surgeon should evaluate the sutures to ensure that the inferior epigastric pedicle has not been inadvertently included within a suture and that the sutures have not been placed too close together laterally, which could devascularize the central rectus muscle. In some patients, a posterior sheath release approximately 2 cm lateral to the midline can reduce vascular congestion, particularly if the congestion is related to rectus sheath constriction.

▲ The appropriate number of mesh inset sutures must be placed at the proper intervals. Too few sutures or too long an interval between consecutive sutures may result in herniation and/or insufficient mechanical strength to withstand the forces of the abdominal wall musculature. Too many sutures or too small an interval between consecutive sutures may compromise the vascularity of the central rectus complex, potentially leading to poor wound healing, musculofascial necrosis, and subsequent failure of the defect repair.

▲ The surgeon should perform a complete release of the musculature from near the pubis to superior to the costal margin to enable maximal medialization of the rectus complex. The surgeon also should perform a complete dissection between the internal and external oblique muscles to the lateral axillary line. Together, these two maneuvers facilitate the primary fascial closure of very large defects in the epigastric region without undue tension.

Selected References

Baumann DP, Butler CE: Abdominal wall wounds. In Marsh J, Perlyn C, editors: *Decision-Making in Plastic Surgery*. St. Louis, MO: Quality Medical Publishing, In Press.

Breuing K, Butler CE, Ferzoco S, Franz M, Hultman CS, Kilbridge JF, Rosen M, Silverman RP, Vargo D: Incisional ventral hernias: review of the literature and recommendations regarding the grading and technique of repair, *Surgery.* Epub ahead of print, March 19, 2010: In Press.

Butler CE: *Ciné Clinic I: Plastic Surgery: Minimally invasive component separation with inlay bioprosthetic mesh (MICSIB)*, San Francisco, CA, October 13, 2008, American College of Surgeons 94th Annual Clinical Congress.

Butler CE, Langstein HN, Kronowitz SJ: Pelvic, abdominal, and chest wall reconstruction with AlloDerm in patients at increased risk for mesh-related complications, *Plast Reconstr Surg* 116:1263–1275, 2005.

Campbell K, Butler CE. Minimally Invasive Component Separation with Inlay Bioprosthetic Mesh (MICSIB) for Complex Abdominal Wall Reconstruction. *Plast Reconstr Surg.* In Press.

CHAPTER 11

Endoscopic Component Separation

Michael J. Rosen, MD, FACS

1. Clinical Anatomy

- ▲ The rectus muscle can be fairly wide, up to 8 to 10 cm, and therefore the initial cut down for the balloon dissector must be performed in the lateral abdominal wall to avoid inadvertently placing the balloon in the rectus sheath.
- ▲ Understanding the anatomic characteristics of the external and internal oblique muscles is critical to ensuring accurate placement of the balloon dissector when performing an endoscopic component separation. The external oblique is primarily fascialike on the lower to midabdomen and is more muscular laterally and cephalad. The internal oblique is primarily muscular except for the most medial 2 to 3 cm of fascia just before its insertion into the linea semilunaris.
- ▲ Clearly identifying the linea semilunaris is important to safely performing a component separation. Inadvertently transecting the linea semilunaris during a component separation will result in a full thickness defect of the lateral abdominal wall and a troublesome hernia to repair.
- ▲ The external oblique muscle inserts 5 to 7 cm above the costal margin and should be dissected off the ribs to maximize medialization.

2. Preoperative Considerations

1. Optimization of Comorbidities

- ▲ Abdominal wall reconstruction is a major surgical procedure requiring careful preoperative clearance. Smoking cessation is mandatory, weight loss is strongly encouraged, nutritional status is optimized, and cardiac status is stratified.

2. Anatomic Considerations

▲ Skin Considerations

- ▲ Skin ulcerations and peristomal excoriations are carefully prepared preoperatively to maximize healing potential. Because skin flaps are not raised in this technique, skin preservation is very important.
- ▲ The primary advantage of an endoscopic component separation is the elimination of lipocutaneous skin flaps. This reduces wound infections and flap ischemia. In cases where excess skin must be resected or skin flaps will be necessary to mobilize the skin to the midline, the endoscopic component separation should not be used. In these cases an open component separation or concomitant panniculectomy is performed as described in other chapters.

▲ Musculofascial Considerations

- ▲ Ideal characteristics for an endoscopic component separation include a relatively wide, well-preserved rectus muscle. With a wide rectus muscle, a large mesh typically can be placed in the retrorectus position as an underlay (as described in Chapter 5 without a skin flap).
- ▲ Component separation techniques have limitations. Large defects, >20 cm in width, and multiple recurrent hernias with fixed noncompliant abdominal walls often cannot be medialized with this technique. In addition, patients with transverse incisions should not be approached with an endoscopic technique.

▲ Reconstructive Considerations

- ▲ The surgeon should consider whether skin flaps will be necessary to place the mesh. The absence of skin flaps can create technical challenges in placing a large sheet of mesh as an underlay. If appropriate mesh placement requires large skin flaps, I perform an open technique.
- ▲ If the mesh must be placed in an intraperitoneal position without skin flaps and wide coverage, laparoscopic assistance is helpful as described in the following section.

3. Operative Steps

1. Equipment

- ▲ Equipment needs include a 10-mm, 30-degree laparoscope; bilateral inguinal hernia balloon dissector (Covidien, Norwalk, CT); 30-mL balloon-tipped trocar (Covidien, Norwalk, CT); laparoscopic trocars; and an ultrasonic dissector or LigaSure™ device (Covidien, Norwalk, CT) (Fig. 11-1).
- ▲ Patients receive appropriate preoperative antibiotics and invasive monitoring as needed, and epidural catheters are routinely placed for postoperative pain control.

Chapter 11 • Endoscopic Component Separation 187

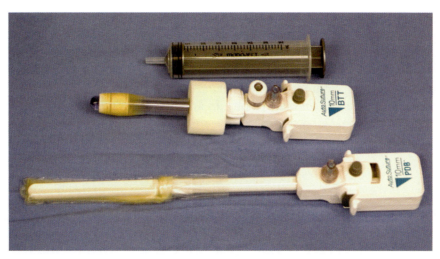

Figure 11-1.

▲ **Patient Positioning**

- ▲ Patients are placed in the supine position with both arms abducted. Access to the posterior axillary line is important to place the lateral abdominal trocar during the endoscopic component separation and can be limited if the arm is tucked at the sides.

▲ **Trocar Strategy**

- ▲ Figure 11-2 shows trocar positioning, with lines showing the linea semilunaris, external oblique fascia, and costal margin
- ▲ The endoscopic component separation is typically performed first to avoid introducing any contamination from the midline wound into the lateral abdominal space. Given that these are closed spaces and no lymphatics are divided, drains are not routinely placed at the component separation sites.

▲ **Endoscopic Component Separation Operative Steps**

- ▲ A cut-down incision is performed off the tip of the eleventh rib. It is critical that this incision is made lateral to the linea semilunaris to avoid placing the balloon in the rectus sheath. This port should be placed lateral enough to allow space between the linea semilunaris and the trocar, enabling complete cephalad dissection. In my opinion, this is the most important step in the operation, and the anatomy must be clearly identified. Therefore, in obese patients I extend this incision to the appropriate size to permit clear identification of the fibers of the external oblique. The subcutaneous tissue and Scarpa fascia are bluntly separated, and the external oblique is grasped with Kocher clamps.
- ▲ Depending on how far lateral you have performed your cut down, the external oblique can be only fascia or fascia and muscle. It is important to confirm this anatomy, to avoid cutting too deep into the internal oblique. The external oblique fibers are split and bluntly separated. An **S** retractor gently creates the plane underneath the external oblique and above the internal oblique heading in a caudal direction (Fig. 11-3).

Chapter 11 • Endoscopic Component Separation 189

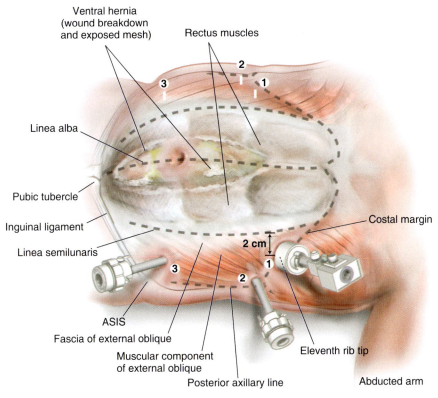

Figure 11-2.

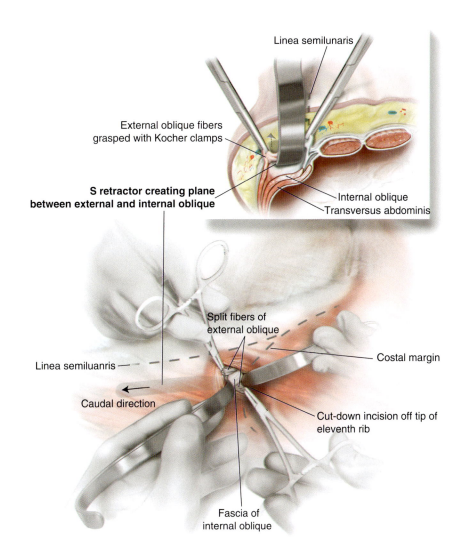

Figure 11-3.

- ▲ A standard bilateral inguinal hernia balloon dissector is placed underneath the external oblique and passed inferiorly to the pubic tubercle (Fig. 11-4). This balloon should be guided laterally to avoid injuring the linea semilunaris. If prior transverse incisions are encountered, the balloon might not be able to traverse the scar tissue and should be aborted and the intermuscular space created under direct vision.
- ▲ The balloon is insufflated under direct vision, and the orientation of the external oblique fibers ("hands in pockets"), internal oblique fibers ("hands on the hips"), and the linea semilunaris are identified (Fig. 11-5).

Chapter 11 • Endoscopic Component Separation 191

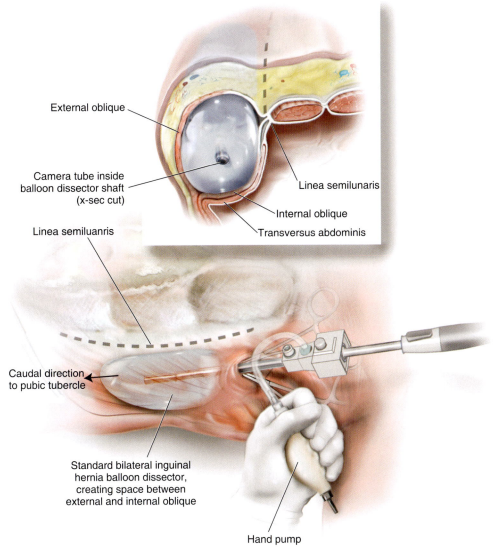

Figure 11-4.

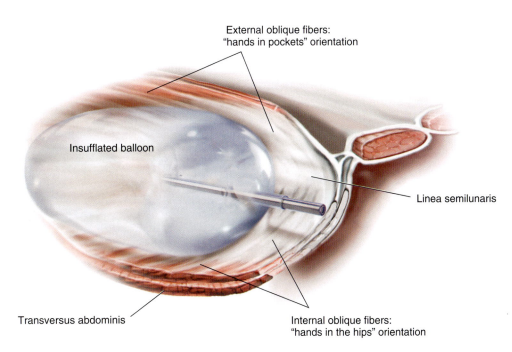

Figure 11-5.

- ▲ The shape of the standard bilateral inguinal hernia balloon dissector does not permit cephalad dissection of the external oblique off the costal margin. Therefore, the balloon is removed, and a finger is placed in the intermuscular space, and the dissection is bluntly carried out over the costal margin using a sweeping motion (Fig. 11-6). If this space is not created at this point, the dissection planes can be confusing laparoscopically and may result in a technical error. Remember the external oblique inserts 5 to 7 cm above the costal margin and should be cleared off the costal margin to permit the muscles to slide medially.
- ▲ A balloon tipped trocar is secured in the space to prevent air leakage. One should avoid the use of a triangular shaped structural balloon at this point because it can result in obliteration of the dissection space. Insufflation pressures of 10 to 12 mm Hg are used.
- ▲ The inferior space can be bluntly created with a 30-degree, 10-mm laparoscope to complete the dissection of the intermuscular space to the posterior axillary line and inguinal ligament.
- ▲ The second port is placed in the posterior axillary line. This port is placed as far laterally as possible to provide the appropriate angle to release the external oblique, 2 cm lateral to the linea semilunaris.
- ▲ Using scissors with cautery, in the posterior axillary port, and the camera in the cut-down port, the external oblique is incised from as cephalad as possible, to the inguinal ligament/pubic tubercle (Fig. 11-7). Great care should be taken to complete the release lateral to the linea semilunaris.
- ▲ Extra release can be achieved by continuing the dissection superficially through Scarpa fascia. The majority of the blood supply runs superficial to this layer and won't be disturbed.
- ▲ The third port is placed through the released external oblique in the lower abdomen. This port is placed medial to the original cut-down port in the line that the external oblique will be transected when going over the costal margin. This orientation is important because the cephalad portion of the dissection can be challenging as it is performed in a reverse camera orientation.

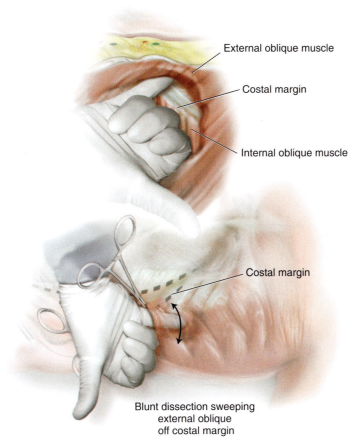

Figure 11-6.

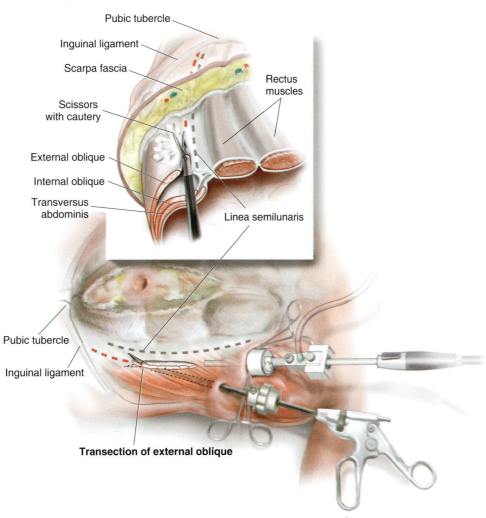

Figure 11-7.

▲ The camera is then placed in the lower abdominal trocar and the scissors are placed in the lateral port, and the cephalad dissection is completed separating the external oblique off the costal margin (Fig. 11-8). The external oblique is carefully separated off the costal margin to provide a clear plane and trajectory when transecting the external oblique. This avoids releasing the linea semilunaris or dissecting underneath the costal margin.

▲ Once the dissection of the external oblique is completed, the camera is positioned in the lateral port and the LigaSure™ ultrasonic dissector is placed in the inferior port (Fig. 11-9). Since the external oblique is fairly muscular at the cephalad portion, I prefer to use LigaSure™, as simple cautery can result in troublesome bleeding.

Chapter 11 • Endoscopic Component Separation   195

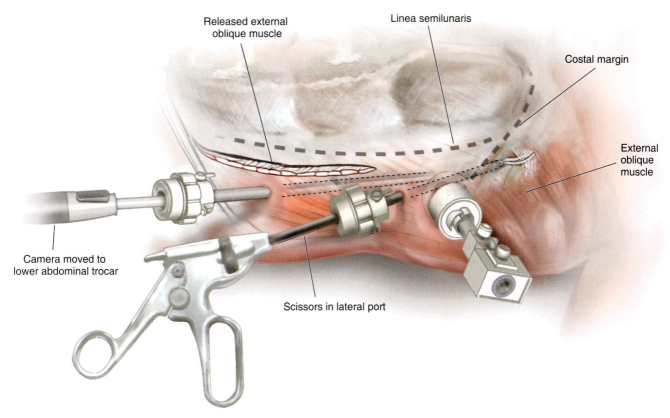

Figure 11-8.

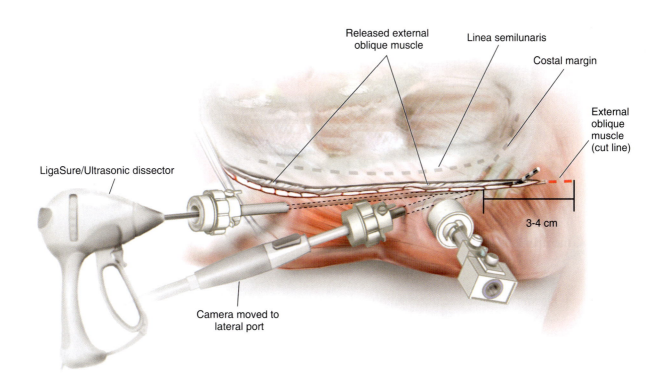

Figure 11-9.

- ▲ The external oblique is transected several centimeters above the costal margin (Fig. 11-10). The exact cephalad extent of the transection of the external oblique is variable, but it should be at least 5 cm above the superior extent of the hernia defect, and likely, at least 3 to 4 cm above the costal margin.
- ▲ A bilateral component separation is preferred in most patients to provide symmetric distribution of tension on the closure.
- ▲ Midline laparotomy is performed, and bowel work is completed as necessary.

▲ Mesh Placement

- ▲ In general, mesh should be placed under appropriate physiologic tension, using transfascial fixation sutures to aid in medialization of the rectus muscles. These sutures allow the forces of the abdominal closure to be redistributed to lateral abdominal wall. If the mesh is placed in a completely tension-free manner, and the fascia is reapproximated in the midline, the mesh will buckle, and this likely leads to seroma formation, poor integration, and mesh sepsis.

▲ Retrorectus Placement

- ▲ My preferred space for mesh placement is in the posterior rectus space. By using this technique as described in Chapter 5 skin flaps are not necessary for wide mesh overlap. Drains are routinely placed above the mesh and below the rectus muscle. Although some authors describe continuing the dissection through the linea semilunaris into the lateral abdominal plane during a retrorectus repair, this should be avoided if a component separation has been performed. If the external oblique is released and then the transversus abdominis is intentionally or unintentionally released, the lateral abdominal wall is only supported by the internal oblique, which likely will result in at least a bulge if not a hernia. Therefore, if the rectus muscle seems too narrow to place a wide enough piece of mesh, the surgeon has several alternative options. A standard open component separation can be performed, allowing large skin flaps and easier mesh placement

▲ Intraperitoneal Placement

- ▲ Placing a large piece of mesh in the intraperitoneal position without a skin flap is technically challenging. Alternatively, laparoscopic visualization can be used to fixate the mesh. In this approach, the abdominal portion of the procedure can be completed in an open fashion. Before closing the midline incision, the mesh can be placed intraperitoneally and secured with several transfascial fixation sutures (Fig. 11-11). Several laparoscopic ports can be placed in the lateral abdominal wall under direct visualization. The midline

Chapter 11 • Endoscopic Component Separation 197

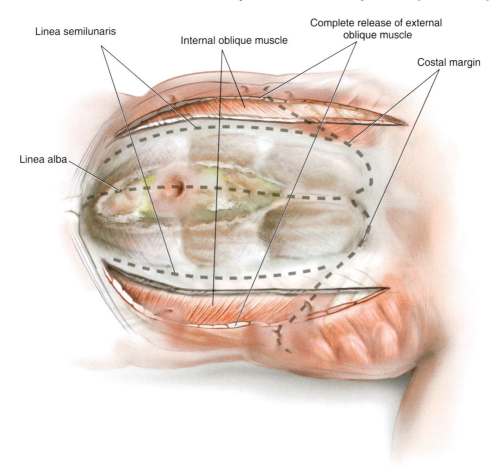

Figure 11-10.

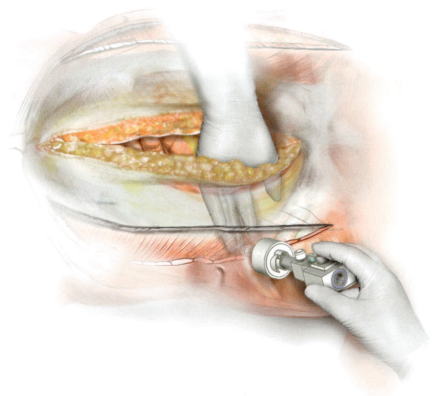

Figure 11-11.

incision is then closed to allow for insufflation of the peritoneal cavity. The mesh can then be secured using various laparoscopic fixation devices, including tackers or transfascial sutures (Figs. 11-12 and 11-13).

4. Postoperative Care

- ▲ Not all defects can be closed with a component separation. If excessive tension is necessary to reapproximate the midline fascia, a bridging type repair is indicated. Careful monitoring of hemodynamic physiology and changes in airway pressure are undertaken. All patients undergoing complex abdominal wall reconstructions remain intubated overnight if there is a rise of greater than 5 mm Hg in plateau airway pressures after fascial closure.
- ▲ It should be noted that the full effect of a component separation is typically not seen until 24 to 48 hours later, and defects can often be closed under moderate tension and allow the abdominal wall to completely expand.
- ▲ Epidural catheters are maintained until patients are tolerating a diet and have full return of bowel function.
- ▲ Diets are not advanced until patients have return of bowel function. While early postoperative feeding has shown promise in other fields of surgery, early postoperative retching and vomiting can lead to disruption of the surgical repair in complex abdominal wall reconstruction. Routine nasogastric tube decompression is avoided.
- ▲ Drains are maintained until outputs are <30 mL/drain/day.
- ▲ Antibiotics are only continued for up to 24 hours unless otherwise indicated.

Chapter 11 • Endoscopic Component Separation 199

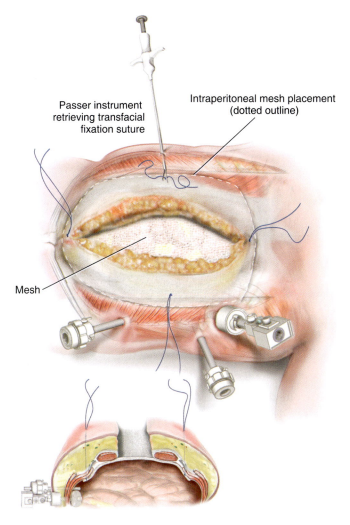

Figure 11-12.

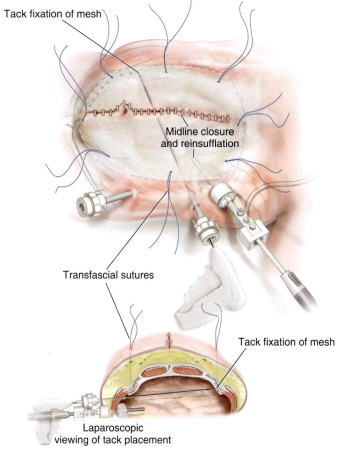

Figure 11-13.

5. Pearls/Pitfalls

- ▲ Realize the limitations of this operation.
- ▲ Medial advancement is difficult to achieve with defects at the xiphoid and suprapubic region of the abdominal wall. These should be avoided early in one's experience.
- ▲ Large defects, >20 cm, and noncompliant fixed abdominal wall defects often cannot be medialized to completely reconstruct the linea alba.
- ▲ Realistic expectations for patients, families, and surgeons as to the severity of the operation, including risks, and the ability to reconstruct a normal abdominal wall are critical to the success of this procedure.
- ▲ Endoscopic component separation is ideal in circumstances where a stoma is present. If the stoma is through the rectus muscle, a component separation can be performed endoscopically without undermining the skin around the stoma and risking peristomal skin necrosis and a floating stoma.
- ▲ Component separation should be performed bilaterally in most cases to redistribute the tension symmetrically during closure.
- ▲ Endoscopic component separation does not achieve the same release as an open component separation. Typically 85% of the fascial release can be achieved without a skin flap.
- ▲ If the exposure cannot be achieved laparoscopically for the cephalad part of the release of the external oblique, the skin incision can be enlarged, and using lighted retractors, the release can be completed using an open technique.

Selected References

Harth KC, Rosen MJ: Endoscopic versus open component separation in complex abdominal wall reconstruction, *Am J Surg* 199(3): 342–346, 2010 Mar:discussion 346–347.

Rosen MJ, Fatima J, Sarr MG: Repair of abdominal wall hernias with restoration of abdominal wall function, *J Gastrointest Surg* 14(1):175–185, 2010 Jan.

Rosen MJ, Jin J, McGee M, Marks J, Ponsky J: Laparoscopic component separation in the single stage treatment of infected abdominal wall prosthetic removal, *Hernia* 11(5):435–440, 2007 Oct.

Rosen MJ, Reynolds HL, Champagne B, Delaney CP: A novel approach for the simultaneous repair of large midline incisional and parastomal hernias with biological mesh and retrorectus reconstruction, *Am J Surg* 199(3):416–420, 2010 Mar:discussion 420–421.

Rosen MJ, Williams C, Jin J, McGee M, Marks J, Ponsky J: Laparoscopic versus open component separation: A comparative analysis in a porcine model, *Am J Surg* 194(3):385–389, 2007 Sep.

SECTION V

Other Abdominal Wall Procedures

CHAPTER 12

Panniculectomy and Abdominal Wall Reconstruction

Maurice Y. Nahabedian, MD, FACS

1. Clinical Anatomy of the Anterior Abdominal Wall

1. Relevant General Anatomy

- ▲ When considering panniculectomy in the setting of abdominal hernia repair, the underlying musculature, aponeurotic layers, and adipocutaneous structures are important. The three components are interrelated and should be addressed systematically in order to optimize outcomes following panniculectomy.

2. Relevant Muscular Anatomy

- ▲ The rectus abdominis and the internal, external, and transverse oblique musculature contribute to the support and contour of the anterior abdominal wall (Fig. 12-1).
- ▲ The perforating vasculature to the adipocutaneous component of the anterior abdominal wall emanates from the intramuscular vascular network (Fig. 12-2). The majority of significant perforators arise from the deep inferior epigastric system. Other blood vessels contributing to the perforating system include the superficial inferior epigastric artery, superficial circumflex iliac artery, and the deep circumflex iliac artery. All of these perforators converge at the dermis, forming the subdermal plexus.
- ▲ Prior abdominal operations associated with undermining can disrupt this perforating vascular network. However, secondary perforators can evolve over time and may be preserved. In addition, as a compensatory mechanism, the remote vascularity will acclimate to the new perfusion patterns and perfuse the undermined tissue.

Chapter 12 • Panniculectomy and Abdominal Wall Reconstruction

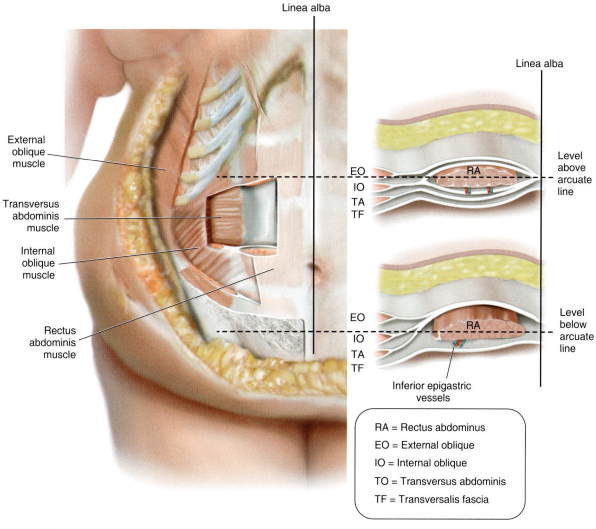

Figure 12-1.

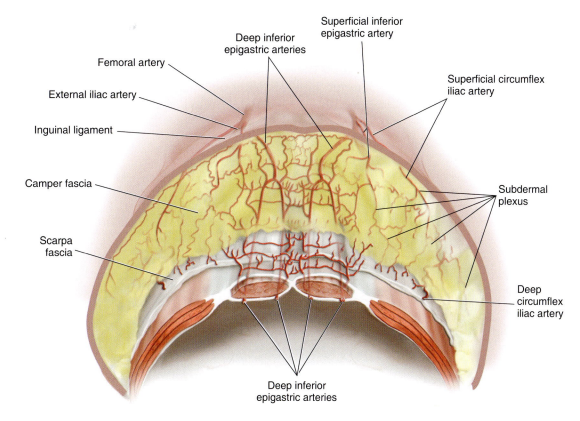

Figure 12-2.

3. Relevant Aponeurotic Anatomy

- ▲ The aponeurotic layers of the anterior abdominal wall include the linea alba, anterior rectus sheath, posterior rectus sheath, and the external oblique fascia (Fig. 12-3).
- ▲ The anterior rectus sheath and linea alba are composed of collagen fibers arranged in an interwoven lattice. The width and thickness of these structures vary along the surface of the anterior abdominal wall. These measurements fluctuate at various regions of the anterior abdominal wall and are related to the distance from the umbilicus. With respect to the linea alba, its width ranges from 11 to 21 mm between the xiphoid process and the umbilicus and then decreases from 11 to 2 mm from the umbilicus to the pubic symphysis. The thickness of the linea alba ranges from 900 to 1200 μm between the xiphoid and the umbilicus and increases from 1700 to 2400 μm from the umbilicus to the pubic symphysis. With respect to the anterior rectus sheath, the thickness ranges from 370 to 500 μm from the xiphoid to the umbilicus and then increases to 500 to 700 μm from the umbilicus to the pubic symphysis. The posterior rectus sheath, on the other hand, is slightly thicker than the anterior rectus sheath above the umbilicus, ranging from 450 to 600 μm, but then it drops off precipitously from the umbilicus to the arcuate line to 250 to 100 μm.

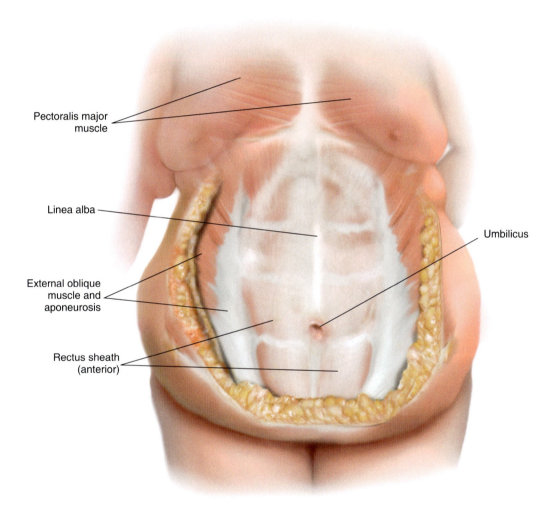

Figure 12-3.

- ▲ Perforating vessels pierce the anterior rectus sheath and external oblique fascia as they course through the adipose layer, until contributing to the subdermal plexus of vessels (Figs. 12-4 and 12-5).

4. Relevant Adipocutaneous Anatomy

- ▲ In the patient with an abdominal pannus, the overlying skin may be thickened and indurated. Ulcerations may be present with associated infections.
- ▲ The thickness of the pannus is variable and depends on body habitus and body mass index (BMI). The adipose component may be edematous with very large fatty lobular tissue.

2. Preoperative Considerations

- ▲ As with all operations, proper patient selection is important. A careful assessment of the risks and benefits of panniculectomy must be made, and the patient must be informed of the risks. These risk factors can increase the risk of postoperative morbidity and complications.

1. Preoperative Imaging

- ▲ Preoperative imaging is important when considering panniculectomy. Computed tomography (CT) or magnetic resonance imaging (MRI) delineate the size of the hernia defect and provide information regarding the thickness of the abdominal pannus (Fig. 12-6). The abdominal musculature also is appreciated. MRI also permits visualization of the larger arteries and veins that course through the pannus.

2. Assessment of Risk Factors

- ▲ Systemic risk factors that require optimization include but are not limited to diabetes mellitus, obesity, hypertension, pulmonary disease, poor nutritional status, cardiac disease, connective tissue disorders, abdominal aortic aneurisms, and immunosuppression. Local risk factors include but are not limited to prior soft tissue or cutaneous infections, fistula, indurated skin, lymphedema, and ulcerations.

Chapter 12 • Panniculectomy and Abdominal Wall Reconstruction

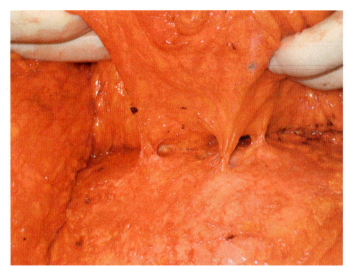

Figure 12-4.

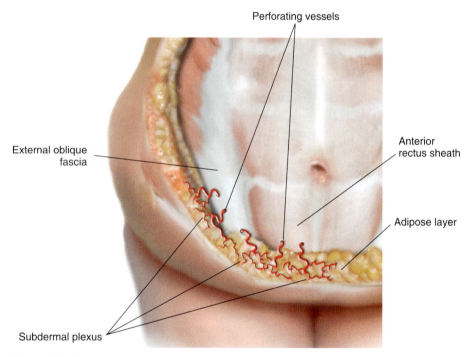

Figure 12-5.

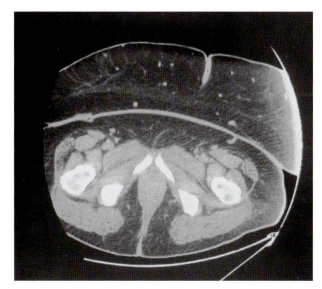

Figure 12-6.

▲ In patients with an elevated BMI (>35), uncontrolled diabetes mellitus, and poor nutritional status, the incidence of complications such as delayed healing, incisional dehiscence, soft tissue necrosis, infection, and prolonged drainage are likely to be increased. The anticipated length of the operation may influence the timing of the panniculectomy, immediate or delayed.

3. Prior Hernia Surgical History

▲ Prior studies have demonstrated an increased risk of infection in patients with an abdominal hernia. Although, many of these operations appear at first glance to be "clean" operations, they are, in fact, more susceptible to infection. Many of these infections manifest in the skin and subcutaneous fat. The incidence of soft tissue infection is approximately 10-fold higher in patients with a hernia (16% vs. 1.5%). In patients with a prior abdominal hernia repair, the risk of infection continues to increase (42% vs. 12%). Surgeons should be cognizant of these statistics when considering panniculectomy.

▲ In general, prior vertical midline incisions are preferred because a fleur-de-lis pattern can be used. With this pattern, excess skin and fat can be excised in both the horizontal and vertical planes. When the prior incisions are transverse in orientation, problems related to blood supply can occur, especially when the incisions are located in the mid- and upper abdominal areas. Low transverse abdominal incisions are usually fine because this is where the transverse incisions are usually made for panniculectomy.

3. Operative Steps

▲ Preparing for panniculectomy is in many ways similar to preparing for abdominoplasty. The principles and concepts for the two are similar. Design patterns for skin excision must consider the vascularity of the skin. This will be related to the location of the prior incisions, the thickness of the soft tissues, and the degree of undermining. The degree of soft tissue undermining must include an appreciation for the thickness of the pannus because this can impact the perfusion of the adipocutaneous component.

1. Design Patterns for Panniculectomy

▲ There are several design patterns for abdominal panniculectomy. These include the horizontal incision; vertical incision; and a horizontal and vertical incision, also known as a fleur-de-lis pattern (Fig. 12-7). The specific pattern depends on the location of excess tissue and the location of prior incisions. Most patients with abdominal hernias will have a prior vertical midline incision. Incorporating this into the excision pattern is useful and does not usually result in additional scars.

Chapter 12 • Panniculectomy and Abdominal Wall Reconstruction 211

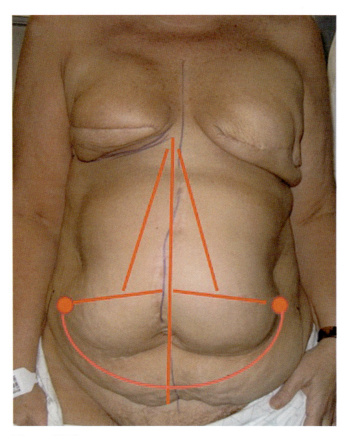

Figure 12-7.

2. Technique of Perforator Sparing

- ▲ In patients with abdominal hernias and excess abdominal skin and fat, some degree of soft tissue undermining is usually necessary in order to adequately close and contour the abdominal wall. The undermining is always at the junction of the fascia and fat. All of the perforators supplying the skin and fat pierce the fascia (see Fig. 12-5). Preservation of one or more perforators improves the vascularity of the adipocutaneous layer and minimizes the incidence of delayed healing or skin necrosis.
- ▲ Undermining can be performed using electrocautery or blunt dissection techniques. A blunt, tapered-point surgical scissor or clamp can be used to separate the perforator from the surrounding fat. An alternative approach is to use a low-voltage electrocautery device with a fine-tip surgical clamp.
- ▲ In general, smaller perforators (<1 mm) are usually cauterized. Larger perforators (1.0 to 2.5 mm) can be preserved. The presence of a palpable pulse in the perforator is recommended when considering preservation.
- ▲ The number of perforators to be spared is also variable and depends on the body habitus and the thickness of the abdominal pannus. Personal experience has demonstrated that preservation of a single perforating vessel on each side of the hemiabdomen is usually adequate. Surgeons also should be aware that in some patients with multiple hernia repairs, perforating vessels may no longer be present.

3. Technique of Skin/Fat Excision

- ▲ Preoperative markings are important. With the patient in the standing position, the amount of excess skin is approximated by grasping and elevating the pannus (Fig. 12-8). The markings typically include the incision for the hernia repair and the incisions for the panniculectomy (Fig. 12-9).
- ▲ Before the operative incisions, measures to control and limit blood loss may be considered. One such maneuver is to place tumescent fluid into the soft tissues of the pannus. The typical tumescent solution consists of 1 ml of 1:1000 epinephrine solution per liter of lactated Ringer solution.
- ▲ Typically, the panniculectomy is performed after the hernia has been completed. This is important in order to better assess the exact amount of skin and fat to be excised. In cases where an open component separation has been performed, it is important to preserve perforators when possible to optimize skin perfusion.
- ▲ Once the hernia repair is complete, the soft tissues are further undermined off of the anterior rectus sheath, and the amount of excess skin and fat is determined (Fig. 12-10). The degree of undermining depends on the thickness of the adipocutaneous tissues, location of scars, and assessment of skin vascularity. Vertical skin excisions are performed by elevating

Chapter 12 • Panniculectomy and Abdominal Wall Reconstruction 213

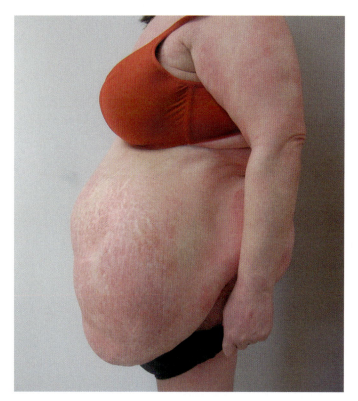

Figure 12-8.

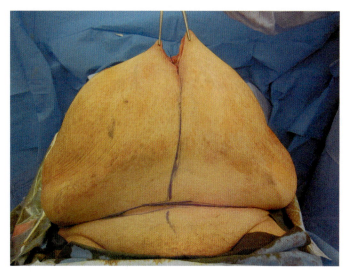

Figure 12-9.

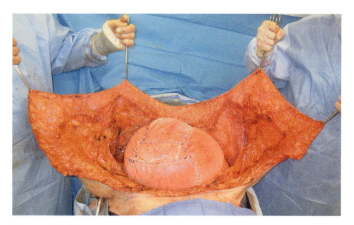

Figure 12-10.

the adipocutaneous flaps and redraping one side over the other (Fig. 12-11). The overlapping areas are marked before excision (Fig. 12-12). Vertical and horizontal skin excisions proceed, incorporating the vertical and horizontal incisions (Fig. 12-13). It is important to excise any abnormal or thickened skin. The vascularity of the remaining skin flaps is based superolaterally. In patients with a very large or thick pannus, it is important to avoid extensive undermining that may compromise vascularity.
- ▲ In cases where the hernia is extremely large and associated with a loss of domain in which the hernia sac is lining the deep fat layer, the sac or scar is excised because it may be a nidus for infection. The skin flaps are then elevated and redraped in order to determine how much will be excised. Skin excision is performed sharply to minimize any thermal damage to the edges.

Chapter 12 • Panniculectomy and Abdominal Wall Reconstruction 215

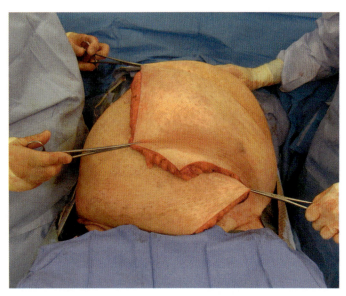

Figure 12-11.

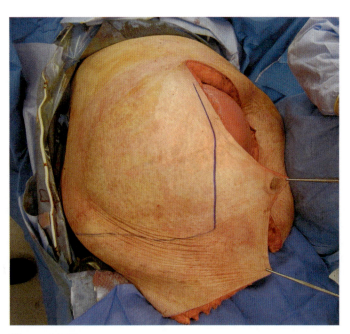

Figure 12-12.

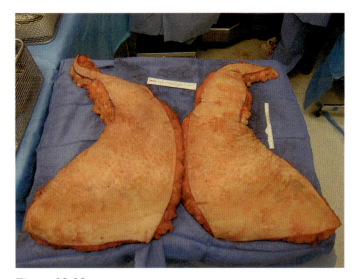

Figure 12-13.

▲ An alternative technique for skin pattern design and excision is the "Mercedes" approach (Figs. 12-14 and 12-15). This technique is indicated in patients in whom a vertical and horizontal skin excision is necessary. The advantage of this pattern is that it will preserve vascularized tissue at the trifurcation point and potentially minimize the delayed healing and skin necrosis that often occurs there. In preparation for this technique, the vertical midline and transverse horizontal patterns are delineated much like the standard techniques. The unique feature of this design is that an equilateral triangular pattern is delineated just below the umbilicus extending to the horizontal markings. The lengths of these triangular limbs are usually 15 to 20 cm and vary, based on body habitus and the dimensions of the pannus. This triangular skin is not excised with the panniculectomy. It is preserved as a caudally based flap that is advanced in the cephalad direction following the central and lateral skin excisions.

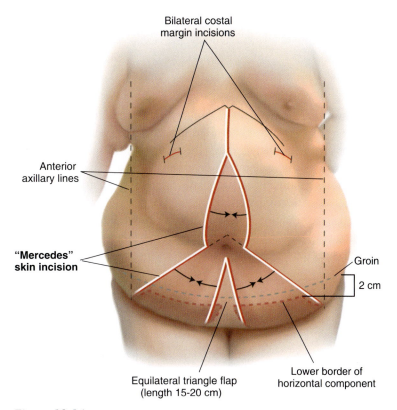

Figure 12-14.

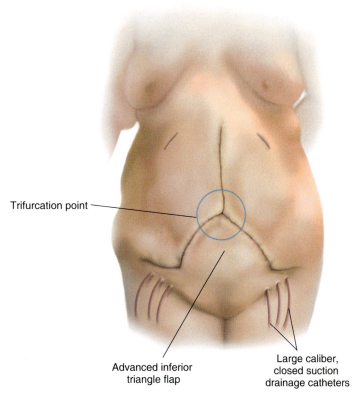

Figure 12-15.

4. Closure Techniques

- Before skin closure, the wounds are copiously irrigated with an antibiotic solution. Closed suction drains are placed in the lateral gutters and as needed for the hernia repair. These drains are usually large caliber and can be inserted through the incision or via a remote skin site. The closure is completed in layers using absorbable sutures in the Scarpa layer and the dermis. The cutaneous closure can be performed using staples or sutures, depending on the perceived risks of infection, delayed healing, and incisional dehiscence.
- In some cases, the incision is not closed completely and a negative pressure wound therapy device is applied (Fig. 12-16). The reasoning for this is to minimize potential fluid collections and soft tissue edema. Once stable, this device can be removed and the wound closed secondarily.

4. Postoperative Care

1. Hospital Care

- **Antibiotics:** Postoperatively, patients are continued on intravenous antibiotic. In some centers, antibiotic coverage is delivered during the perioperative period (24 hours). However, personal experience has been favorable with a 1-week duration. This may be prolonged in the setting of a postoperative infection.
- **Drains:** The duration of the drains is variable and based on quantity of fluid and the need for prolonged suction to promote tissue adherence. Typically, drains are removed when the output is <30 mL/drain/day and usually left in place for 1 to 2 weeks.
- **Venous thromboembolism (VTE):** All patients following hernia repair and panniculectomy will require VTE prophylaxis in the form of pneumatic compression devices and chemoprevention using pharmaceutical agents such as Lovenox or subcutaneous heparin. Pulmonary consideration may be relevant because the added pressure on the diaphragm from the hernia repair and the panniculectomy may increase airway resistance. Incentive spirometry and early ambulation are encouraged to improve pulmonary status and circulation.
- **Nutrition:** Nutritional status is assessed and diets are advanced as tolerated once bowel function has returned. In some situations when enteral feeding is not possible early, parenteral feeding is advised.
- **Length of stay:** The length of hospital stay is variable and depends on various factors. These include but are not limited to return of bowel function, development of complications, and patient compliance. Reid and Dumanian (2005) have determined that the average length of stay in patients who have component separation repair of an abdominal hernia with panniculectomy was 7.7 days.

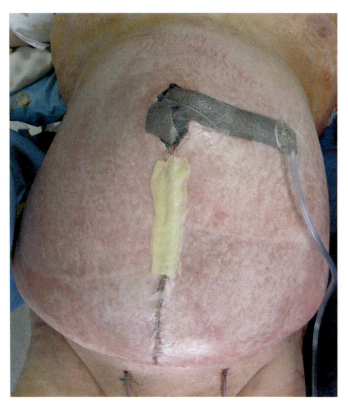

Figure 12-16.

2. Home Care

▲ Following hernia repair and panniculectomy, patients are instructed to minimize strenuous activities for 6 weeks. The use of an abdominal binder is appropriate once it is known that tissue viability is certain. Patients may shower and get the incision wet on day 3 following surgery, if possible. Most patients will require a convalescence period of 1 to 2 months following surgery.

5. Management of Complications

▲ When performing panniculectomies in patients with abdominal hernias, one should not be surprised in the event of complications. In the majority of cases, complications are infection, soft tissue necrosis, and delayed healing or incisional dehiscence. Studies have demonstrated that the incidence of a major postoperative wound complication in increased sixfold when the BMI is greater than 35, and that those patients are 5 times more likely to undergo reoperation.

▲ **Infection:** Postoperative wound infections typically manifest within a few days and may present with cellulitis or drainage (Fig. 12-17). Appropriate cultures and sensitivities are obtained. Infectious disease consultation is recommended and based on surgeon comfort and extent of disease. Causative organisms are variable and may include staphylococcus, streptococcus, *Escherichia coli,* and others. Surgical incision and drainage procedures may be necessary.

▲ **Soft tissue necrosis:** Impaired vascular circulation, increased tension, or soft tissue infection may result in tissue necrosis (see Fig. 12-17). Surgical debridement is necessary. The debridement must include all necrotic tissue and extend to viable, bleeding tissue. Closure immediately following debridement is usually not performed. Local wound measures are implemented and may include wet to dry dressings or enzymatic measures. Secondary closure is considered when all signs of infection and necrosis are cleared.

▲ **Incisional dehiscence:** Dehiscence can occur because of tension or abnormal forces being placed upon the incision. In the event of a pure dehiscence, secondary closure may be indicated, However, in the event of contamination, local wound measures may be indicated for a period of time, followed by delayed secondary closure.

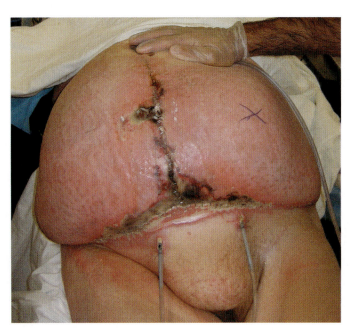

Figure 12-17.

6. Pearls and Pitfalls

- ▲ **Set expectations:** Before any of these procedures, it is important to set expectations during the initial and subsequent preoperative consultations. Complications are common, and patients with abdominal hernias, pannus formation, and associated comorbidities must be aware of the potential adverse events.
- ▲ **Avoid the "hand-in-glove" fit:** When excising excess skin, it is tempting to maximally excise to obtain optimal contour. Avoid this temptation. Postoperative soft tissue edema may result in increased tension. In addition, postoperative complications such as dehiscence or soft tissue necrosis may result in an inability to achieve closure when desired. Leaving a small amount of skin redundancy is not a problem. It can be easily corrected a few months later once all healing is complete.
- ▲ **Negative pressure wound therapy:** In some situations where the risk of soft tissue infection or delayed healing is considered high, it may be advantageous to leave a portion of the incision open. The application of a negative pressure wound therapy device is advised in these situations. The benefits include controlling edema, reducing tension on the incision line, and serving as an exit portal for excess fluid.
- ▲ In situations where the thickness of the abdominal pannus is extreme (>6 cm), excision of the loose fat to the level of Scarpa fascia is appropriate and can facilitate closure.
- ▲ In morbidly obese patients (BMI >40) with a large abdominal pannus, weight loss measures are advised when possible. This may potentially decrease the postoperative complications that are likely in this population.
- ▲ In complicated patients requiring hernia repair and panniculectomy, a multidisciplinary approach is recommended. Early consultation with plastic surgery is advised.
- ▲ Inverted "T" incisions can have a high propensity for delayed healing and incisional dehiscence. In situations where this is likely, recommendations include conservative skin excision, perforator preservation, a Mercedes type incision pattern, or a delayed panniculectomy.

Selected References

Askar OM: Surgical anatomy of the aponeurotic expansions of the anterior abdominal wall, *Ann R Coll Surg Engl* 59:313–321, 1977.

Axer H, v. Keyserlingk DG, Prescher A: Collagen fibers in linea alba and rectus sheaths: I. General scheme and morphological aspects, *Journal of Surgical Research* 96:127–134, 2001.

Axer H, v. Keyserlingk DG, Prescher A: Collagen fibers in linea alba and rectus sheaths II. Variability and biomechanical aspects, *Journal of Surgical Research* 96:239–245, 2001.

Borud LJ, Grunwaldt L, Janz B, Mun E, Slavin SA: Components separation combined with abdominal wall plication for repair of large abdominal wall hernias following bariatric surgery, *Plast Reconstr Surg* 119:1792, 2007.

Butler CE, Reis SM: Mercedes panniculectomy with simultaneous component separation ventral hernia repair, *Plast Reconstr Surg* 125:94, 2010.

Cooper CM, Paige KT, Beshlian KM, Downey DL, Thrilby RC: Abdominal panniculectomies: High patient satisfaction despite significant complication rates, *Ann Plast Surg* 61:188–196, 2008.

Houck JP, Rypins EB, Sarfeh IJ, Juler GL, Shimoda KJ: Repair of incisional hernia, *Surg Gynecol Obstet* 169:397, 1989.

Korenkov M, Beckers A, Koebke J, et al: Biomechanical and morphological types of the linea alba and its possible role in the pathogenesis of midline incisional hernia, *Eur J Surg* 167:909–914, 2001.

Nahabedian MY, Manson PN: Contour abnormalities of the abdomen following TRAM Flap breast reconstruction: A Multifactorial Analysis, *Plast Reconstr Surg* 109:81–87, 2002.

Nahabedian MY, Dooley W, Singh N, Manson PN: Contour Abnormalities of the abdomen following breast reconstruction with abdominal flaps: The role of muscle preservation, *Plast Reconstr Surg* 109:91–101, 2002.

Reid RR, Dumanian GA: Panniculectomy and the separation-of-parts hernia repair: A solution for the large infraumbilical hernia in the obese patient, *Plast Reconstr Surg* 116:1006, 2005.

Saulis AS, Dumanian GA: Periumbilical rectus abdominis perforator preservation significantly reduces superficial wound complications in "separation of parts" hernia repairs, *Plast Reconstr Surg* 109:2275, 2002.

CHAPTER 13

Tissue and Fascial Expansion of the Abdominal Wall

Daniel A. Medalie, MD

1. Introduction and Clinical Description

The abdomen lends itself to tissue expansion in patients of all ages and a multitude of clinical problems. Both congenital and acute defects of the abdominal wall can be addressed by the sequential expansion of adjacent tissues. These include the treatment of giant congenital nevi, tumors, burn scar contracture, posttraumatic defects, and loss of skin and fascial domain following previous surgery or injury. This chapter addresses the treatment of skin and subcutaneous tissue defects of the abdominal wall by utilizing prosthetic tissue expanders to both create new tissue and recruit tissue from healthy adjoining areas. It also discusses fascial expansion of the abdominal wall by the process of serial excision of a fixed prosthetic mesh. Because the anatomy of the abdominal wall is described elsewhere in this book, it is not repeated here.

1. Typical Skin Defect Requiring Tissue Expansion

Soft tissue expansion is performed by the insertion of a silicone balloon under the skin and subcutaneous tissue. Gradual injection of sterile saline into the expander via a remote or integrated port inflates the skin and subcutaneous tissues over the expander, inducing new growth and recruiting regional tissue via mechanical creep and the viscoelastic properties of skin. The dermis overlying the expander does thin somewhat, but the tissue remains sensate and the vascularity remains the same or even improves. The abdomen is an excellent area for tissue expansion. The overlying expanders have no adverse effect on the viscera, and the donor sites tend to be large with a relatively flat base to support the expander.

The typical defect that lends itself to repair via the insertion of tissue expanders is a well-defined defect that is well healed and stable (Fig. 13-1, *A*). Areas that have been irradiated or subject to diffuse trauma, such as burns and subsequent grafting and scar contracture, are less amenable to expansion. Open wounds or chronically draining wounds are also fraught with problems because of the high incidence of infection and subsequent extrusion of the expander. If a tumor is to be removed, there must be absolute certainty that the tumor is not contiguous with the tissue expanded pocket. In Fig. 13-1, *A*, a patient is shown with a large midline abdominal hernia

Chapter 13 • Tissue and Fascial Expansion of the Abdominal Wall 225

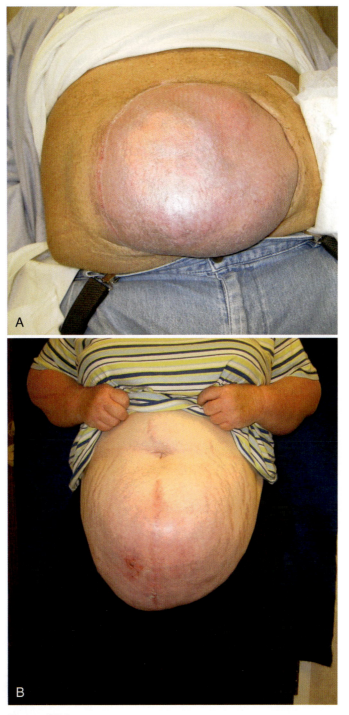

Figure 13-1.

and well-healed skin graft over bowel. The width of the graft is clearly too great to allow primary closure of the adjacent skin and subcutaneous tissues. He also has a large fascial defect, and if this is closed with prosthetic mesh, good skin closure over the mesh will be impossible. The shown defect will respond ideally to progressive expansion of bilateral crescenteric tissue expanders placed on either side of the central defect. The expanders are inserted on top of the abdominal wall fascia and completely underneath all of the skin and subcutaneous tissue lateral to the central graft and hernia. Over the course of several weeks to months, the expanders are filled with sterile saline via remote port. When they are deemed to be adequately expanded, they are removed in the operating room (OR), the central graft is excised, the hernia is repaired, and the skin flaps are advanced to the midline to adequately close the defect (see Figs. 13-2 and 13-5, p. 235).

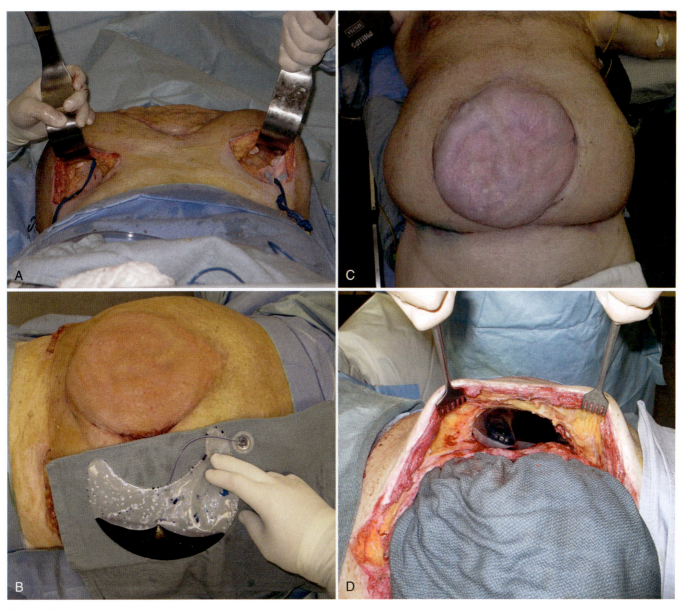

Figure 13-2.

2. Typical Fascial Defect Requiring Fascial Expansion

It is harder to define the typical fascial defect that will require or respond well to expansion via serial excision of prosthetic mesh. Frequently the type of procedure needed to close a fascial defect is not known until the hernia is dissected free during surgery, and the extent of the fascial loss or loss of domain is completely evaluated. In the patient shown in Fig. 13-1, B, on page 225, there is adequate skin coverage of the hernia, but there is a clearly massive hernia with obvious loss of abdominal domain. Approaches to the repair of this hernia include prosthetic or biologic mesh repair, separation of component parts repair, regional or free-flap reconstruction, or a combination of all three procedures. It is this author's opinion that the best approach to abdominal wall reconstruction is to replace like with like and to return anatomic structures to their normal place. Thus, the ideal abdominal wall has innervated rectus abdominis muscles in the midline that contract during forced effort and help to maintain the integrity of the abdominal wall. To achieve this goal, the separation-of-parts procedure is ideal (see Chapter 8). Sometimes, however, the fascial defect is so large that the separation of parts is not sufficient. This is usually true if the defect exceeds 16 cm in width and the lateral abdominal wall is fixed and noncompliant. In this case the surgeon can attempt to bridge the defect with mesh (not an anatomic solution) or perform a staged procedure designed to gradually decrease the width of the fascial defect and reacquire abdominal domain. This multistage surgery involves three main components. The first is the initial operation where the hernia is dissected free, and the fascial defect is analyzed. At this time, a piece of nonadherent Gore-Tex mesh is sewn to the fascial edges completely bridging the defect under moderate tension. Ideally the skin is closed over the Gore-Tex and drains are placed. The second stage is a series of multiple operative trips to serially excise the central piece of Gore-Tex (usually no more than 4 cm in width). This process gradually pulls the rectus muscles and the fascia back to the midline. In the final operation, the last piece of Gore-Tex is removed, a separation of parts is performed, the closure is usually reinforced with mesh underlay or overlay, and the skin is closed on top (see Figs.13-7, p. 237; 13-8, p. 239; and 13-12, p. 243)

2. Tissue Expansion

1. Indication for and Analysis of Soft Tissue Defect

Tissue expansion may be indicated in any defect that cannot be closed primarily without threatening necrosis of tissues or wound dehiscence. The patient needs to be made aware that the process is long and involves multiple outpatient visits to the doctor for the expansion. It is also temporarily cosmetically deforming. Sometimes, with patients who have responsible family members, I have allowed them to perform expansions themselves (after careful instruction on sterile technique). This is useful in cases where the patient lives at a distance from the doctor's office and lets them participate in their own care. It should be reiterated that patients with open wounds, draining incisions, or irradiated wound beds are not good candidates for expansion. There is no absolute contraindication for the process, rather the incidence of infection or implant extrusion rises to a level where the risks may outweigh the benefits. It is generally recommended to overinflate the expander by about 20% and then allow it to settle with no expansion for 3 months before the definitive operation. This helps prevent tension and possibly skin necrosis at the wound margins.

2. Choice of Tissue Expander Size, Shape, and Location

Fortunately today there are many options for tissue expansion. Multiple companies have premade expanders of all shapes and sizes and also have the ability to custom fabricate expanders of almost any desired dimensions. Most of the expanders come with remote ports, but several are also fitted with integrated ports. These ports are all composed of self-sealing silicone rubber backed by stainless steel and can be located by magnetic sensing devices placed over the skin. The length of the expander must match the length of the wound, and the height of the expander ideally should match the width (or when opposing symmetric expanders are placed, the height should match half the width). I prefer rectangular expanders for most defects except in the case of circular or elliptical defects where there is a large discrepancy in the width of the wound at the center versus either end. In those cases, a crescenteric expander is the ideal choice. Fill volume is not extremely important because the expanders are designed to tolerate overfilling by several times the official recommended volume. The placement location of the expander in the abdominal wall is not as complicated as it is in scalp expansion (for instance). In most instances, the expander or expanders will be adjacent to the long access of the defect. Care must be taken to visualize the final closure of the wound in order to properly place the expanders and subsequently close the defect with a minimum of disfiguring scars.

3. Operative Steps

1. Tissue Expansion and Closure of Abdominal Wall Skin

▲ *Insertion of Tissue Expanders*

After the abdominal wall has been analyzed and the expanders chosen and ordered, the first operation for insertion of the expanders is performed (Fig. 13-2, *A-D* and Fig. 13-3). The patient is asked to bathe with antimicrobial soap the night before the surgery (if practical). On the day of surgery, intravenous (IV) antibiotics are administered, and sequential compression devices are applied before induction. The wound should be prepped with alcohol and chlorhexidine because this provides the most effective antimicrobial barrier and the longest duration of action.

It is a natural instinct to place the incision for the expander at the edge of the wound to be closed. While this may work, it also subjects the incision to the forces of expansion and can lead to wound dehiscence and expander extrusion. I thus prefer to make a separate incision perpendicular and lateral to the long axis of the wound (see Fig. 13-2, *A*, and Fig. 13-3). The incision is subsequently incorporated into the final closure by acting as a release for the expanded flap. If this is deemed too impractical, then I recommend keeping the incision for the expander as small as possible to minimize the forces upon it. A pocket is dissected along the wound using a lighted retractor to visualize and create an appropriate space. The pocket lies completely under the skin and subcutaneous fat of the abdominal wall (including Scarpa fascia). It should rest on the anterior fascia of the rectus and external oblique (Fig. 13-2, *A*). Several authors have described placing the expanders under the anterior rectus and external oblique fascia to create an expanded fasciocutaneous flap. This has the advantages of maintaining excellent blood supply to the tissues and strength. It is a more complicated operation and should be approached with care, especially so as not to damage the rectus muscle.

Once the pocket is made large enough to just fit the completely flat expander, it is irrigated with a triple antibiotic irrigation. I use 1 L of saline mixed with 1 g of cefazolin (Ancef), 80 mg of gentamicin, and 50,000 units of bacitracin. This mixture has a broad spectrum and minimal tissue toxicity. Excellent hemostasis must be achieved before the placement of the expander. The expander is then opened on the field and left in its plastic container. All gloves are changed, and fresh towels are applied around the wound. The abdominal wall is cleansed again with alcohol. The antibiotic solution is then added topically to the expander in its container, and the expander is lightly pressed to see if any air bubbles leak out (it comes prefilled with air). Depending on where the port is located (integrated or remote), the expander should then be accessed with a 23-gauge butterfly needle and all remaining air removed. Sixty to 100 mL of saline with methylene blue are then added to the expander to prevent distortion and allow it to lay flat (see Fig. 13-2, *B*). All remaining air (bubbles floating on the saline) is then removed from the expander. The expander is rolled into a tube and gently placed into the pocket with minimal contact with the outside skin. A finger that has been dipped in the antibiotic solution is then used to smooth the expander out and ensure that it completely fills the pocket and lays flat.

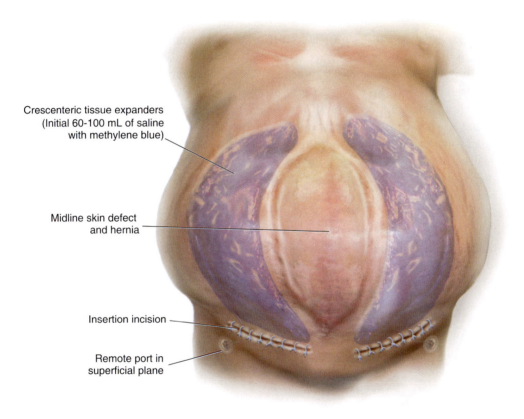

Figure 13-3.

The patient shown in Figure 13-3 is lying prone with paired crescenteric tissue expanders inserted lateral to the midline abdominal skin defect and hernia. The insertion incisions are perpendicular to the long axis of the defect and will be incorporated into the final closure as back cuts used to help advance the skin flaps. If a remote port is being used, a tunnel and small pocket need to be created several inches away from the expander so that they can be easily accessed (see Fig. 13-3). It is very important not to kink the tubing and also to place the port in a relatively superficial plane (especially if the patient is obese). If the port is too deep, it may not be easily felt or accessed. If it is too close to the expander, then there is a risk of damaging the expander. If the tube is kinked, then the expansion is impossible and another procedure will need to be performed. The methylene blue is useful because sometimes a seroma forms around the expander and port. The blue ensures that the surgeon knows that he has indeed accessed the expander and not just the seroma cavity. I recommend a remote port in all obese patients because an integrated port may be difficult to locate through the thick tissue, even with the magnetic finder provided by the manufacturer. Although I do not like closed suction drains touching the expander, I also do not like seromas and feel that a drain is usually warranted for several days. I try to remove them as soon as possible and keep the patient on oral antibiotics for as long as the drains are in and then 48 hours after they are removed. The wound is closed with deep and superficial absorbable monofilament sutures, and Dermabond is applied. I then access the port and test it to make sure that it works. At that time, I may choose to inject more saline into the expander, depending on how tight the closure was. I like to use an abdominal binder to prevent tension on the wound for the first 7 to 10 days.

▲ Progressive Fill of Expanders

Two weeks after the initial operation, the drains should be out and the wound well sealed. I then begin inflation of the expander (or expanders as the case may be). The skin is prepped with alcohol, and a long butterfly needle is used to access the port. A 60-mL syringe filled with saline is attached to the needle, and the plunger is pulled back until methylene blue is seen in the butterfly needle tubing. I then feel confident to push the 60 mL of saline into the expander (Fig. 13-4). The amount to be injected varies by patient and size of expander. I like to feel the skin over the expander and also listen to the patient's subjective report of tightness. It is always better to inject less than theoretically possible in order to minimize the risk of wound dehiscence or breakdown.

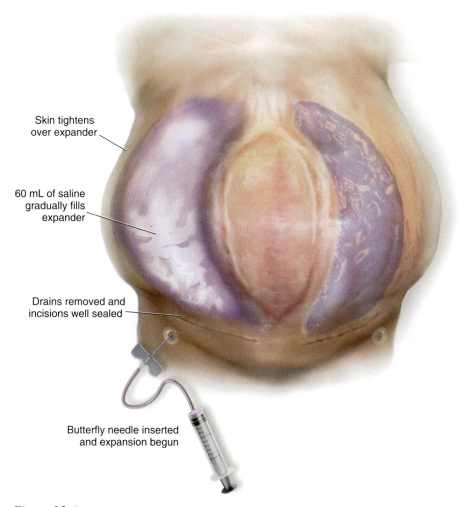

Figure 13-4.

▲ Removal of Expanders and Closure of Skin Defect

When the expanders have been inflated to their desired amount, the final operation is planned (see Fig. 13-2, C). The same antiseptic measures are taken, and then the wound is completely excised. In the example shown, the skin graft is removed from the bowels, and the intervening tissue between the tissue expanders and the defect is incised (see Fig. 13-2, D). The expanders and ports are removed (Fig. 13-5, A). This creates ready access to the lateral edge of the rectus muscle, facilitating a separation-of-parts procedure. After the fascial defect is closed and reinforced with biologic mesh (Fig. 13-5, B), the expanded skin and subcutaneous tissue are advanced to the midline (Fig. 13-6). The body forms a capsule around the tissue expander and this capsule contributes to the blood supply of the overlying skin. In general it is advisable to leave the capsule alone, but frequently the edges of the capsule and sometimes the skin need to be incised perpendicular to the line of the defect to allow easy advancement of the flap. The capsule also may be serially scored to create an accordion effect and allow flap advancement. The surface of the abdominal wall on which the tissue expander rests also is covered by capsule, and it is recommended to abrade this surface with electrocautery to generate adhesions between the abdominal wall and the overlying flap of skin and fat. This helps limit postoperative seromas. Drains are always placed and left in until total drainage is less than 30 mL/24 hours. An abdominal binder is placed, and the patient is advised to wear it at all times for 3 months (this is also to take tension off of the hernia repair). The patient in Figure 13-5 is shown at 3 months with good reduction of the hernia and closure of the skin defect (see Fig. 13-5, C and D).

4. Pearls/Pitfalls

1. Managing the Infected or Extruded Tissue Expander

If the expander extrudes or becomes infected early in the expansion, then it is recommended to remove it, allow the wound to heal for at least 6 weeks, and then try again. Ideally 3 months should go by between efforts. Sometimes the wound breaks open, but there is no infection present. In this case, I have sometimes attempted to take the patient to the OR, clean the wound, irrigate the pocket with antibiotic, and then close the wound while leaving the expander in place. Much of the volume is removed from the expander to allow easy closure of the dehiscence. When this works, I feel lucky, not skilled. In the setting of infection, I do not believe it is possible to rescue the expander.

If the expansion is almost complete and the skin breaks down to reveal the expander, I place the patient on antibiotics; have them apply topical mafenide acetate (Sulfamylon), a powerful topical antimicrobial, to the wound; and plan to electively take them to the OR for expander removal and definitive closure of the defect. If the expander becomes infected, I perform the same procedure but take them to the OR as soon as possible.

Chapter 13 • Tissue and Fascial Expansion of the Abdominal Wall   235

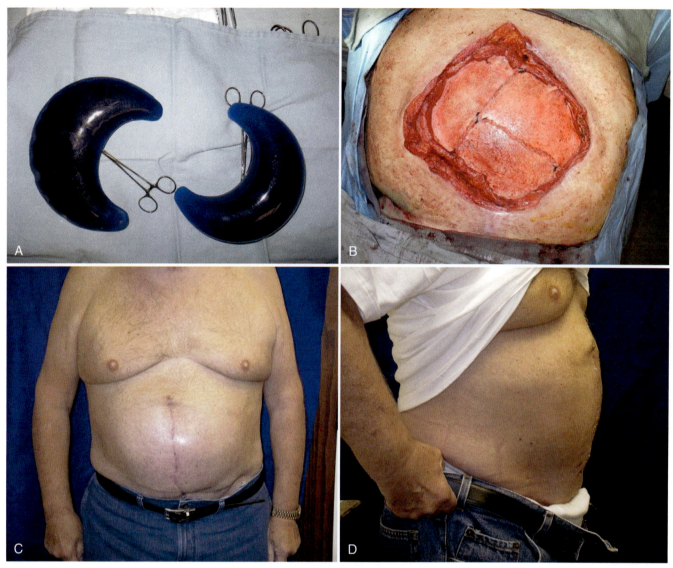

Figure 13-5.

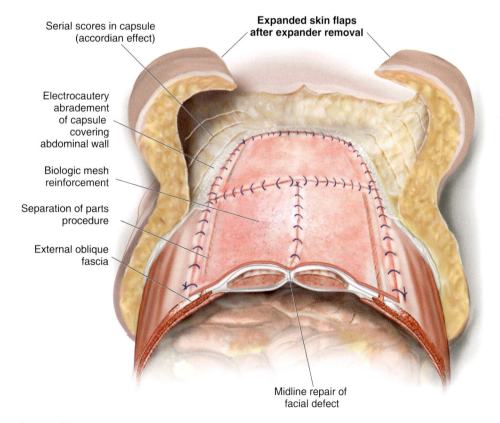

Figure 13-6.

2. Estimating When Skin Expansion Is Adequate

There is no magic rule for determining when the tissue expansion is complete, but in general, the height of the expander or expanders must equal the width of the defect. The height is difficult to gauge, especially since some have argued that the height should include both the edge adjacent to the defect and the opposite edge. One way of estimating is to take a tape measure and place it at the base of the lateral edge of the expander, pass it over the maximum projection of the dome, and measure to the edge of the advancing edge of expanded tissue. The base width of the expander is then subtracted from this arc length to estimate the degree of advancement. Ultimately it is better to err on the side of overexpansion. Excess tissue can always be removed and will facilitate a tension-free closure.

5. Fascial Expansion

1. Indication and Analysis of Fascial Defect

As mentioned previously, it is difficult in some cases to determine preoperatively whether a patient will require serial excision of mesh to facilitate closure of the fascial defect. In some patients the defect is so large, the need is obvious (see Fig. 13-1, *B* and Fig. 13-7, *A* and *B*). As outlined in Chapter 8, the best method of closure of large fascial defects is the separation of component parts of the abdomen with biologic or prosthetic mesh reinforcement. At the time of the initial take down of the hernia, the decision is made as to whether to proceed with definitive repair or to stage the repair. It is important not to perform the separation of parts until the final procedure. The patient should be informed preoperatively and give consent to any and all staged procedures necessary to close the fascial defect.

I find that the best response to reverse fascial expansion is in patients who have had midline incisions with loss of abdominal domain. Patients who have lost fascia and or parts of the rectus abdominis musculature due to trauma, infection, or cancer have less of a response to the expansion. Additionally, the fascial closure is less secure, and the risk of recurrence is greater because the paired innervated rectus muscles are not symmetric and in the midline. If one rectus is gone, then it is the edge of the external and internal obliques that are being pulled to the midline. While it is possible to do this, the muscles are not oriented in the same direction as the opposing rectus, and the forces working to pull the fascial repair apart are greater.

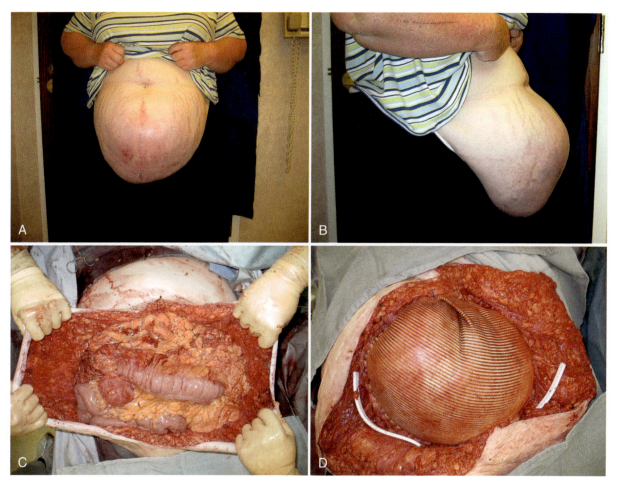

Figure 13-7.

2. Fascial Expansion and Closure of Abdominal Wall Midline Defect

Once the decision to perform serial closure of the fascia is made, the defect is carefully measured and photographed. The hernia is completely separated from the overlying abdominal wall, and a large sheet of Gore-Tex Dual mesh (WL Gore and Associates, Flagstaff, AZ) is sewn under moderate tension to the edges of the defect (see Fig. 13-7, *C* and *D*). Ideally the skin is viable and healthy enough to close over the Gore-Tex. If the skin is of poor quality, then the Gore-Tex can be covered by a VAC (vacuum-assisted closure) (see accompanying video). In this case the skin and the fascia must be advanced together, and the risk of skin necrosis and wound dehiscence is much higher. One way to approach this is to begin to undermine the skin edges at the level of the fascia during each subsequent operation with the ultimate goal of elevating it beyond the lateral edge of the rectus muscles. This is necessary anyway to perform the final separation-of-parts repair. Care should be taken to identify rectus perforators to the skin and preserve them as much as possible. This gradual process of elevating the skin acts to "delay" the skin flap, meaning that the ultimate blood supply is augmented by virtue of the body's response to mild ischemia. This technique is tricky to perform, and it is easy to develop skin edge necrosis by going too fast.

The patient is kept in the hospital and no further surgery is performed until normal bowel function returns. At that time it can be decided whether to perform the subsequent operations as an inpatient or outpatient. A typical operative sequence is every Monday, Thursday until the defect is ready for definitive closure.

The second phase of the surgery involves the serial excision of the Gore-Tex in the midline with moderate to tight closure. The patient is brought to the OR and the skin is opened (or VAC removed, as the case may be). The Gore-Tex is assessed for tightness, and a pinch test is performed in the midline with the patient paralyzed (see video). Unless the closure was very loose at the initial operation, I do not recommend removing more than a 4-cm wide strip of central Gore-Tex. The two edges of the cut Gore-Tex are then sewn together with a running locking permanent suture, such as a #1 Prolene. The skin is then closed securely with deep stitches and superficial staples (drains are always placed), and a binder is applied. One trick I sometimes perform is to take a large adhesive, occlusive sheet and use it to take tension off of the skin closure. This is done by applying the adhesive sheet to the lateral aspect of one side of the abdomen, manually pushing the skin towards the midline, and then draping the sheet over the incision to the other side of the abdomen. The patient in Figure 13-8 has been taken back to the OR for serial excision of the Gore-Tex mesh. Figure 13-8, *A* shows the patient just before her first excision with a measured 30-cm fascial defect. In Figure 13-8, *B*, a midline 4-cm strip of Gore-Tex is being removed. The cut ends of the Gore-Tex are reapproximated with a running locking suture (*C*). Figure 13-8, *D* shows the patient now with a 21-cm wide defect, having undergone another excision of Gore-Tex. The excisions will proceed until the width of the Gore-Tex is no greater than 4 to 6 cm. Figure 13-9 shows the patient's abdomen with the patient supine. The Gore-Tex mesh has been placed previously and a central strip of Gore-Tex is being removed to allow reduction of the width of the mesh with gradual stretching of the fascia and rectus muscles back to the midline of the abdomen.

Chapter 13 • Tissue and Fascial Expansion of the Abdominal Wall   239

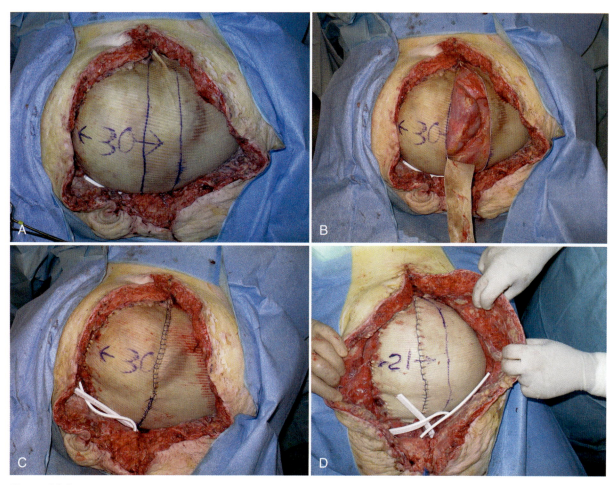

Figure 13-8.

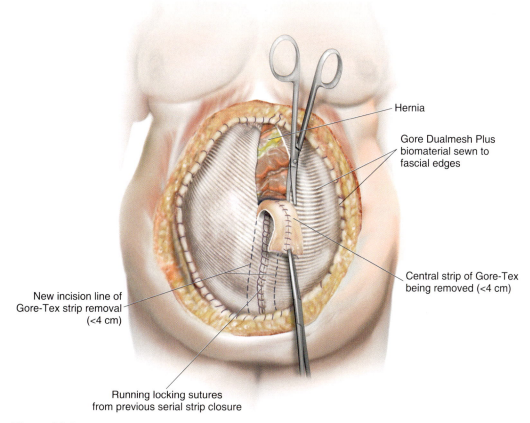

Figure 13-9.

Once the Gore-Tex is down to its last few centimeters, the final operation is planned. The final strip of Gore-Tex is removed, and the bowel is separated from the lateral abdominal wall (Fig. 13-10). You will find that there is a capsule over the bowel where the Gore-Tex was in contact with it. Under the lateral edge of the abdominal wall there is no capsule and the bowel should be freed completely. It is important to break down adhesions on the lateral abdominal wall at each stage of the procedure to prevent fusion of the visceral block to the abdominal wall which will prevent medialization during final reconstruction. A separation of parts is performed, and then an underlay of mesh is placed. The fascial closure can even be further reinforced with an overlay of biologic mesh (Fig. 13-11). Figure 13-12, *A* on page 243 depicts the final operation in which the remaining Gore-Tex is removed, a separation of component parts is performed, and the fascia is closed. The first sheet of biologic mesh has been laid across the repair, and the entire fascial repair has been reinforced by biologic mesh in Fig. 13-12, *B*, p. 243. In Figure 13-12, *C* and *D*, on page 243, the patient is shown 3 weeks after the completion of her repair.

Drains should be placed and left in for a long time to prevent seroma and subsequent infection. An abdominal binder is placed, and the patient is advised to wear it at all times for 3 months or longer.

Chapter 13 • Tissue and Fascial Expansion of the Abdominal Wall 241

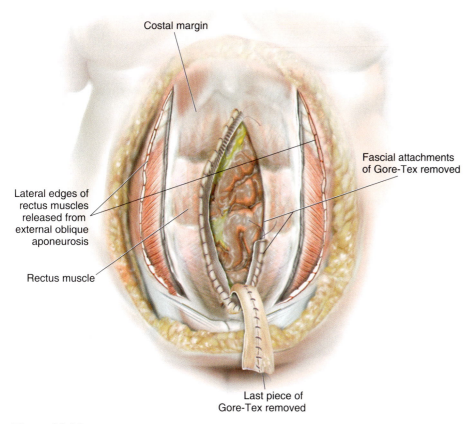

Figure 13-10.

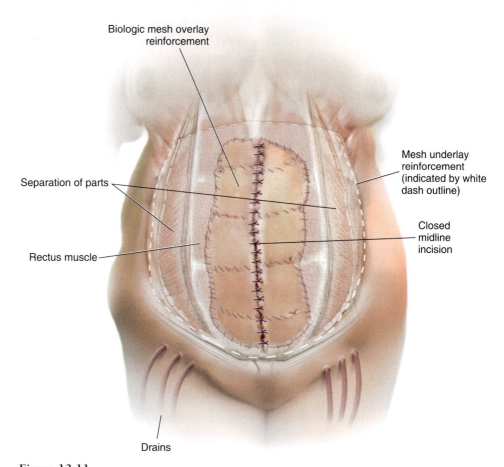

Figure 13-11.

6. Pearls/Pitfalls

1. Assessing the Rapidity of the Fascial Expansion

This is a very difficult and laborious series of operations to perform. It is almost always on a patient who has lost all hope of repair. The most important advice is to be slow and methodic. Do not rush the Gore-Tex excision and prepare the patient for the extreme nature of the approach. The surgeries have a high complication rate and a high risk of infection, seroma, skin necrosis, and recurrent hernia. Unless the situation is acute, I prefer using tissue expansion to facilitate skin closure as opposed to performing simultaneous Gore-Tex excision with VAC closure of the skin.

The patient usually tolerates the smaller serial removal of Gore-Tex procedures well. I do recommend that the patient be extubated deeply (if possible), so as to limit coughing and bucking as the patient wakes up. The Gore-Tex can rip with heavy pressure and the previous gains are quickly lost.

2. Preventing Skin Necrosis in the Final Abdominal Wall Closure

The separation-of-parts procedure can result in skin necrosis if the skin and subcutaneous tissue are elevated completely off of the fascia beyond the lateral edge of the rectus muscles. Perforators to the skin cluster around the umbilicus but extend along the entire length of the rectus muscles. There are medial and lateral row perforators. Not all need to be preserved. I try to preserve two to three lateral row perforators on each side. This is done by identifying one and using a Kelly clamp to dissect it free with a large cuff of subcutaneous tissue. The other perforators will be in roughly the same line as the first one. Even one perforator can make a huge difference and prevent skin flap necrosis. This is important, especially in the case of a tight skin closure. Exposure of the midline closure and mesh can seriously compromise all of the previous efforts.

Selected References

Argenta LC, Austad ED: Principles and techniques of tissue expansion. In McCarthy JG, editor: *Plastic Surgery*, 1990, W.B. Saunders Co, pp 475–507.

Carlson GW, Elwood E, Losken A, Galloway JR: The role of tissue expansion in abdominal wall reconstruction, *Ann Plas Surg* 44:147, 2000.

Hobar PC, Rohrich RJ, Byrd S: Abdominal wall reconstruction with expanded musculofascial tissue in a posttraumatic defect, *Plas Recon Surg* 94(2):379–383, 1994.

Jacobsen WW, Petty PM, Bite U, Johnson C: Massive abdominal-wall hernia reconstruction with expanded external/internal oblique and transversalis musculofascia, *Plas Recon Surg* 100(2):326–335, 1997.

Lipman J, Medalie DA, Rosen MJ: Staged repair of massive incisional hernias with loss of abdominal domain: a novel approach, *Am J Surg* 195(1):84–88, 2008.

Mander EK: Reconstruction using soft tissue expansion. In Cohen M, editor: *Mastery of plastic and reconstructive surgery*, ed1, 1994, Little, Brown and Co, pp 201–215.

Paletta CE, Huang DB, Dehghan K, Kelly C: The use of tissue expanders in staged abdominal wall reconstruction, *Ann Plas Surg* 42:259, 1999.

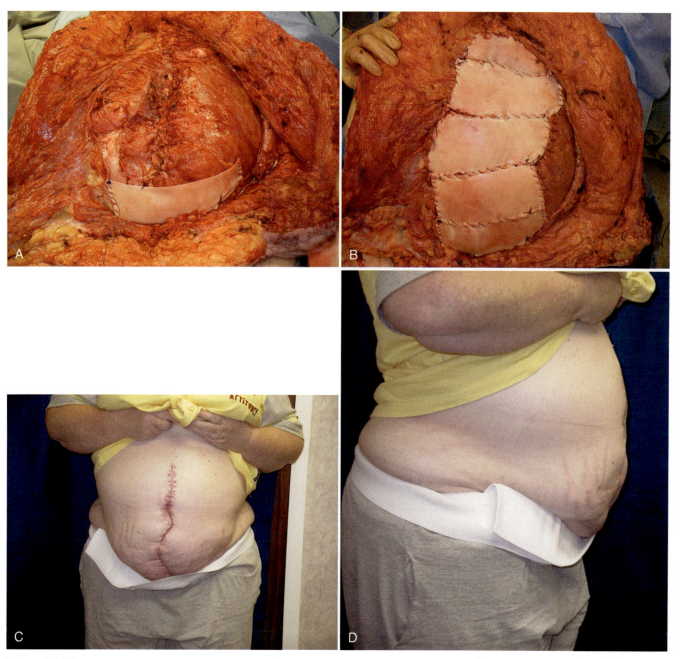

Figure 13-12.

CHAPTER 14

PROGRESSIVE PREOPERATIVE PNEUMOPERITONEUM FOR HERNIAS WITH LOSS OF ABDOMINAL DOMAIN

Alfredo M. Carbonell, DO, FACS, FACOS

1. Clinical Anatomy

1. Features/Characteristics of the Defect

▲ *Definition of Loss of Abdominal Domain*

- ▲ There is no consensus in the literature on the definition of loss of abdominal domain. Determination of this condition is subjective and typically refers to massive hernias with a significant amount of intestinal contents that have herniated through the abdominal wall into a hernia sac that forms a secondary abdominal cavity. On physical exam, the inability to reduce the herniated contents below the level of the fascia when the patient is lying supine should raise suspicion of the diagnosis. Although the surgeon can often make the assumption that a patient has loss of domain on physical exam, we utilize computed tomography (CT) to determine the true nature of the hernia.

2. Measuring Loss of Domain

- ▲ We define a loss of abdominal domain on CT scan as greater than 50% of the intestinal contents lying outside the native abdominal cavity in the hernia sac. This may be more accurately defined when the ratio of the volume of the hernia sac to the volume of the abdominal cavity is ≥0.5.
- ▲ A sagittal reconstruction of the CT scan is used to measure the length of the hernia sac from the top to the bottom of the sac. The length of the abdominal cavity is measured from the top of the diaphragm to the inferior aspect of the symphysis pubis (Fig. 14-1, *A*).
- ▲ Axial reconstructions are used to measure the width of the hernia sac and abdominal cavity at their widest point. The height of the hernia sac is measured from an imaginary line drawn across the hernial orifice to the apex of the hernia sac at its tallest portion. The height of the abdominal cavity is measured from the anterior portion of the fourth lumbar space to an imaginary line drawn across the hernial orifice (see Fig. 14-1, *B*).

Chapter 14 • Progressive Preoperative Pneumoperitoneum 245

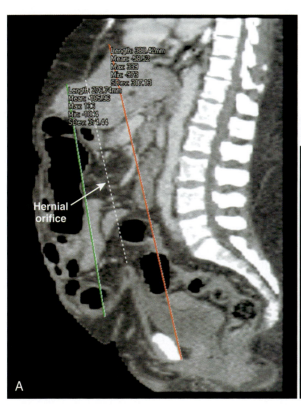
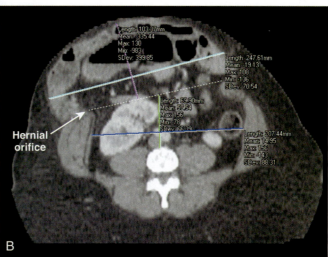

Figure 14-1.

▲ Using the formula to measure the volume of an ellipsoid (V = 4/3 × π × r1 × r2 × r3), the hernia sac and abdominal cavity volumes can be measured and compared. To simplify the ellipsoid volume equation, multiply the length, height, and width measurements of the cavities times a factor of 0.52 (V = 0.52 × L × H × W). Loss of domain exists when the ratio of the volume of the hernia sac to the volume of the abdominal cavity is ≥0.5.

▲ *Physiology of Hernias with Loss of Abdominal Domain*

▲ In patients with loss of abdominal domain, the bowels reside outside the abdominal cavity. As intraabdominal pressure decreases to approach atmospheric pressure, abdominal viscera become edematous and their vasculature becomes engorged. This makes simple hernia reduction nearly impossible. In addition, respiratory function is altered secondary to the loss of diaphragmatic support, and anterior spinal support fails, leading to lordosis.

4. Physiology of Progressive Preoperative Pneumoperitoneum

▲ The immediate reintroduction of viscera and abdominal reconstruction in patients with loss of domain can result in a significant increase in intraabdominal pressure, which can lead to abdominal compartment syndrome and its resultant ill effects. Progressive preoperative pneumoperitoneum (PPP) attenuates the adverse physiologic effects associated with ventral hernia repair in patients with a loss of abdominal domain.
▲ Insufflation of the abdominal cavity acts as an intraperitoneal pneumatic tissue expander and lengthens the abdominal wall musculature, increasing the volume of the abdominal cavity. This allows for adequate accommodation for the herniated contents.
▲ The pneumoperitoneum also dissects throughout the intraperitoneal cavity providing a pneumatic lysis of adhesions aided by gravity as the bowels are suspended by their adhesions within the hernia sac.
▲ Physiologically, PPP slowly creates a chronic abdominal compartment syndrome. With decreased diaphragmatic excursion, the patient is forced to overcome the inherent decreased inspiratory capacity. Additionally the adverse cardiovascular effects of acute abdominal compartment syndrome are attenuated by the slow introduction of intraperitoneal air.

2. Preoperative Considerations

1. Physical Examination

▲ The physical exam alone is often helpful in determining whether a patient has loss of domain. With the patient lying supine on the examination table, the surgeon should attempt to reduce the herniated contents below the fascia. If the hernia does not reduce because of the amount of herniated contents, the patient likely has loss of domain

▲ The abdominal wall should be examined for elasticity. Although some massive hernias may be irreducible, the patient's abdominal wall musculature may have such laxity and elasticity that it could accommodate the herniated contents easily at the time of surgery. This finding would obviate the need for PPP because single stage repair may be feasible.

▲ The quality of the skin should be examined to determine if any adjunctive maneuvers will be required to obtain safe skin closure at the time of hernia repair.

▲ Wide thin scars, ulcerated skin, thin subcutaneous tissue with tense and immobile skin, and large pannus flaps should all raise concern over skin closure. Consultation with a plastic surgeon may help determine the need for preoperative tissue expanders, panniculectomy, or complex skin closure at the time of hernia repair.

2. Computed Axial Tomography

▲ As previously described, the volume of the hernia sac and abdominal cavity are calculated and compared. A volume ratio of the hernia sac to the abdominal cavity of ≥0.5 should raise the suspicion of loss of abdominal domain.

▲ Other attributes of the abdominal wall should be examined on CT because they may determine the utility or futility of preoperative pneumoperitoneum.

▲ In our experience, patients with small defects and a significant amount of herniated contents benefit the most from preoperative pneumoperitoneum.

▲ Patients with round-shaped abdominal cavities and thick, robust rectus abdominis and oblique muscles may experience less muscle lengthening with preoperative pneumoperitoneum compared to those with a more ellipsoid appearance to the abdominal wall and thin atrophic musculature.

▲ Patients with "open book" abdomens, such as those with significant loss of abdominal wall substance (missing abdominal wall musculature) and hernia defects that span the entire abdominal wall, may not benefit anatomically from preoperative pneumoperitoneum because there may not be enough abdominal wall musculature to stretch. The physiologic benefits may still be realized however.

3. Planning Abdominal Wall Reconstruction

▲ *Weight Loss*

▲ Most patients with massive hernias and loss of domain are obese. Every effort should be made to have the patient lose weight preoperatively.

▲ There is no standard rule, however, a weight loss of 20 to 30 pounds can make a large difference in the ability to obtain fascial closure and complete abdominal wall reconstruction

▲ Our patients undergo a 4 to 8 week preoperative physician-observed meal replacement program, which consistently achieves our target weight loss goal.

▲ *Contaminated Abdominal Wall*

- ▲ Patients with enteral or urinary stomas or enterocutaneous fistulas are candidates for PPP. Attention should be paid to the stoma to ensure ischemia does not develop during insufflation.
- ▲ Patients with infected mesh and massive hernia with loss of domain pose a special problem. Although still candidates for preoperative pneumoperitoneum, serious consideration should be given to mesh removal and skin closure first followed by PPP at a second stage. An abdominal wall with infected mesh will be indurated and edematous; as a result, little muscle lengthening will occur with PPP. Additionally, mesh removal will undoubtedly damage some abdominal wall, making the immediate reconstruction all the more difficult.

3. Operative Steps

1. Stage I

▲ *Placement of Percutaneous Vena Cava Filter*

- ▲ PPP significantly elevates the intraabdominal pressure and creates a chronic abdominal compartment syndrome. As a result, venous return through the vena cava is decreased, and patients are at risk for thromboembolic events.
- ▲ Percutaneous vena cava filters protect patients from life-threatening pulmonary emboli. They do not, however, prevent deep venous thrombosis.
- ▲ We place patients on thrombotic chemoprophylaxis with heparin sodium.
- ▲ Despite these aggressive measures, we have still had patients develop significant deep venous thrombosis and near caval occlusion. Full-dose anticoagulation may be indicated in patients who are more at risk.

▲ *Exploratory Laparoscopy with Placement of Percutaneous Catheter System*

- ▲ Exploratory laparoscopy allows for minimally invasive access to the abdominal cavity for direct visualization and placement of a percutaneously placed intraperitoneal catheter system for the pneumoperitoneum.
- ▲ We use a 5-mm optical viewing trocar placed at the lateral hypochondrium (Fig. 14-2).
- ▲ A peritoneal dialysis catheter is placed under direct vision, using the Seldinger technique with a percutaneous, tear-away introducer sheath (Fig. 14-3).

Chapter 14 • Progressive Preoperative Pneumoperitoneum 249

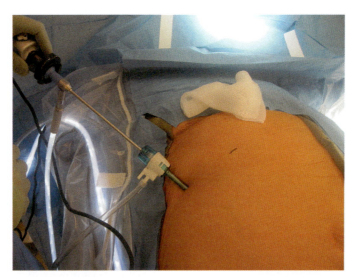

Figure 14-2.

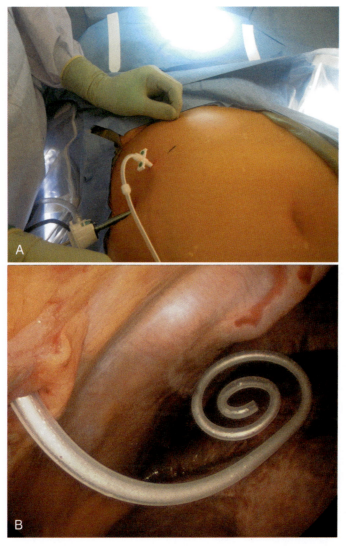

Figure 14-3.

- ▲ The catheter cuff is placed into the subcutaneous tissue and the catheter is sutured in position (Fig. 14-4).
- ▲ The pneumoperitoneum is evacuated, and the trocar site incision is closed with an absorbable subcuticular suture.

▲ Patient Care Plan

- ▲ The patient is admitted to a step-down unit for close monitoring of pulse oximetry and all vital signs
- ▲ Chemothromboprophylaxis is begun postoperatively.
- ▲ A full liquid diet with protein supplementation is started immediately.
- ▲ The patient is instructed to utilize incentive spirometry and ambulate daily.

2. Stage II

▲ Progressive Preoperative Pneumoperitoneum

- ▲ Peritoneal insufflation begins on the first postoperative day, and is performed daily.
- ▲ Laparoscopic insufflation tubing is utilized to connect the air hose at the patient's bedside to the peritoneal dialysis catheter (Fig. 14-5).
- ▲ The air is turned on slowly to begin insufflation. The patient is closely monitored for signs of distress.
- ▲ The insufflation proceeds and the patient will begin to complain of abdominal tightness followed by mild flank discomfort. Once the patient begins to experience some shortness of breath or mild anxiety, the insufflation is stopped. There is no specific volume of air that should be injected nor the intraperitoneal pressure measured. The endpoint of insufflation is always the patient's level of discomfort.
- ▲ The skin should be moisturized daily as pneumoperitoneum can lead to skin dryness and cracking.
- ▲ If at any point during this process the patient becomes hemodynamically unstable or develops decreased urine output the pneumoperitoneum can be evacuated by wall suction aspiration.

Chapter 14 • Progressive Preoperative Pneumoperitoneum 251

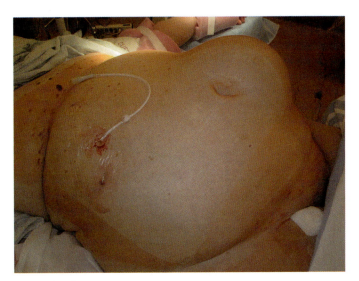

Figure 14-4.

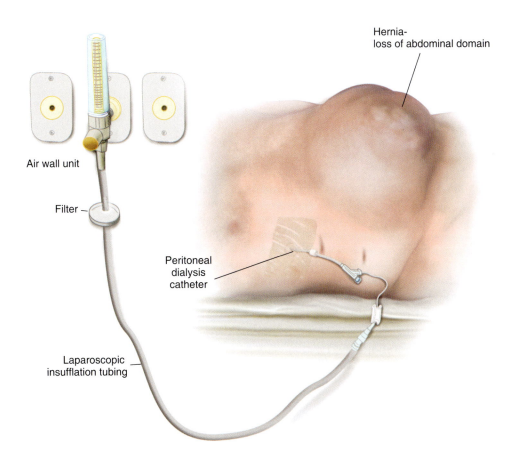

Figure 14-5.

▲ Repeat CT Scan to Determine Suitability for Stage III

- ▲ After 7 days of daily PPP, a CT scan is performed to determine the suitability of the abdominal wall for repair.
- ▲ The CT should demonstrate that the herniated contents have fallen back into the native abdominal cavity and now lie below an imaginary line drawn across the hernial orifice (Figs. 14-6 to 14-9).
- ▲ If the bowel has not fallen back into the abdominal cavity and the volume of the abdomen does not look to have increased significantly, then pneumoperitoneum should continue for 4-5 more days and a repeat CT performed. If at this point there is no change, it is unlikely PPP will work as a pneumatic tissue expander and consideration should be given to either saline tissue expansion or myofascial pedicled flap closure of the abdominal wall.

3. Stage III

▲ Abdominal Wall Reconstruction

- ▲ Once the patient is ready for reconstruction, the surgeon should use the technique with which he or she is most comfortable.
- ▲ Every effort should be made to ensure rectus abdominis reapproximation in the midline with ventral fascial closure overtop the mesh.
- ▲ Our preferred method for abdominal wall reconstruction in these patients is the Rives-Stoppa retromuscular hernia repair technique with or without the addition of a posterior components separation (PCST).

Chapter 14 • Progressive Preoperative Pneumoperitoneum 253

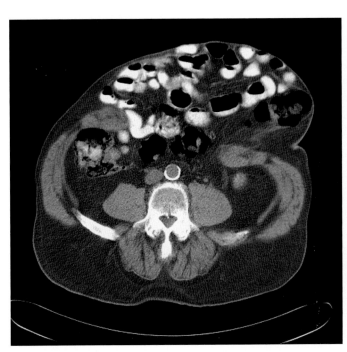

Figure 14-6.

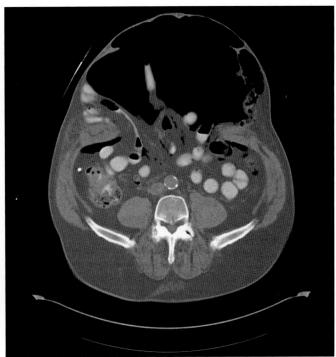

Figure 14-7.

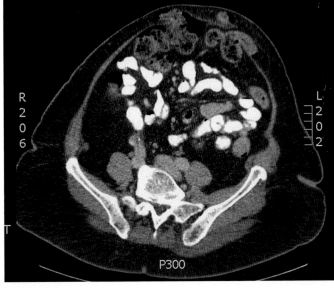

Figure 14-8.

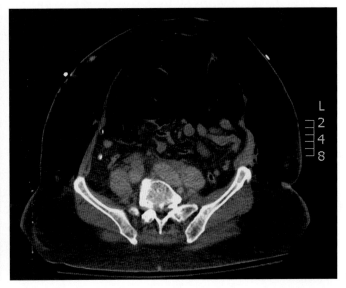

Figure 14-9.

▲ **Rives-Stoppa with PCST**

- ▲ After a complete lysis of adhesions a towel is placed intraperitoneally to protect the underlying viscera.
- ▲ The posterior rectus sheath is divided vertically 1 cm or less from the edge of the linea alba and the division continues 5 cm cephalad to the hernia defect edge and 5 cm caudal to it (Fig. 14-10).
- ▲ The posterior rectus sheath is reflected posteriorly under tension and the rectus muscle is gently dissected off the ventral aspect of the sheath (Fig. 14-11).
- ▲ A similar dissection is performed on the contralateral side.
- ▲ If it does not appear that the posterior rectus sheath will reapproximate in the midline under little to no tension, a posterior components separation technique (PCST) will be required.
- ▲ For the PCST, the dissection is carried to the lateral most extent of the rectus sheath. With a Richardson retractor reflecting the rectus laterally at this lateral extent, a subtle ridge becomes evident. This ridge is formed by the rolled over anterior leaf of the internal oblique aponeurosis as it fuses with the transversus abdominis aponeurosis to form the posterior rectus sheath (Fig. 14-12).
- ▲ By incising the fascia 1 to 2 mm medial to this ridge, the interparietal plane between internal oblique and transversus abdominis muscle is accessed, and the incision is continued for the entire length of the skin incision and beyond (Fig. 14-13).
- ▲ The interparietal plane is dissected far out laterally. This dissection disconnects the transversus abdominis muscle from the anterior components, allowing medial advancement of the posterior rectus sheath for complete peritoneal closure and medial rectus advancement for total abdominal wall reconstruction. PCST provides a well-vascularized and wide space for mesh placement with similar advancement to the Ramirez component separation without the need for a subcutaneous skin dissection and its attendant morbidity.
- ▲ The protective towel, which was placed intraperitoneally, is removed now, and the posterior rectus sheath is reapproximated in the midline with a slow-absorbing monofilament suture.
- ▲ The synthetic mesh is placed in the retromuscular space and fixated with full-thickness permanent transabdominal sutures utilizing the Reverdin needle (Fig. 14-14).
- ▲ The anterior sheath is closed in the midline ventral to the mesh, using a slow-absorbing monofilament suture and a 4:1 suture-to-wound-length ratio.

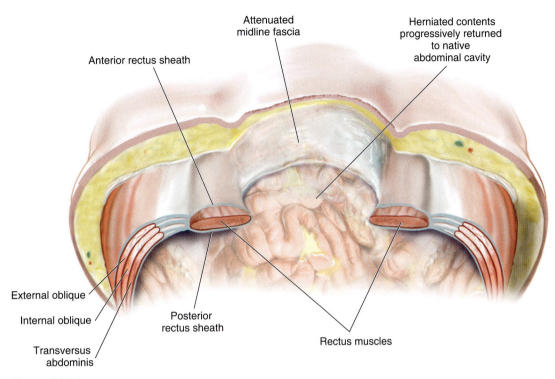

Figure 14-10.

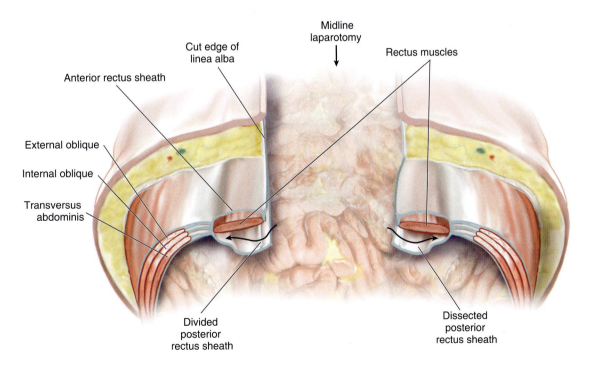

Figure 14-11.

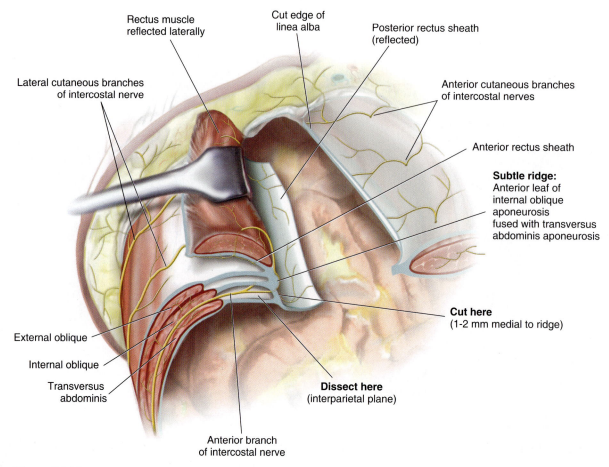

Figure 14-12.

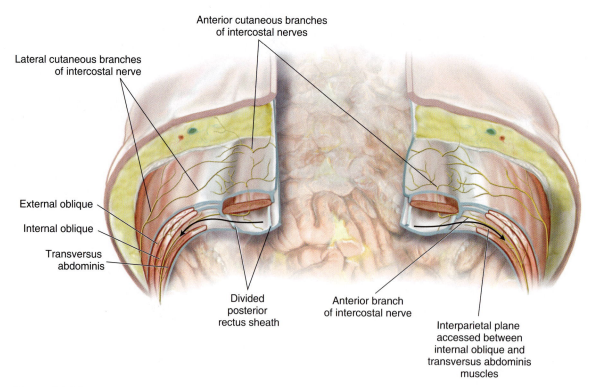

Figure 14-13.

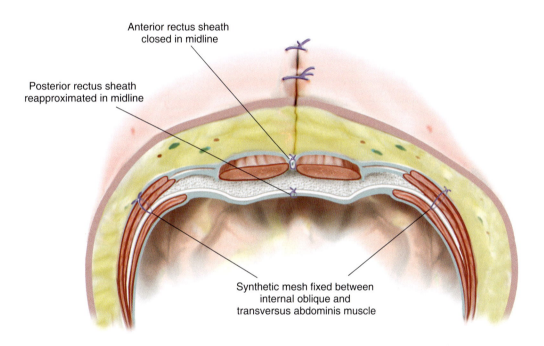

Figure 14-14.

▲ *Intraperitoneal Onlay of Mesh (IPOM) Repair*

- ▲ If the retromuscular space is inaccessible because of inflammation, fibrosis, or rectus muscle absence, then an alternate technique for abdominal wall closure should be employed.
- ▲ To ensure medial rectus reapproximation, a traditional Ramirez components separation may be performed.
- ▲ A tissue-separating mesh is deployed in the intraperitoneal position, and suture-fixated circumferentially with a wide overlap (greater than 5 cm) utilizing full-thickness permanent transabdominal sutures, placed with the Reverdin needle.
- ▲ The anterior sheath is closed in the midline ventral to the mesh, using a slow-absorbing monofilament suture and a 4:1 suture-to-wound-length ratio.

4. Pearls/Pitfalls

- ▲ Not identifying loss of abdominal domain preoperatively can place the surgeon in a difficult position intraoperatively where they may be unable to relocate the herniated contents back into the abdominal cavity and close the hernia defect.
- ▲ The Silo technique with sequential mesh excision can be helpful in the aforementioned scenario.
- ▲ A large piece of Dualmesh (W.L. Gore, Elkton, MD) is circumferentially sewn to the fascial edge of the hernia defect, and the skin is closed temporarily over the top of the mesh.
- ▲ Every 3 days, the patient returns to the operating room where a central ovoid shape of the mesh is excised and the cut mesh edges reapproximated. This technique slowly pulls the abdominal wall muscles to the midline.
- ▲ Once the remaining fascial gap is less than 5 cm, the mesh is completely excised and a Ramirez components separation is performed with fascial reinforcement (synthetic, biologic, or bioabsorbable) for complete abdominal wall reconstruction
- ▲ **Subcutaneous emphysema:** Subcutaneous emphysema occurs almost uniformly in patients undergoing PPP because air leaks out along the tract of the insufflation catheter into the subcutaneous tissue. This is self-limited and, in our experience, has not required any intervention.
- ▲ **Nutrition:** Patients undergoing PPP typically experience early satiety and even anorexia as a result of their increased intraabdominal pressure. Although every attempt should be made to encourage enteral alimentation, parenteral nutrition may be necessary while the patients are hospitalized for their insufflations.
- ▲ **Physiologic collapse during pneumoperitoneum:** It is possible that a patient may become hemodynamically unstable during PPP. For this reason patients are kept in a close observation unit while they undergo insufflation, and vital signs are monitored closely. Should physiologic collapse occur at any point, the pneumoperitoneum may be promptly evacuated from the catheter, using wall suction.

Selected References

Carbonell A, Cobb WS, Chen SM: Posterior components separation during retromuscular hernia repair, *Hernia: the journal of hernias and abdominal wall surgery* 12(4):359–362, 2008.

Mcadory RS, Cobb WS, Carbonell AM: Progressive preoperative pneumoperitoneum for hernias with loss of domain, *The American surgeon* 75(6):504–508, 2009:discussion 508–509.

Moreno: Chronic eventrations and large hernias. Preoperative treatment by progressive pneumoperitoneum-original procedure, *Surgery* 22:945–953, 1947.

Tanaka EY, Yoo JH, Rodrigues AJ, Utiyama EM, Birolini D, Rasslan S: A computerized tomography scan method for calculating the hernia sac and abdominal cavity volume in complex large incisional hernia with loss of domain, *Hernia* 14(1):63–69, 2010.

CHAPTER 15

Rotational and Free Flap Closure of the Abdominal Wall

Christopher G. Zochowski, MD and Hooman Soltanian, MD, FACS

1. Preoperative Considerations

1. Comorbidities

- ▲ Skin and subcutaneous fat may be of varying thicknesses and qualities in patients because of body habitus, scarring, steroid use, malnutrition, advanced age, and other factors.
- ▲ Bleeding tendencies should be addressed preoperatively.
- ▲ Conversely, a thrombogenic state will put any flap at risk and may warrant a hematologist to assist in the pre- and postoperative care.

2. Open Wound Management

- ▲ The timing of the closure of abdominal wounds is on a case-by-case basis.
- ▲ Appropriate dressings should be applied to the wound before surgery to prevent desiccation of the soft tissues and intraabdominal contents.
- ▲ Negative pressure dressings allow for easier management of large abdominal wounds, but the wound must be monitored closely when the dressing is applied over exposed bowel.
- ▲ Some wounds require frequent debridements to determine the extent of viable tissue and clearance of infection.
- ▲ Open wounds increase the nutritional and fluid requirements of the patient.
- ▲ Chronic open wounds should be converted to acute clean wounds before closure.

3. Timing

▲ Optimize the patient before closure of the abdominal wall in regard to nutrition, cardiovascular status, and pulmonary function. The closure may lead to prolonged intubation, and this risk is increased in patients with chronic obstructive pulmonary disease (COPD) and smokers.
▲ Closure should be timed after bowel edema has subsided (stage if needed).
▲ Avoid intraoperative nitrous oxide use. Consider a nasogastric tube.

4. Defect Assessment and Flap Selection

▲ Assess the extent of missing or aberrant structures and define the anatomical region of the tissue loss.
▲ Assess the quality of remaining structures and loss of domain.
▲ Take note of an ostomy position if present.
▲ Assess for enterocutaneous fistulae.
▲ Rule out previous damage to the blood supply of any potential flaps.
▲ Pedicled flaps are limited by their arc of rotation and the size and location of the defect.

2. Muscular Flaps (Table 15-1)

TABLE 15-1. Flap Types

			MUSCLE FLAPS			
FLAP	TYPE OF FLAP	REGION OF COVERAGE	PARTS	SIZE	ARTERY	VARIANTS
Gracilis	Muscle or myocutaneous Pedicled or free	Lower quadrant	Muscle, skin		Ascending branch of medial circumflex femoral artery (profunda femoris)	Functional flap (anterior branch of obturator nerve) Sensate flap (anterior femoral cutaneous nerve)
Latissimus dorsi	Muscle or myocutaneous Pedicled or free	Upper quadrant, epigastrium, lower quadrant; delayed can cross midline.	Muscle, skin	Muscle 20 × 40 cm, skin 12 × 20 cm with primary closure	Thoracodorsal (subscapular)	
Rectus abdominis	Muscle or myocutaneous Pedicled or free	Upper and lower quadrants; Less suitable in epigastrum	Muscle, rectus fascia, skin	Muscle 25 × 6 cm and large transverse or vertical skin paddle possible	Superior epigastric artery (internal mammary), deep inferior epigastric artery (external iliac)	Can be superiorly or inferiorly based
Rectus femoris	Muscle or myocutaneous Pedicled or free	Lower quadrant; Umbilicus is superior limit	Muscle, skin	Possible 15 × 40 cm, can be primarily closed if width <7 cm	Descending branch of the lateral circumflex artery (profunda femoris)	Functional muscle flap (motor branch from the femoral nerve), sensate flap (intermediate cutaneous nerve of the thigh)
Mutton chop flap (rectus femoris + fascia of the thigh)	Composite Pedicled or free	Lower quadrant, umbilical, suprapubic, epigastric, upper quadrant	Skin, rectus femoris muscle, medial fascia of the thigh	Similar to RF flap	Descending branch of the lateral circumflex artery (profunda femoris)	
Tensor fascia lata	Muscle or myocutaneous Pedicled or free	Umbilical, suprapubic, and lower quadrant; Costal margin is superior limit; if delayed, can reach all ipsilateral quadrants reliably	Muscle, fascia, skin, external table of iliac crest	Possible 15 × 40 cm, can be primarily closed if width < 10 cm.	Ascending branch of lateral femoral circumflex artery (profunda femoris)	Chimeric flap on a common pedicle with ALT flap or RF Can include outer table of iliac crest as osteomyocutaneous flap Sensate flap (T12 dermatome)
Internal oblique	Muscle or myocutaneous Pedicled or free	Lower quadrant, groin	Muscle	10 × 20 cm	Deep circumflex iliac artery	
External oblique	Muscle or myocutaneous Pedicled or free	Upper quadrant, epigastrum	Muscle, skin		Segmental intercostals (pedicled) 1–2 large branches of the deep circumflex iliac artery (free)	
Vastus lateralis	Muscle or myocutaneous Pedicled or free	Lower quadrant	Muscle, skin		Descending branch of medial circumflex femoral artery (profunda femoris)	
			FASCIOCUTANEOUS FLAPS			
Anterolateral thigh flap	Fasciocutaneous Pedicled or free	Ipsilateral upper and lower quadrants, contralateral lower quadrant	Skin, fascia	8 × 25 cm with primary closure	Septocutaneous perforators from descending branch of the lateral femoral circumflex artery (profunda femoris)	Sensate flap (lateral femoral cutaneous nerve) ALT adipofascial flap ALT fascial Flap
Deep inferior epigastric- based (island)	Fasciocutaneous Pedicled or free	Versatile	Skin, small portion of muscle and fascia	Variable skin paddle, similar size to VRAM	Deep inferior epigastric artery (external iliac)	Many designs of skin paddle
Groin flap	Fasciocutaneous Pedicled or free	Lower quadrant, (upper if delayed)	Skin	Pinch test to determine, 10 × 25 cm	Superior circumflex iliac artery (external iliac/SFA)	

(Continued)

Table 15-1. Flap Types—cont'd

			MUSCLE FLAPS—cont'd			
FLAP	**TYPE OF FLAP**	**REGION OF COVERAGE**	**PARTS**	**SIZE**	**ARTERY**	**VARIANTS**
Iliolumbar	Fasciocutaneous Pedicled or free	Lateral, middle third	Skin	Pinch test to determine	Circumflex iliac artery and lumbar artery	
Thoracoepigastric	Fasciocutaneous	Upper quadrant	Skin, fascia	Width 10–15 cm (with primary closure), up to 30 cm in width	Musculocutaneous perforators of the superior epigastric artery	
Superficial inferior epigastric	Fasciocutaneous Pedicled or free	Lower quadrant	Skin	Depends n the abdominal wall skin laxity	Superficial inferior epigastric artery	
			OTHER FLAPS			
Omentum		All	Fat, connective tissue, lymphatics	Large surface area available	Right omental artery (right gastroepiploic artery), or left gastroepiploic artery	

ALT, Anterolateral thigh; *RF*, rectus femoris; *TFL*, tensor fasciae lata; *VRAM*, vertical rectus abdominis myocutaneous.

▲ Figure 15-1 shows the cross-sectional anatomy of the thigh demonstrating the possible muscles for coverage of abdominal wall defects

1. Tensor fascia lata

▲ *Anatomy*

- ▲ The flap can be musculocutaneous.
- ▲ Sensory innervation includes the lateral cutaneous branch of the twelfth thoracic nerve and the lateral cutaneous sensory nerve of the thigh (L2 and L3). Motor innervation is supplied by the distal branch of the superior gluteal nerve (L4 and L5).
- ▲ Arterial blood supply is from the ascending branch of the lateral femoral circumflex artery, which is 1.5 to 2.5 mm diameter. The vein is slightly larger than the artery when traced to the origin on the lateral femoral circumflex.
- ▲ Pedicle length can be up to 10 cm. The pedicle enters the tensor fasciae lata (TFL) muscle at the level of the junction of the proximal and middle thirds of an axis drawn from the anterior superior iliac spine (ASIS) to the lateral aspect of the patella. It emerges from beneath the rectus femoris muscle, anterior to the vastus lateralis and enters the muscle via the deep surface medially 6 to 8 cm from the ASIS.
- ▲ The descending branch of the lateral femoral circumflex artery continues beyond the TFL muscle to supply the skin of the anterolateral midthigh and the lower thigh. It can be harvested with the anterolateral thigh skin to enlarge the perfused vascular territory.

Chapter 15 • Rotational and Free Flap Closure of the Abdominal Wall

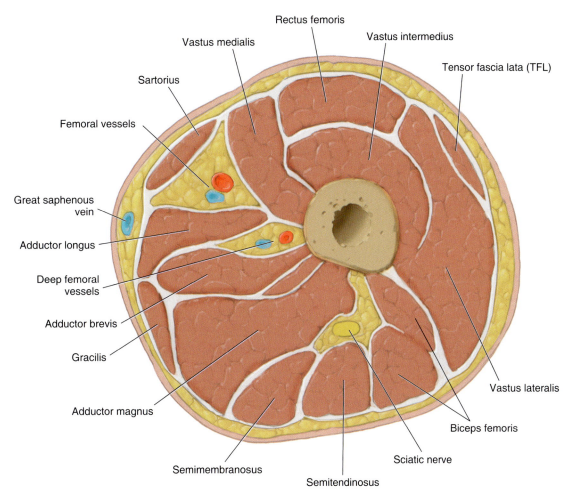

Figure 15-1.

▲ The TFL muscle (Fig. 15-2) is a short, flat muscle that is approximately 12 to 15 cm long. It acts as an accessory flexor and medial rotator of the thigh. It originates from the anterior iliac crest and the deep surface of the fascia lata. At the origin, it lies between the gluteus medius and sartorius, and superficial to the vastus lateralis. It inserts into the iliotibial tract, which inserts distally on Gerdy's tubercle on the lateral aspect of the tibia.
▲ The fascia lata is the deep fascia of the thigh. It thickens to form the iliotibial tract laterally and attaches distally to the lateral condyle of the tibia. The TFL muscle is enclosed by the fascia lata, and distally, the muscle fibers coalesce with the iliotibial tract in the middle third of the thigh. The thickness of the fascia lata over the TFL muscle makes it a strong fascial donor site suitable for reconstructing abdominal wall defects.

▲ *Flap Design*

▲ Skin territory can be up to 15 × 40 cm. A line from the ASIS 10 to 15 cm posteriorly marks the origin of the TFL muscle, with the skin territory extending 2 cm cranial to this line (Fig. 15-3). The lower skin territory is 8 cm above the lateral femoral condyle. Posterior skin territory is a line drawn from the greater trochanter to the fibular head or approximately along the axis of the femur. The anterior border is a line drawn from the ASIS to the lateral aspect of the patella.
▲ The entry point of the pedicle is at the level of the junction of the proximal and middle third of the line or 6 to 8 cm from the ASIS.
▲ The rotation arc of the pedicled flap reaches the costal margin if the tensor muscle is completely detached from its origin and raised as an island flap.

Chapter 15 • Rotational and Free Flap Closure of the Abdominal Wall

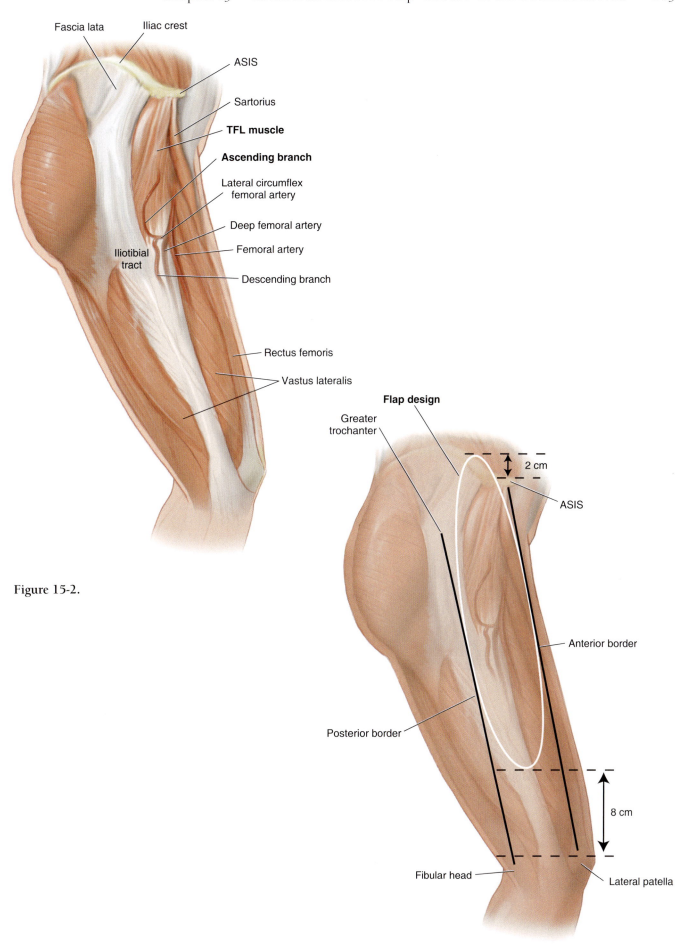

Figure 15-2.

Figure 15-3.

▲ **Marking and Dissection**

- ▲ The flap is marked as an ellipse over the axis of the TFL muscle and to incorporate the pedicle proximally.
- ▲ The patient is prepped and draped supine with a bump under the ipsilateral hip.
- ▲ The flap is elevated from distal to proximal.
- ▲ The skin and deep fascia are incised together in a plane deep to the iliotibial tract fascia.
- ▲ As dissection proceeds cranially, the space between the rectus femoris and vastus lateralis is retracted with a self-retaining retractor to identify the descending branch of the lateral femoral circumflex artery.
- ▲ The ascending branch is then identified as one proceeds in a superior direction (Fig. 15-4).
- ▲ With the ascending branch identified, its course to the TFL can be isolated
- ▲ The proximal flap is then divided by electrocautery while protecting the pedicle.
- ▲ The pedicle can be traced to the origin of the lateral femoral circumflex vessels to gain length.
- ▲ If more length is needed, flex the patient at the hip.

▲ **Variations**

- ▲ Variations include a free flap, chimeric flap, and an osteomusculocutaneous flap.
- ▲ Chimeric flaps are on a common pedicle with the anterolateral thigh and/or the rectus femoris flap.
- ▲ In an osteomusculocutaneous flap, a portion of the external table of iliac crest can be harvested with the proximal flap.

▲ **Postoperative Care**

- ▲ The donor site can be closed primarily if planned appropriately. Skin graft may be needed for larger flaps including skin.
- ▲ Close the donor site in layers over closed suction drains.
- ▲ Ambulation can begin postoperatively.

▲ **Pitfalls**

- ▲ This procedure results in a long incision on the leg.

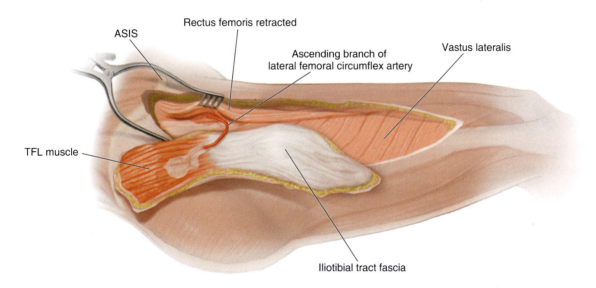

Figure 15-4.

2. Latissimus dorsi

▲ The latissimus dorsi can be used to as a functional free flap, muscle flap, or myocutaneous flap.
▲ The latissimus dorsi is the largest muscle in the body (up to 20 × 40 cm), but it is quite thin (<1 cm thick). It acts as a humeral adductor and internal rotator, and no significant functional deficit results from harvest. It has six origins, from the lower six thoracic spines and supraspinatus ligaments, posterior layer of lumbar fascia, tendinous attachments of the iliac crest, strips of muscle interdigitating with the external oblique, muscular slips from lower four ribs, and muscular slips from the scapula. The upper and anterior borders are free. The latissimus is deep to the trapezius. It inserts at the floor of bicipital groove of the humerus behind the tendon of the long head of the biceps. The latissimus forms the posterior fold of the axilla with the subscapularis tendon.

▲ Innervation

▲ Motor innervation is supplied by the thoracodorsal nerve, a branch of the posterior cord of the brachial plexus (C7); this nerve closely accompanies the thoracodorsal artery.

▲ Blood Supply

▲ Arterial blood is supplied through a terminal branch of the subscapular artery (2 to 5 mm diameter), a branch of the axillary artery.
▲ After 5 cm, the subscapular artery gives off the circumflex scapular branch posteriorly and the thoracodorsal artery (2 to 4 mm diameter) (Fig. 15-5).
▲ The thoracodorsal artery courses along the posterior aspect of the axilla for 8 to 14 cm and gives off 1 to 2 branches to the serratus before it enters the latissimus dorsi muscle on its deep surface. The serratus branch can be kept to include the serratus as part of a chimeric flap. The artery divides in the substance of the muscle into vertical and transverse branches and can facilitate a split flap.
▲ Thoracic intercostal and lumbar perforating arteries enter the deep surface of the muscle 8 cm from the posterior midline at the level of the seventh, ninth, and eleventh vertebral spines. They perfuse the inferior and medial latissimus.
▲ There is usually a single vena comitans with the artery that is slightly larger than the artery.
▲ If the pedicle is based on the subscapular artery; a length of five to 10 cm is possible.

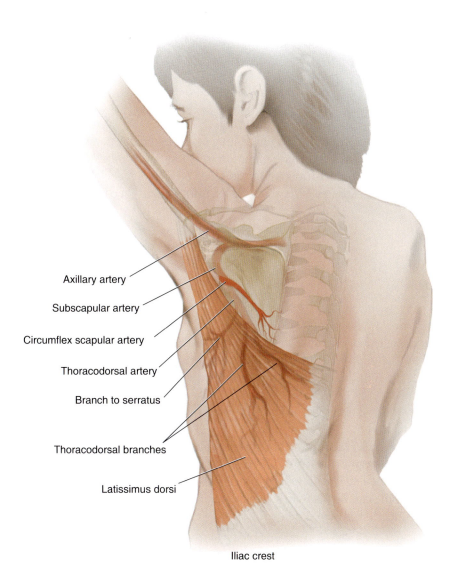

Figure 15-5.

▲ Contraindications

- ▲ There is no absolute contraindication as long as the pedicle is patent.
- ▲ Relative contraindications include radiation to the site, prior axillary dissection, a patient who is reliant on shoulder function for crutches or who is wheelchair bound, or if a functioning spinal accessory nerve is absent from prior neck dissection.

▲ Flap Design

- ▲ The flap design can cover ipsilateral abdominal defects. If raised as an "extended" variant, it can cross the midline by incorporating the rim of supragluteal fascia.
- ▲ If based at the muscle insertion, the pivot point is at the level of the midposterior axillary line.
- ▲ If the insertion is incised, the island flap pivot point is 1.5 to 2 cm inferior to the pectoral humeral junction.
- ▲ The skin paddle can be 12 × 20 cm and may allow for primary closure of the donor site.
- ▲ The skin paddle can be as large as 5 cm anterior and inferior to the muscle without delay and can be made larger with a delay procedure.
- ▲ The skin paddle can be made in a transverse or oblique fashion in women so that the scar is hidden under a brassiere.

▲ *Marking and Dissection*

- ▲ The outline of the anterior and superior edges of the muscle is made. This can be facilitated by having the patient contract the latissimus.
- ▲ If a muscle only flap needed, the incision is marked extending from the posterior axillary fold, then inferiorly and posteriorly over the anterior boarder of the latissimus muscle as dictated by the length of the muscle.
- ▲ If it is a myocutaneous flap, the skin island can be designed anywhere over the muscle.
- ▲ The upper two thirds of the latissimus dorsi muscle contain a higher density of myocutaneous perforators
- ▲ The donor site can be usually closed primarily if the skin paddle width is less than 10 cm.
- ▲ To determine location of the skin island, the distance from the surgical defect to the pectoral-humeral junction is measured.
- ▲ A line is then drawn from the anterior border of the latissimus dorsi to its origin along the posterior iliac crest, and the prior distance is transferred to this line.
- ▲ The patient is placed in a lateral decubitus position on a beanbag, with an axillary roll. The ipsilateral arm is prepped completely and left in the operative field abducted and resting on a Mayo stand, placed anterosuperiorly to the patient.
- ▲ After incision, anterior and posterior flaps are raised superficial to the muscle to expose the latissimus. The flaps are elevated enough to gain adequate exposure for the required muscular harvest.
- ▲ The superior edge of the latissimus is identified at the inferior angle of the scapula and is then elevated. The serratus muscle can be identified, and dissection deep to it should be avoided. This areolar plane is easy to dissect, and some perforators are encountered and ligated.
- ▲ The dissection continues toward the midline, and the areas of origin of the muscle are divided.
- ▲ The dissection proceeds inferiorly, freeing the medial muscle origin. At the inferior/terminal portion of the muscle, there is not a clear plane, and the muscle must be divided with electrocautery.

- ▲ Dissection then proceeds toward the axilla in the areolar plane (Fig. 15-6).
- ▲ The pedicle can be approached directly by dissecting the latissimus from the axilla, or it can be found by following the undersurface of the muscle in a distal to proximal approach.
- ▲ As the axilla is neared, the branch to serratus is ligated and the circumflex scapular branch can be as well if more length is needed.
- ▲ The thoracodorsal nerve is divided, and the artery and vein can be ligated and divided when the recipient area is ready if a free flap is being used.
- ▲ Closure is in layers and over drains. Mattressing sutures can be used to coapt the potential space in addition to drains.
- ▲ The ipsilateral arm can be used postoperatively.
- ▲ Postoperative inspection must be vigilant for seroma or hematoma formation. Drains often remain for a relatively long time. If a clinical seroma develops, aspiration should be done.

▲ Free Flap

- ▲ The procedure for the free flap proceeds similarly as described previously.
- ▲ The pedicle is completely isolated, and the flap elevation completed before ligating the pedicle.
- ▲ The positioning in the lateral decubitus position makes a two-team approach difficult in preparing the recipient site.
- ▲ Deep inferior epigastric, omental vessels, right and left gastroepiploic vessels have been used as recipient vessels.
- ▲ The use of bilateral latissimus dorsi muscles as pedicled flaps or free flaps provides a substantial surface area for coverage.

3. Rectus Femoris

▲ Anatomy

- ▲ **Blood supply:** The descending branch of the lateral circumflex artery (1.5 to 2 mm diameter) (Fig. 15-7) from the profunda femoris is located 8 cm below the inguinal ligament and enters the muscle on its deep surface. It also supplies the tissue of the anterolateral thigh flap.
- ▲ Three to four musculocutaneous perforators are at the proximal portion of the muscle, and fasciocutaneous perforators from the intermuscular septum supply the skin. There are usually two venae comitantes.
- ▲ **Muscle:** It is the most anterior muscle of the quadriceps group. One can harvest muscle flap with tendinous portions both proximally and distally.
- ▲ Its origin is the anterior inferior iliac spine and the ilium just superior to the acetabulum. It inserts at the patellar tendon along with Vastus muscles.
- ▲ Function is the terminal 20 degrees of knee extension.
- ▲ **Nerve:** Motor innervation is supplied by a branch of the femoral nerve, which enters the muscle at the same point as the artery. It can be >20 cm long.

Chapter 15 • Rotational and Free Flap Closure of the Abdominal Wall

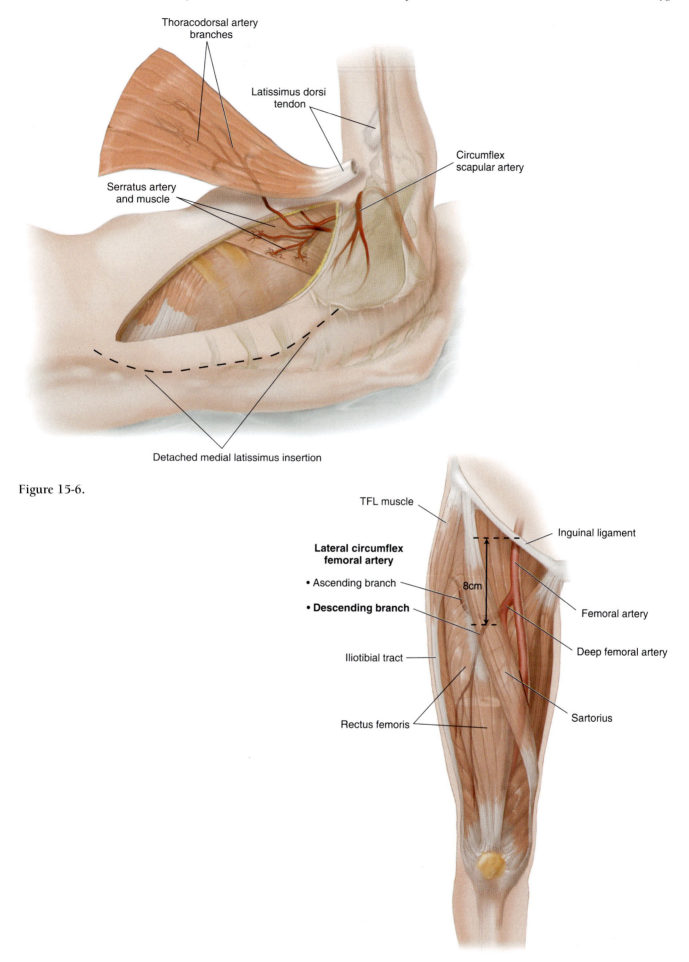

Figure 15-6.

Figure 15-7.

- ▲ It has been described as a functional flap with anastomosis to an intercostal nerve for abdominal wall reconstruction. The native innervation can be maintained and the vascular pedicle trasnferred to recipient vessels closer to the abdominal wall defect (e.g. deep inferior epigastric vessels)
- ▲ Sensory innervation to the skin is by the intermediate cutaneous nerve of the thigh.

▲ Flap Design

- ▲ The flap reconstructs the lower abdominal wall, with the umbilicus as the superior limit.
- ▲ The design can be a muscle flap, myocutaneous flap, functional flap, or sensate flap.
- ▲ Flaps as large as 15 × 40 cm have been described.
- ▲ The donor site can be closed primarily with a myocutaneous flap if the skin paddle is <7 cm wide. The skin paddle is designed directly over the muscle, keeping in mind the proximal perforators.
- ▲ The pivot point is at the entrance of the neurovascular pedicle 8 cm below the inguinal ligament. This low pivot point limits the use of the muscle in abdominal reconstruction as a pedicled flap. This limitation can be overcome by using the muscle as a free flap.

▲ Marking and Dissection

- ▲ The muscle falls on a line drawn from the ASIS to the middle aspect of the patella and terminates approximately 6 cm superior to the patella (Fig. 15-8).
- ▲ A proper skin flap is drawn, keeping in mind the limitations described previously.
- ▲ A pinch test may demonstrate the ability to close primarily before incision.
- ▲ If muscle only, the incision is made in a lazy "S" or a longitudinal fashion down to muscular fascia.
- ▲ The rectus femoris and sartorius muscles are identified deep to the muscular fascia.
- ▲ The sartorius is retracted medially and away from the leg to expose the areolar plane underneath and to identify the lateral femoral circumflex vessels. The femoral nerve and branches are also identified at this level.
- ▲ If a skin paddle is to be used, the skin edges of the myocutaneous flap are sutured to the fascia to prevent shearing during harvest. Cutaneous perforators can be determined with the pencil Doppler.
- ▲ The pedicle can be located by measuring 8 cm from the inguinal ligament or just proximal to the junction of the proximal and middle thirds of the muscle (Fig. 15-9).
- ▲ Ensure that the proper muscle is releasd from the other muscles conjoining at the patellar tendon, usually 6 cm proximal to the patella.
- ▲ The musculotendinuous unit should be elevated from distal to proximal and from lateral to medial.
- ▲ Once the pedicle is identified on the deep surface, the muscle can then be divided proximal to the pedicle.
- ▲ The nerve to the muscle is ligated and divided, as needed.
- ▲ The muscle can either be rotated or turned over for coverage.
- ▲ The muscle fascia can be split or "pie crusted" for further advancement of the flap.
- ▲ The wound is closed in layers over a suction drain.

Chapter 15 • Rotational and Free Flap Closure of the Abdominal Wall 275

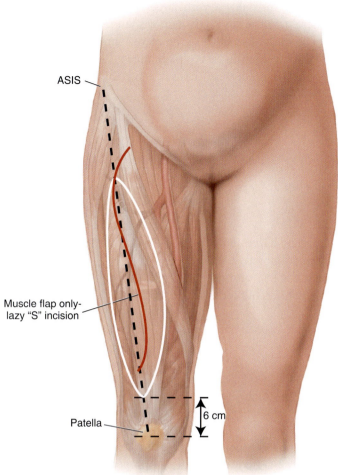

Figure 15-8.

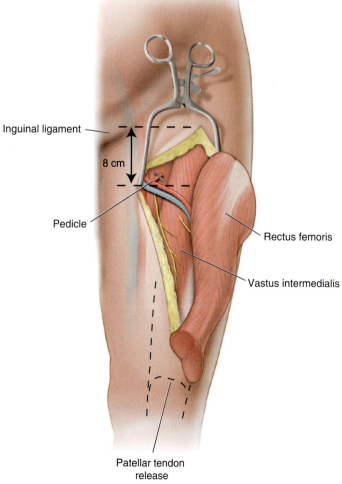

Figure 15-9.

- ▲ The remaining musculotendinuous junctions are medialized with larger figure-of-eight sutures. Suture vastus medialis and vastus lateralis to the cut rectus femoris tendon. Redirecting the remaining muscles will replace some of the lost force of the rectus femoris.
- ▲ Ambulation is allowed according to the protocol for the muscle recipient area.
- ▲ A knee immobilizer is used for approximately 2 weeks. Physical therapy is usually needed for strengthening of the knee extensors.

▲ Extended Rectus Femoris Flap ("Mutton Chop Flap")

- ▲ An extended area of the anterior thigh fascia can be harvested with the rectus femoris. This would allow for coverage of larger defects with autologius tissue.
- ▲ The disadvantage of harvest from this donor site is loss of muscle strength of the thigh.
- ▲ Some report weakness in terminal extension of the knee, but more recent studies denounce this.

3. Fasciocutaneous Flaps (Fig. 15-10, see Table 15-1)

- ▲ Many flaps can be created in the trunk and torso. As depicted in Figure 15-10, on the right side of the torso are axially based flaps, including the deltopectoral, thoracoepigastric, groin, and hypogastric flaps. On the left side of the torso are depictions of bipedicled and laterally based cutaneous flaps.

1. Groin flap

▲ Anatomy

- ▲ Blood is supplied by the superficial circumflex iliac artery (SCIA) from the external iliac/superficial femoral artery at the level of the inguinal ligament (Fig. 15-11). The artery may arise directly from the femoral vessel or from the trunk of a parent vessel supplying the SCIA and the deep circumflex iliac artery (DCIA). The artery also can arise from a common trunk that gives off the superficial inferior epigastric artery (SIEA).
- ▲ The SCIA, which is 1 to 2 mm in diameter, pierces the fascia just lateral to the fossa ovalis at or close to the lateral border of the sartorius muscle and runs in the subcutaneous plane cranially and laterally 2 to 3 cm below the inguinal ligament. This course is maintained to the level of the ASIS and has many connections with branches of the superficial epigastric artery (SEA), DCIA, and lateral femoral circumflex artery.
- ▲ The superficial epigastric artery (SEA) runs parallel to the SCIA and may be dominant. If this is the only vessel delineated by Doppler, design the flap to incorporate this vessel.
- ▲ It is drained by the cutaneous vein to the saphenous system, which is usually a discrete vein along with artery as it courses medially. The vein will arise from the saphenous vein or from a branch off the superficial femoral vein.
- ▲ Pedicle length depends on size and position of the skin paddle and can range from 2 to 5 cm.

Chapter 15 • Rotational and Free Flap Closure of the Abdominal Wall 277

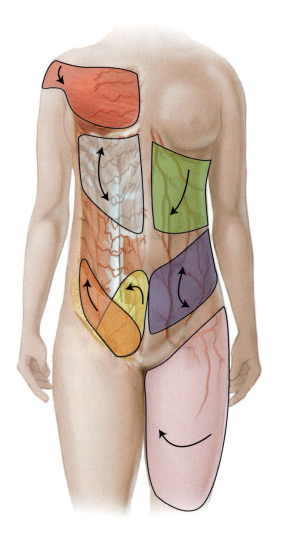

Figure 15-10.

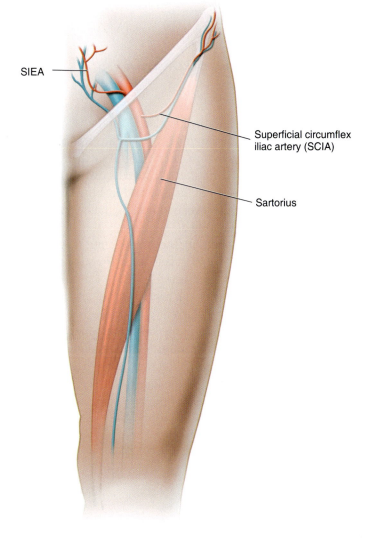

Figure 15-11.

▲ *Flap Design*

- ▲ The sartorius muscle, inguinal ligament, and iliac crest are all identified and marked.
- ▲ Doppler is used to localize the arterial pedicle, usually approximately a fingerbreadth below the inguinal ligament. If not present, seek the SEA by passing the Doppler probe superior to the inguinal ligament.
- ▲ The medial aspect of the flap is marked at the lateral border of the sartorius.
- ▲ The upper and lower borders can be 5 cm above and below the axis of the vessel, but the maximum width of the design is determined by pinching the skin.
- ▲ The length is determined by the defect to be covered.
- ▲ A non-delayed groin flap will survive even with the distal tip placed 5 cm beyond the ASIS. This will cover most ipsilateral lower abdominal defects. If the upper abdomen needs coverage, then the groin flap may require a delay procedure.

▲ *Marking and Dissection*

- ▲ The patient is placed supine.
- ▲ A bump under the ipsilateral hip may be used if the skin paddle extends far laterally.
- ▲ Dissection can be begun medially or laterally.
- ▲ The incision is carried down to the deep fascia and the dissection begun over the deep fascia, identifying and ligating perforating vessels as one proceeds medially.
- ▲ At the level of the ASIS, the interval between the tensor fascia lata and the sartorius muscle is identified.
- ▲ In addition, the lateral femoral cutaneous nerve (LFCN) of the thigh is identified as it exits the deep fascia to enter the subcutaneous tissue in its inferior course. The LCFN may need to be transected.
- ▲ At the lateral aspect of the sartorius, the muscular fascia is incised along the lateral aspect, and the flap elevation plane is now conducted deep to the muscular fascia.
- ▲ Proceeding medially, the superficial circumflex iliac vessels become visible in the plane above the sartorius heading into the muscular fascia.
- ▲ Branches to the muscle are ligated. At the medial aspect of the sartorius, the fascial plane around the pedicle is incised, and the artery and vein are dissected free to their origin (Fig. 15-12).

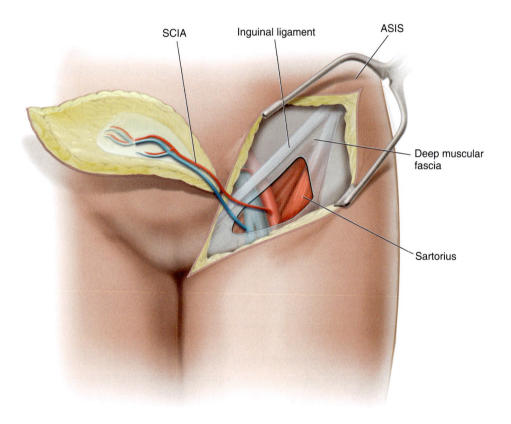

Figure 15-12.

- ▲ The flap is mobilized on the vascular pedicle.
- ▲ The donor area is closed after slight undermining superficial to the deep fascia.
- ▲ Layered closure is used over suction drains.
- ▲ If there is tension on the closure, slight hip flexion may be needed.

2. Extended Deep Inferior Epigastric Perforator Flap

▲ *Anatomy*

- ▲ The course and connections of the deep inferior epigastric artery (DIEA) have been previously covered.
- ▲ If the DIEA is dissected free from the rectus abdominis muscle, a pedicle of 10 to 15 cm is possible. The pedicle can be dissected to the takeoff at the external iliac artery (Fig. 15-13).
- ▲ It usually has two venae comitantes (2-3 mm in diameter).
- ▲ The greatest concentration of perforating vessels is in the periumbilical region. These usually radiate cranially and laterally.
- ▲ The diameter of DIEA is approximately 2-3 mm at its proximal end.

▲ *Flap Design*

- ▲ Borders are the groin and anterior axillary fold.
- ▲ A large skin paddle can be designed on the perforating vessel.
- ▲ A muscle flap alone can be used with a split thickness skin graft after insetting.
- ▲ An axial skin flap can be designed in any direction with its base at the umbilicus, but the longest can be obtained along a line from the umbilicus to the inferior angle of the scapula.
- ▲ The width of the flap can be determined by a "pinch test" based on the laxity of the skin.

▲ *Markings and Dissection*

- ▲ The markings are determined by the defect, with the length of the pedicle obtainable; many variations of shape and size are possible, as long as perforators are included.
- ▲ Incision and dissection in the areolar layer on the deep surface of the subcutaneous fat begins at the distal end of the flap.

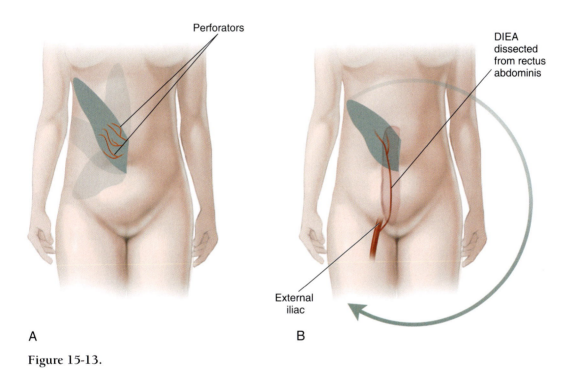

Figure 15-13.

- ▲ Dissection proceeds until the lateral border of the rectus abdominis.
- ▲ Care is taken to protect desirable perforators leading to the designed skin paddle.
- ▲ Then a disk of the rectus abdominis and its sheath that encircle the perforators are isolated.
- ▲ The sheath and muscle at the superior border are divided and the connections to the superior epigastric system are ligated.
- ▲ A sparing amount of muscle and fascia is taken to facilitate closure and reduce donor site morbidity.
- ▲ Care is taken to incise the sheath above the arcuate line.
- ▲ The sheath is then incised longitudinally and the rectus abdominis is dissected free.
- ▲ The DIEA is dissected from the undersurface of the muscle.
- ▲ The pedicle will then course inferolaterally to the external iliac and is ligated at this level.
- ▲ The rectus sheath is repaired to prevent hernia formation or bulge.

3. Thoracoepigastric Flap

▲ *Anatomy*

- ▲ The DIEA supplies the majority of the major perforating vessels leaving the rectus abdominis muscle and running laterally to the area of the latissimus in a suprafascial plane.
- ▲ The superior epigastric artery is smaller than the DIEA, but it supplies the upper abdominal and thoracic flaps (Fig. 15-14, A).
- ▲ The superior epigastric is derived mainly from the internal mammary artery but receives contributions from the terminal branches of the intercostals and the SIEA.

▲ *Flap Design*

- ▲ The flap includes skin, subcutaneous tissue, and muscular fascia of the lateral thoracic and upper abdomen.
- ▲ It can be delayed for larger flaps (Fig. 15-14, B).
- ▲ The base of the flap is the lateral border of the rectus sheath, and this is the point of rotation.
- ▲ The lateral border is the posterior axillary line or anterior edge of the latissimus dorsi muscle. A delayed flap may extend to 5 cm within the dorsal midline.
- ▲ The upper limit in men is the base of areola; in women, the upper limit is the inframammary fold (IMF).
- ▲ The base can be moved cranially or caudally as long as a perforator is included.
- ▲ Flap width can be 10- to 15 cm, with some descriptions of up to 30 cm.
- ▲ The donor site can be closed with a width of 16 cm in an obese patient and 10 cm in a thin patient.

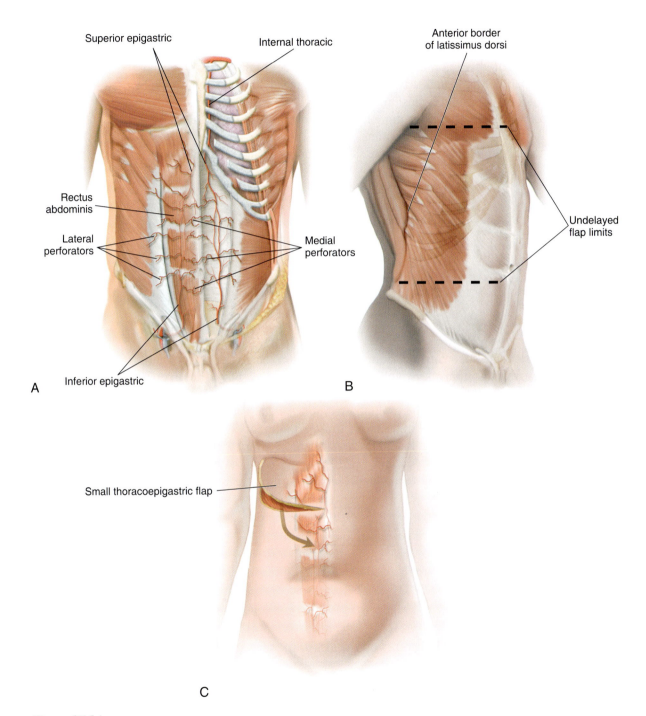

Figure 15-14.

▲ *Marking and Dissection: (Fig. 15-14 C)*

- ▲ The lateral border of the rectus abdominis is palpated and marked.
- ▲ The flap is elevated in a lateral to medial fashion.
- ▲ At the lateral aspect, the muscular intercostal perforators (usually over the serratus anterior) are divided.
- ▲ The elevation from axillary line to the lateral border of the rectus is in a subfascial plane to protect the perforators.
- ▲ There is no dissection medial to the lateral border of the rectus.
- ▲ The perforating vessels may not ever be visualized, and a Doppler may be used for confirmation of perforator inclusion.
- ▲ Posterolaterally, the flap is more random and can be suprafascial.
- ▲ Closure is layered and over drains.
- ▲ If the donor site cannot be closed, a split thickness skin graft can be used.

4. Anterolateral Thigh

▲ *Anatomy*

- ▲ The skin and subcutaneous fat in the anterolateral thigh (ALT) can be thin.
- ▲ The artery's anatomy is variable with size ranging from 1 to 3 mm in diameter. The pedicle can be as long as 7 or 8 cm. It is supplied by the descending branch of the lateral femoral circumflex artery from the profunda femoris. The descending branch travels deep within the space between the rectus femoris muscle and the vastus lateralis muscle.
- ▲ The major draining vein is slightly larger than the artery. Two venae accompany the artery and merge into one at their apex.
- ▲ A major branch of the lateral cutaneous nerve of the thigh enters the flap at the superior aspect.

▲ *Flap Design*

- ▲ The anterolateral thigh flap lies on the axis of the septum dividing the vastus lateralis and the rectus femoris muscles.
- ▲ The skin paddle can be as large as 8 × 25 cm with possible primary closure.

▲ *Marking and Dissection*

- ▲ The axis of the septum between the rectus femoris and the vastus lateralis is marked by a line connecting the ASIS and the lateral patella (Fig. 15-15).

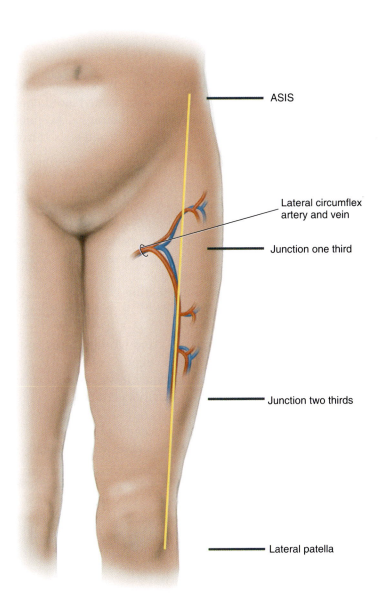

Figure 15-15.

- This line is divided into thirds. The junction of the proximal and middle third is often the site of a perforator that pierces the TFL. It is incorporated for the rare circumstance when the distal perforators are of poor quality or injured during dissection.
- The junction of the middle and distal third is marked and is also incorporated into the flap (Fig. 15-16).
- The middle third of the axis line generally encompasses all substantial perforating vessels.
- A pencil Doppler exam can confirm that perforators are present.
- The anterior flap is elevated first, noting any vessels perforating the rectus femoris. Vessels near the septum are preserved until the posterior flap is elevated.
- Two perforators are found and preserved. The superior perforators may arise from the rectus femoris muscle. The inferior perforators may arise either via the septum or through the medial aspect of the vastus lateralis muscle.
- The posterior flap is elevated toward the septum only after localization of a substantial perforator. If there is no usable perforator or if it is damaged during dissection, the flap is sutured back down to the donor bed.
- The lower perforator can be seen to travel through the vastus and should be dissected toward the descending branch of the lateral circumflex femoral artery (LCFA).
- The septum is identified and any septal perforators are noted. If an adequate perforator is noted, then the flap can be based upon it. Anterior elevation can continue until the septum is isolated both medially and laterally.
- If the blood supply is entirely septal, the descending branch of the LCFA is found at the base of the septum between the rectus femoris and vastus lateralis and dissected proximally (Fig. 15-17).
- If the perforator courses in a transmuscular course, it must be dissected through to the descending branch.
- A light circumferential pressure dressing can be applied to the thigh postoperatively.
- Closed suction is used.
- The patient is allowed to ambulate as soon as clinically indicated for the flap reconstruction.

Chapter 15 • Rotational and Free Flap Closure of the Abdominal Wall 287

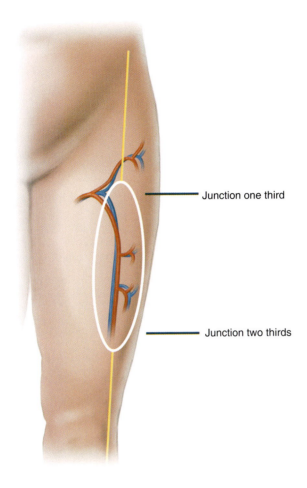

Figure 15-16.

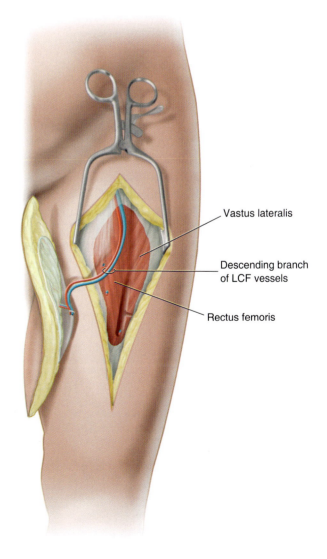

Figure 15-17.

▲ **Flap Variations**

▲ Flap variations include an anterolateral thigh adipofascial flap and an anterolateral thigh fascial flap.

4. Postoperative Care

▲ Patients are allowed to ambulate at differing times, depending on the type of flap used. Free tissue transfer may preclude earlier ambulation to protect the anastomosis.
▲ Support by an abdominal binder may be used if applied properly. A binder that is too tight may cause perfusion problems.
▲ Diets are advanced as tolerated, based on the amount of intestinal manipulation required during opening of the hernia and lysis of adhesions.
▲ Drains are maintained until their drainage is <20 to 30 mL per drain per 24-hour period depending on the site.
▲ The patient may require monitoring in an intensive care unit for free tissue monitoring and increased pulmonary restriction after decreasing the abdominal volume. In addition, many patients requiring closure of the abdominal wall have other severe comorbidities.

5. Pearls/Pitfalls

- ▲ If a pedicled flap is not adequate, then free tissue transfer may be the next step.
- ▲ As previously stated, not all the described pedicled flaps are good options for free tissue transfer. There are limitations in vessel match, length of pedicle, size and type of tissue to be transferred.
- ▲ For perforator based flaps, such as the ALT flap, the size and location of the perforator determines whether an additional vessel is needed.
- ▲ Vessels can be temporarily clamped with micro clamps to determine inflow dominance.
- ▲ Closure of the abdominal defect with a combination of flap and synthetic or biologic mesh may be required.
- ▲ Each flap choice needs to be assessed for potential morbidity.

Selected References

Gottlieb JR, Engrav LH, Walkinshaw MD, Eddy AC, Herman CM: Upper abdominal wall defects: immediate or staged reconstruction? *Plast Reconstr Surg* 86(2):281–286, 1990.

Mansberger AR Jr, Kang JS, Beebe HG, Le Flore I: Repair of massive acute abdominal wall defects, *J Trauma* 13(9):766–774, 1973.

Mathes SJ, Steinwald PM, Foster RD, Hoffman WY, Anthony JP: Complex abdominal wall reconstruction: a comparison of flap and mesh closure, *Ann Surg* 232(4):586–596, 2000.

Rohrich RJ, Lowe JB, Hackney FL, Bowman JL, Hobar PC: An algorithm for abdominal wall reconstruction. *Plast Recon Surg* 105(1):202–216.

Steinwald PM, Mathes SJ: Management of the complex abdominal wall wound, *Adv Surg* 35:77–108, 2001.

Strauch B, Vasconez LO, Hall-Findlay EJ, editors: *Grabb's Encyclopedia of Flaps*, ed 2, Philadelphia, 1998, Lippincott-Raven.

Yeh K, Saltz R, Howdieshell T: Abdominal wall reconstruction after temporary abdominal wall closure in trauma patients, *Southern Medical Journal* 89(5):497–502, 1996.

CHAPTER 16

Managing the Open Abdomen

Daniel Vargo, MD

1. Clinical Anatomy

Management of the open abdomen does not depend so much on recognition of the anatomy of the abdominal wall but on the maintenance of the anterior peritoneal space (Fig. 16-1). If this space is maintained, there is the potential to continue to work toward closure of the abdominal wall. If this space is lost, then the surgeon must move on to protecting the viscera from the external environment and trying to obtain skin closure over the bowel.

2. Preoperative Considerations

1. Resuscitation

Patients who require open abdomens usually fall into one of two categories: those who still have an acute process ongoing (Fig. 16-2) and those who are in the stable phase and are in the process of having their abdomens closed (Fig. 16-3).

Those in the acute phase need to have physiologic abnormalities—acidosis, hypothermia, and coagulopathy—corrected. Providing crystalloid and blood products will accomplish this, although volume resuscitation can itself have adverse effects, specifically on intraabdominal pressure and the development of abdominal compartment syndrome (ACS). Even if the abdomen has a temporary covering in place, intraabdominal pressures need to be monitored. This is typically done with monitoring of bladder pressure. If bladder pressure is elevated or if the patient is clinically developing ACS, then the closure that was placed on the abdomen needs to be loosened to allow the viscera to expand and take pressure off of the vena cava, kidneys, and lungs.

Chapter 16 • Managing the Open Abdomen 291

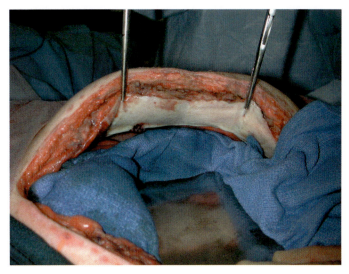

Figure 16-1.

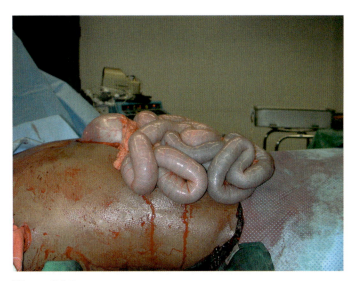

Figure 16-2.

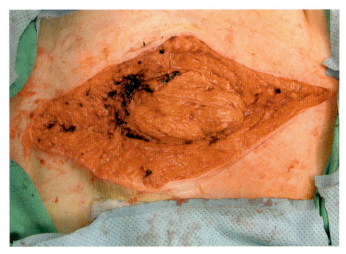

Figure 16-3.

2. Pharmacologic Management

Whether or not a patient who has an open abdomen needs to remain paralyzed and intubated has been questioned. Obviously, if the patient is critically ill or if there are other reasons why intubation and paralysis are necessary, these will take precedence over the open abdomen. If, however, the patient does not have acute physiologic derangements, then weaning of paralysis and just maintaining the patient on sedation is reasonable. Whereas some would extubate these patients, in this author's experience, extubation is not warranted for patients who are going back to surgery frequently and who also usually have other medical issues that are being addressed.

The other pharmacologic question is that of antibiotic use. There have been no randomized controlled trials and very few case-control series using antibiotics with an open abdomen if there is no gross contamination or infection. Thus, antibiotics in clean and clean-contaminated cases cannot be justified beyond 24 hours. If the wound is contaminated or infected, then prophylactic/therapeutic antibiotics should be administered. The length of time depends on the severity of contamination or infection and the patient's other comorbidities. One final issue is the abdomen that has laparotomy pads in place to control bleeding. These patients should be placed on prophylactic antibiotics because of an increased incidence of intraabdominal abscess.

Nutrition also can be considered a pharmacologic intervention. There is no contraindication to enteral nutrition just because the abdomen is open. Although there may be other reasons not to institute enteral feedings, the presence of an open abdomen is not one of them.

3. Planned Open Abdomen

There is a subset of incisional hernia patients for whom it is known before surgery that the patient will need to have an open abdomen after the initial operation. Candidates include hernias with loss of domain, significant abdominal wall infection, and multiple abdominal wall fistulae. With infection and fistulae, definitive hernia repair often has to wait until there is decontamination of the abdominal wall. With loss of domain, the abdominal domain often has to be "reclaimed" by stretching the rectus and lateral abdominal complexes, and this requires the patient to have an open abdomen.

3. Operative Steps

1. Decision to Leave the Abdomen Open

The decision to leave an abdomen open depends on the clinical scenario, as previously stated. It does not matter if the patient's condition is acute or chronic; anatomy and physiology are what drive the decision. Once the decision is made, the steps are similar no matter the reason.

2. Technique

The focus of the technique is to maintain the anterior abdominal domain, and, if a fistula is present, to control effluent while still providing for visceral protection.

All visceral surgery should be completed, if possible. Once this is done, a temporary coverage for the intestine is fashioned. This can be a plastic drape, iodine-impregnated drape (Figs. 16-4 to 16-9), or a commercially available visceral drape (Figs. 16-10 to 16-13). The key point is to get the drape under the abdominal wall and passed all the way laterally to the paracolic gutters. The author believes that some sort of support of the visceral drape is needed to accomplish this. The Barker technique, in which an operative towel is sandwiched between two iodine-impregnated drapes, is favored. This provides enough support such that the covering will not shift once placed.

After the visceral coverage is in place, drains are placed over the cover in the abdominal wound. For a midline laparotomy, these drains are not placed in the gutters of the wound but instead looped in the superior and inferior recess of the wound. This is where most leakage occurs and thus is where the drains need to be.

A blue operative towel is placed over the drains and is then covered by another sheet of iodine-impregnated plastic. Before placing this final sheet of plastic, the drains are connected to wall suction and maintained on wall suction until just before transfer out of the operating room.

Chapter 16 • Managing the Open Abdomen   295

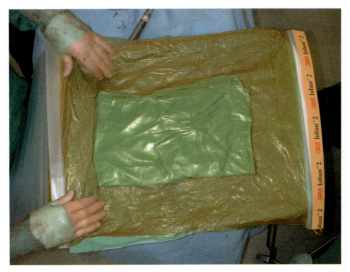

Figure 16-4.

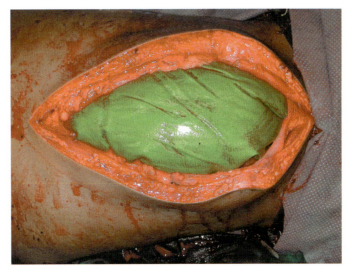

Figure 16-5.

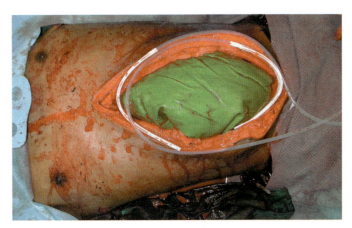

Figure 16-6.

296 Section V • Other Abdominal Wall Procedures

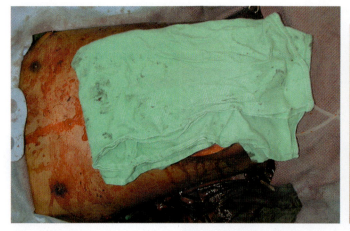

Figure 16-7.

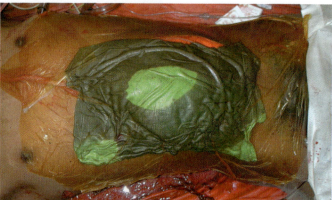

Figure 16-8.

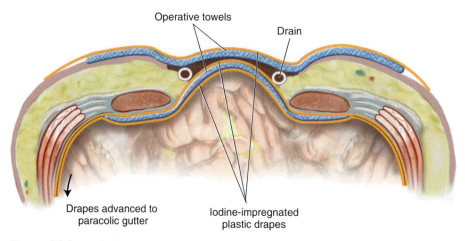

Figure 16-9.

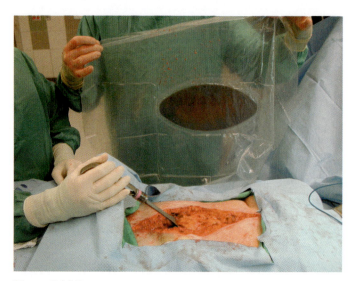

Figure 16-10.

Chapter 16 • Managing the Open Abdomen 297

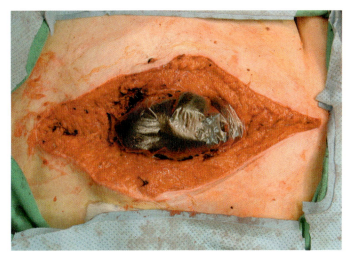

Figure 16-11.

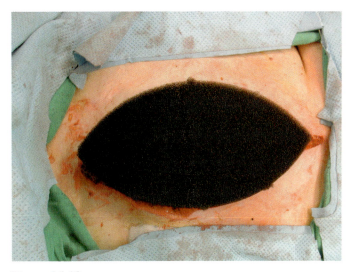

Figure 16-12.

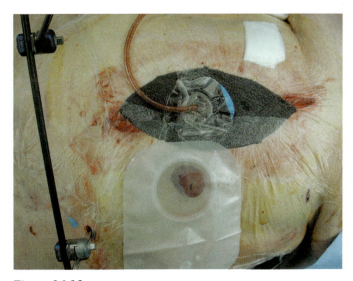

Figure 16-13.

3. Fascial Closure

While none of these patients are candidates for complete fascial closure, most patients can have part of their abdominal wall reapproximated at each operation (Figs. 16-14 to 16-16). Every time a patient goes to the operating room, an attempt should be made to bring at least some of the fascia back together. This may be just one or two stitches, but in the end, it is progress, and progress is what is needed in these difficult patients.

4. Postoperative Care

1. General Care Issues

General postoperative care is used in all patients. Ensuring adequate resuscitation, appropriate antibiotic therapy, and nutritional support are critical. These patients have very large wounds, and they need all of the aforementioned in place to allow for healing.

Most patients are admitted to an intensive care unit. As previously stated, management of paralysis and intubation are made on a case-by-case basis, depending on what other issues are present.

Another aspect of postoperative care is maintaining the dressing. The drains should be kept to low continuous wall suction. This keeps fluid from building up under the dressing and dissecting the dressing away from the abdominal wall, leading to leakage from the dressing. This leakage is bad in that it does not allow for quantification of fluid from the abdomen, in addition to leading to maceration of the skin.

2. Reoperation

Patients should be taken to surgery whenever it is felt that more progress can be made with regards to their closure. Usually this means every day or every other day. At the time of these procedures, every attempt should be made to reapproximate some fascia.

Chapter 16 • Managing the Open Abdomen 299

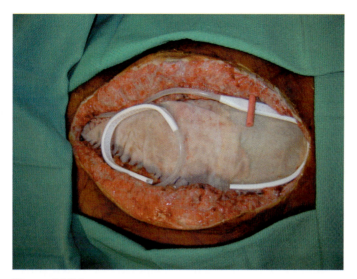

Figure 16-14.

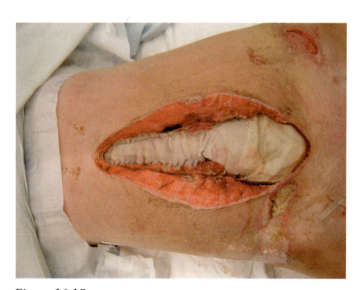

Figure 16-15.

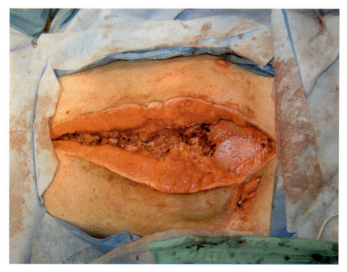

Figure 16-16.

3. Complications

The main complication unique to this patient population is enteroatmospheric fistula. While surgeons are used to managing enterocutaneous fistulae, this fistula is present in the middle of a large visceral block of tissue. Early identification and management of the fistula effluent is critical. If there is any question that a fistula has developed, the patient should be taken to the operating room and evaluated. Presence of a fistula usually means the abdomen cannot be entirely closed. However, one can proceed with as much fascial closure as possible, possibly sparing the patient from a very large ventral hernia defect.

5. Pitfalls/Pearls

The major pitfall in management of the open abdomen is giving up too quickly. While it is easier to just place some type of mesh coverage over the abdomen and wait to skin graft, the cost of this to the patient in terms of both lost productivity and dollars has been well documented. With the appropriate dressing in place, patients have been serially closed over the course of three weeks.

If dressings are not applied in such a way that the viscera are protected, then each dressing change can debride away some of the bowel serosa, and this will lead to a fistula. If a negative pressure wound therapy (NPWT) system is being used over the viscera, then it either needs to be covered in plastic, or a nonadherent type sponge needs to be used.

A time will come when the patient is not getting any better, and the reason for this is the open abdomen. This patient has developed tertiary peritonitis, and the only way they are going to get better is to cover the viscera. In this patient, a biologic-type mesh is believed to be the most appropriate closure. It prevents adhesions (good for reoperation at a later date); protects the viscera during dressing changes (lower fistula rate); and in select patients, may function as their definitive closure.

If the fascia is very close to closing, one may be tempted to perform a component separation (CS) to allow for primary reapproximation of the fascia. This is to be discouraged because reherniation in this patient population is high, and if CS has been performed, a major secondary reconstruction option has been eliminated. It is better to bridge with a biologic mesh and save the more complex reconstruction options for a later date.

The exception to the aforementioned is the patient whose CS was planned and the abdominal wall was being staged. This includes abdominal wall infections and loss of domain type hernias. Here, CS can be performed as planned if it is thought the patient may benefit.

Selected References

Brock WB, Barker DE, Burns RP: Temporary closure of open abdominal wounds: The vacuum pack, *Am Surg* 61:30–35, 1995.

Diaz JJ, Cullinane DC, Dutton WD, et al: The management of the open abdomen in trauma and emergency general surgery: Part 1- Damage Control, *J Trauma* 68(6):1425–1438, 2010.

Vargo D, Richardson JD, editors: "Management of the Open Abdomen: From Initial Operation to Definitive Closure," *Am Surg* Vol. 75(2): S1–S22, 2009.

CHAPTER 17

Managing Pediatric and Neonatal Abdominal Wall Defects

Arjun Khosla, MD and Todd A. Ponsky, MD

1. Clinical Anatomy

- ▲ In a patient with an omphalocele (also known as exomphalos) (Fig.17-1), the bowel and viscera, covered by a membrane composed of visceral peritoneum, Wharton jelly, and amnion, herniate through a central defect (≥4 cm) at the umbilical ring. The viscera extend into the base of the umbilical cord and the umbilical cord inserts into the apex of the omphalocele sac. The sac may contain loops of small bowel, large intestine, stomach, and liver (in 50% of cases). These viscera are otherwise functionally normal.
- ▲ Omphalocele is a congenital abnormality and is often associated with other anomalies and syndromes in 60% to 70% of cases. These include Beckwith-Wiedemann syndrome, Cantrell pentalogy, exstrophy of the bladder/cloaca, and chromosomal trisomies such as Down syndrome. The most common anomalies discovered are cardiac and gastrointestinal.
- ▲ In patients with gastroschisis (Fig.17-2), the small bowel freely protrudes, without an overlying sac, through a smaller defect (<4 cm) at the junction between the umbilicus and the skin. The defect is almost always to the right of the umbilicus. The herniated contents may include small bowel, stomach, bladder, fallopian tubes, ovaries, and testes.
- ▲ Unlike omphalocele, gastroschisis is not congenital. It is thought to be related to an in utero vascular accident. For that reason, gastroschisis is associated with small bowel atresias, which also are believed to be caused by in utero vascular accidents.
- ▲ Both omphalocele and gastroschisis are associated with intestinal malrotation, prematurity, and intrauterine growth restriction (IUGR).
- ▲ The incidence of omphalocele is 1 in 5000 live births while that of gastroschisis is 1 in 2500 live births. Furthermore, mothers of infants with omphalocele are, on average, 10 years older than those with gastroschisis.
- ▲ It is important to differentiate a ruptured omphalocele sac, which occurs in 10% to 18% of patients with omphalocele, from gastroschisis because this distinction may affect clinical management. Although the initial treatment for these two entities is the same, the search for other associated conditions is affected.
- ▲ In gastroschisis, due to exposure to amniotic fluid and compromised blood supply, the small bowel may become thick, shortened, edematous, discolored, and covered with fibrinous exudates (also known as a "peel"). This may reduce the malleability of the bowel and make manual reduction more difficult. Furthermore, extensive peel is thought to lead to a prolonged ileus after bowel reduction.

Chapter 17 • Managing Pediatric and Neonatal Abdominal Wall Defects

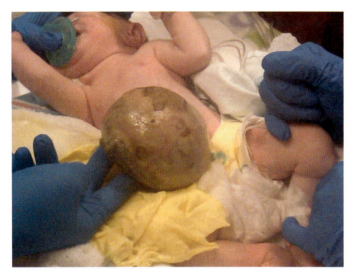

Figure 17-1.

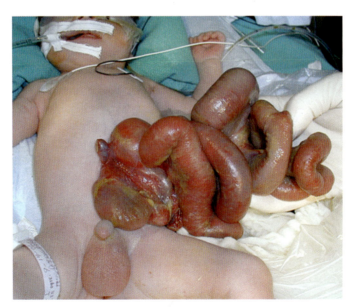

Figure 17-2.

- Omphalocele is due to the primary failure of the developing intestines to return to the abdominal cavity after migration into the umbilical cord during weeks 6 to 12 of gestation. Figure 17-3 depicts a cross-sectional diagram of the anatomy seen in omphalocele. The abdominal muscles are otherwise normally developed.
- Gastroschisis is believed to be caused by involution of the right umbilical vein during the fourth week of development. The resulting ischemia leads to a full-thickness defect in the musculature of the abdominal wall. Figure 17-4 shows a cross-sectional diagram of the anatomy seen in gastroschisis.

2. Preoperative Considerations

- Both omphalocele and gastroschisis may be suspected prenatally with an elevated maternal serum α-fetoprotein (although this level can be normal or elevated because of other conditions) and can be diagnosed readily by prenatal ultrasonography in 75% to 80% of cases (after 14 weeks' gestation when the fetal midgut returns to the abdomen). They can be differentiated sonographically by the presence of a sac, location of the defect, and presence of additional abnormalities. These methods have increasingly led to detection before birth and allow for prenatal education and family counseling.
- If an omphalocele is discovered, it is important to search for associated anomalies by performing an amniocentesis or chorionic villus sampling for karyotype analysis, as well as fetal echocardiography to find structural abnormalities.
- Steps are taken to stabilize the infant immediately following birth. A careful assessment of the oxygenation and ventilation is done because of an association with pulmonary hypoplasia, and the child is intubated if in respiratory distress. A nasogastric tube is placed to decompress the stomach. The patient is placed on the right side to preserve bowel perfusion. The sac is covered with moist gauze and plastic wrap. Care must be taken when handling the viscera because too much pressure can lead to abdominal compartment syndrome and mishandling of the intestines can lead to volvulus. These infants are often hypovolemic and are given aggressive intravenous fluid resuscitation resulting from both evaporative and third-space fluid losses. With gastroschisis (or ruptured omphalocele) prophylactic broad-spectrum intravenous antibiotics are administered. Temperature is controlled with a heating lamp. Routine blood work is ordered and a detailed physical exam is performed.
- With an intact omphalocele sac, surgical repair is not immediately necessary. Conservative treatment allows time for the diagnosis of associated conditions and lowers the risk of increased intraabdominal pressure and wound complications associated with aggressive closure. However, with gastroschisis or a ruptured omphalocele, urgent surgical repair is required.
- With omphalocele, patients can undergo primary closure, staged closure, or nonoperative management with late closure. Those with gastroschisis may similarly undergo primary closure, or, if the abdominal cavity is too small to accommodate the protuberant bowel, staged closure. Infants with gastroschisis also may be able to undergo the recently developed sutureless repair.

Chapter 17 • Managing Pediatric and Neonatal Abdominal Wall Defects 305

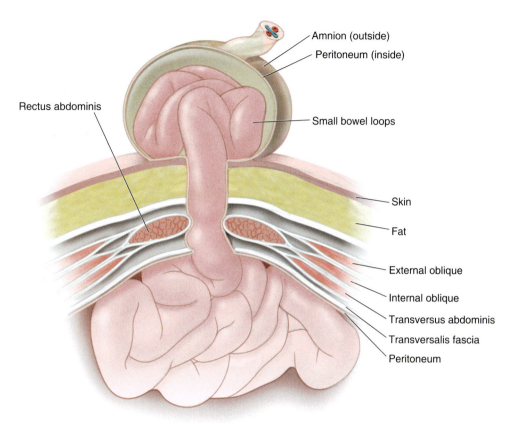

Figure 17-3.

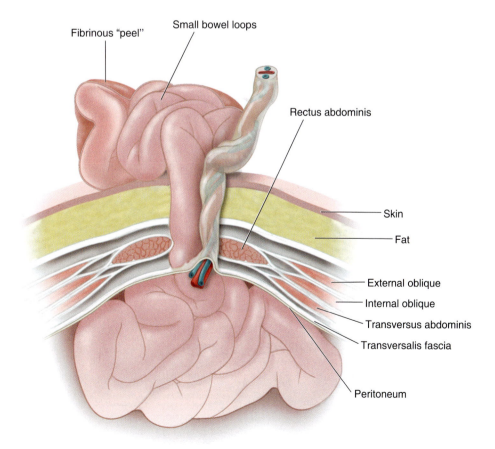

Figure 17-4.

3. Operative Steps

1. Omphalocele

- ▲ When possible, **primary closure** should be performed. This is sometimes possible for small or moderately sized defects. The omphalocele sac is excised (Fig.17-5). The umbilical arteries and vein are identified and ligated. The skin is then undermined enough for a secure fascial closure. The viscera are reduced. And the fascia is closed, usually in a transverse fashion. The skin often can be closed using a purse-string suture to try to recreate an umbilicus (Fig.17-6).
- ▲ Larger defects require gradual reduction of the viscera. There are several methods for **staged closure** of an omphalocele.
- ▲ For the **Gross technique**, developed in 1948, the omphalocele sac is excised. The skin is undermined enough to provide minimal tension. Prosthetic material may be needed to bridge the fascial defect (Fig.17-7). The skin is then closed over the defect (Fig.17-8). The resulting ventral hernia is then repaired at a later time. In recent years, many surgeons who use this approach are using biologic mesh material for closure.

Chapter 17 • Managing Pediatric and Neonatal Abdominal Wall Defects 307

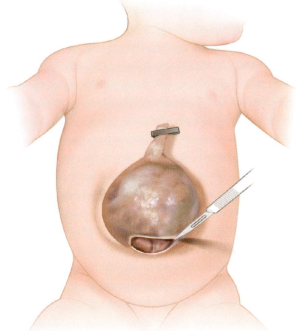

Figure 17-5.

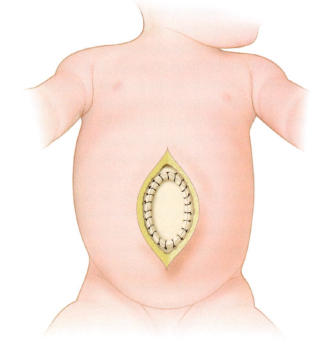

Figure 17-7.

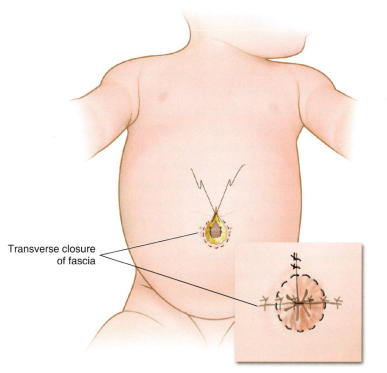

Transverse closure of fascia

Figure 17-6.

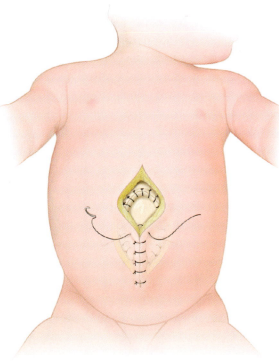

Figure 17-8.

- ▲ The **Schuster technique**, developed in 1967, is particularly useful for large or ruptured omphaloceles. This technique involves using a silo to gradually reduce the herniated viscera over several days to a week. As much of the viscera as possible are returned to the abdomen. A nonabsorbable material such as silastic sheeting can be used as a silo, secured to either the fascia or skin with nonabsorbable suture. The silo is then closed over the top of the viscera and suspended perpendicularly to avoid kinks in the intestine, allowing gravity to pull the viscera back into the abdomen (Fig.17-9). The silo is tightened daily to assist in visceral reduction. Once the viscera are reduced within the abdominal cavity, the silo is removed and the fascia and skin are closed.
- ▲ **Sequential sac ligation** is when the natural omphalocele sac itself is used as a silo. It requires a sac that is strong and not adherent to the viscera. Traction is applied to the sac to slowly reduce its contents. As the viscera are reduced into the abdominal cavity, the sac is twisted and ligated with umbilical ties (Fig.17-10).
- ▲ **Tissue expanders** also have been used successfully in the closure of giant omphaloceles. The tissue expander is placed within the peritoneal cavity and slowly inflated with saline over several weeks, increasing the abdominal domain. The infant is eventually taken to the operating room (OR) for visceral reduction and fascial/skin closure.
- ▲ **Nonoperative (escharotic) therapy** is an option for those patients who are not good candidates for surgical intervention (premature, chromosomal abnormalities, significant congenital heart disease, or pulmonary hypoplasia) and the author's preferred option for giant omphaloceles. The omphalocele sac is painted with an escharotic material, such as silver sulfadiazine. The authors have also used an Aquacel dressing (ConvaTec, Skillman, NJ) for this purpose. These materials prevent infection, form granulation tissue, and allow the sac surface to eventually epithelialize and contract over several months. The resulting ventral hernia is then electively repaired once the underlying cardiac, pulmonary, and/or other conditions have improved.

Chapter 17 • Managing Pediatric and Neonatal Abdominal Wall Defects 309

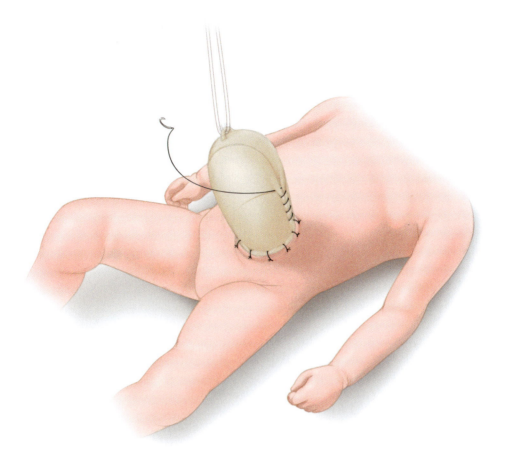

Figure 17-9.

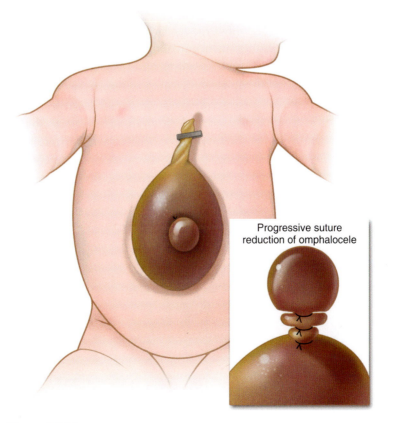

Figure 17-10.

2. Gastroschisis

- ▲ **Primary closure** of gastroschisis is possible in a majority of cases. Muscle relaxation is often used to assist with visceral reduction. Also, decompression of the stomach or bowel may aid in reducing the volume of the intestines. It may be difficult to reduce the herniated contents through a small defect, and thus, the neck of the defect may need to be enlarged superiorly (Fig. 17-11). The bowel must be examined for possible atresias or perforations. The skin is then undermined enough to provide a secure closure. Because the risk of subsequent umbilical hernia is high after gastroschisis repair, the fascia lateral to the umbilical ring should be identified and used for placement of the suture (Fig. 17-12). Care must be taken to avoid abdominal compartment syndrome by putting too much pressure on the reduced intestines. If atresia is noted, the bowel is reduced at the first operation and a second operation is done 4 to 6 weeks later to correct the atresia as the intraabdominal inflammation resolves.
- ▲ As with omphalocele, **staged closure**, can be used when reducing the herniated viscera is too difficult or produces too much intraabdominal pressure. A silo is used to gradually reduce the bowel by decreasing the swelling and rigidity of the inflamed bowel and progressively stretching the abdominal cavity. The silo also prevents electrolyte, fluid, and heat losses. Recently, preformed spring-loaded silos that can be placed at the bedside without sutures or anesthesia have shown to be associated with fewer ventilator days, more rapid return of bowel function, and fewer complications (Fig. 17-13).

Chapter 17 • Managing Pediatric and Neonatal Abdominal Wall Defects 311

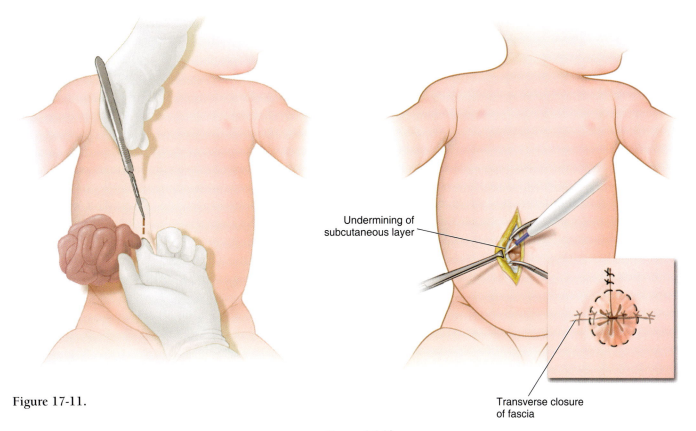

Figure 17-11.

Figure 17-12.

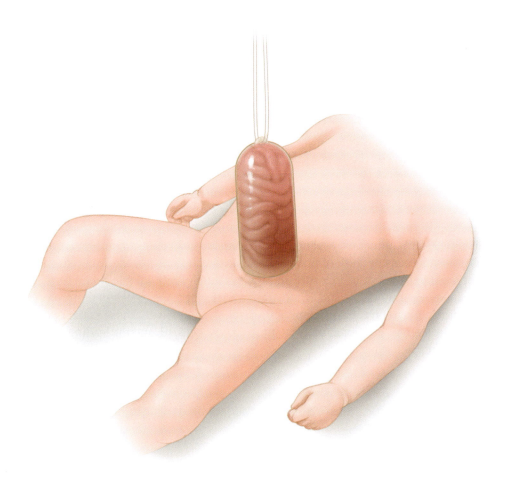

Figure 17-13.

▲ **Sutureless repair**, developed by Sandler et al. (2004), allows the defect to naturally heal over the reduced bowel. The bowel is first manually reduced into the abdominal cavity (Fig.17-14, A, B). The umbilical cord is wrapped into a coil over the defect. The area is covered with a 2 × 2 gauze sponge and Tegaderm dressing (3M, St. Paul, MN) and allowed to heal over several days (Fig.17-14, C, D). This type of repair uses no sutures, eliminates the need for a trip to the OR, and may be cosmetically superior to traditional surgical repair.

4. Postoperative Care

▲ Postoperative care requires the neonatal intensive care unit (NICU). Larger defects require mechanical ventilation for days to weeks. It is important to monitor for signs of abdominal compartment syndrome (hypotension, oliguria, acidosis, intestinal ischemia, liver dysfunction) with intragastric or intravesical catheters. The intraabdominal pressure should not be above 15 to 20 mm Hg.

▲ After repair, ileus is common, resolving more quickly in patients with omphalocele than those with gastroschisis. A nasogastric tube is necessary initially and total parenteral nutrition is started early. In fact, many surgeons place a central venous catheter at the time of operation for this purpose. Once bowel function has returned, enteral feedings can begin. Elemental formula is best tolerated and once the infant's caloric intake is adequate (usually around 3 to 4 weeks without complications) the patient is ready for discharge to home.

▲ Gastroschisis also is associated with morbidity and mortality related to gastrointestinal dysfunction, such as short bowel syndrome and sepsis from intraabdominal, wound, or central line infection.

▲ With omphalocele, the long-term outcome is most dependent on the associated chromosomal/structural abnormalities with an overall mortality of 10% to 30%. Long-term complications include gastroesophageal reflux disease, feeding disorders, and adhesive bowel obstruction, but most of these issues improve over time. Most individuals without severe associated anomalies grow up to live normal lives.

▲ The long-term outcome for patients with gastroschisis has dramatically improved over the past few decades because of improved surgical technique and perioperative management, such as the use of staged closure and the availability of total parenteral nutrition. Overall mortality is now <10%, and is most often associated with intestinal atresia. Prognosis is most dependent on the condition of the exteriorized bowel. Those patients with intestinal atresia undergo additional surgical procedures, delayed enteral feedings, and have prolonged hospital stays.

Chapter 17 • Managing Pediatric and Neonatal Abdominal Wall Defects 313

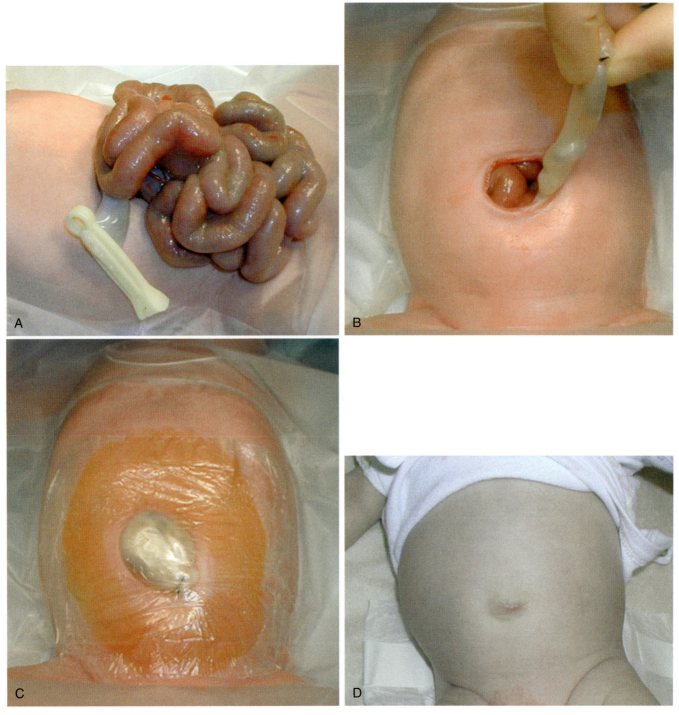

Figure 17-14.

5. Pearls/Pitfalls

- ▲ If a fetus is discovered to have an abdominal wall defect, there is no evidence to suggest that early delivery or cesarean-section is beneficial. The mode and timing of delivery should be determined by fetal well-being and obstetric considerations. Serial ultrasound exams during pregnancy can aid in evaluating the condition of the bowel and whether the fetus is at risk.
- ▲ It is important to differentiate omphalocele from gastroschisis because this distinction greatly affects clinical management. A membranous sac covering the viscera is present in omphalocele (unless ruptured) and absent in gastroschisis. Omphalocele is a central defect, whereas gastroschisis is lateral to (usually to the right of) the umbilicus. The herniated viscera in omphalocele may include bowel, stomach, and liver, whereas gastroschisis may involve bowel, stomach, bladder, and gonads.
- ▲ Omphalocele can be repaired electively, while the presence of associated abnormalities is investigated. However, gastroschisis (and ruptured omphalocele) require urgent surgical repair because these entities leave the infant vulnerable to dehydration, hypothermia, electrolyte abnormalities, and infection.
- ▲ When repairing these abdominal wall defects, care must be taken to avoid too aggressive of a repair, which can potentially lead to abdominal compartment syndrome, causing more complications and putting the remaining bowel at risk. Avoidance of abdominal compartment syndrome decreases the risk of intestinal ischemia, necrotizing enterocolitis, and intestinal perforation, all of which can lead to devastating consequences for a vulnerable infant.

Selected References

Aspelund GLJ: Abdominal wall defects, *Current Paediatrics*:192–198, 2006.
Henrich K, Huemmer HP, Reingruber B, Weber PG: Gastroschisis and omphalocele: treatments and long-term outcomes, *Pediatr Surg Int* 24:167–173, 2008.
Langer JC: Abdominal wall defects, *World J Surg* 27:117–124, 2003.
Ledbetter DJ: Gastroschisis and omphalocele, *Surg Clin North Am* 86:249–260, 2006:vii.
Mann S, Blinman TA, Douglas Wilson R: Prenatal and postnatal management of omphalocele, *Prenat Diagn* 28:626–632, 2008.
Molenaar JC, Tibboel D: Gastroschisis and omphalocele, *World J Surg* 17:337–341, 1993.
Puri PHM, editor: *Pediatric Surgery*, New York, NY, 2006, Springer-Verlag Berlin Heidelberg, pp 153–170.
Sandler A, Lawrence J, Meehan J, Phearman L, Soper R: *J Pediatr Surg* 39(5):738–741, 2004 May.

SECTION **VI**

Mesh Choices

CHAPTER 18

Biologic Mesh Choices for Surgical Repair

Michael G. Franz, MD

1. Indications for the Use of Biologic Mesh Materials

- ▲ The major indication for the use of biologic meshes during abdominal wall surgery is improved wound healing. This most often translates into the minimization of wound complications. Studies have reported wound infection rates of 4% to 16% after incisional ventral hernia repair. The application of synthetic mesh to reinforce abdominal wall repairs significantly reduced recurrence rates, but it introduced an increased risk of complicated wound infections, synthetic mesh infections and erosion into the bowel. Level one data find that recurrence rate and wound infection are related, in that a postoperative wound infection significantly increases the incidence of recurrent incisional hernia. Another inherent limitation with synthetic meshes is shrinkage. It is well measured now in animal models and with human explants that synthetic meshes lose on the average 20% of their surface area following implantation. This is believed to contribute to high hernia recurrence rates. The era of managing traumatized patients with open abdomens expanded the use of biologic mesh based abdominal wall reconstruction. Here there was concern for wound contamination and exposure of synthetic prostheses to the abdominal viscera. Tenuous or insufficient skin coverage also is suggested as an indication for the use of a biologic mesh during abdominal wall repair.
- ▲ The risk of laparotomy wound complications may be graded and wound outcomes predicted based on patient comorbidities and level of contamination. Now long-term experience with synthetic meshes in the abdominal wall raises awareness and concern for acute and chronic infections, as well as intestinal injury. The growing problem of infected mesh explantation also drove increased use of biologic meshes as replacements. Obesity is now a measurable risk factor for increased wound complications following ventral hernia repair.
- ▲ The growing popularity of major reconstructive procedures for large ventral hernias also expanded the use of biologic meshes. The perceived need for reinforcement following component separation procedures and the concern for the implantation of synthetic materials into these large surface area wounds led to this adaptation of biologic mesh. Clinical studies have supported reduced recurrence rates using mesh reinforcement during component separation.

TABLE 18-1. Tissue Source and Properties of Biologic Meshes

PRODUCT	MANUFACTURER	PROPERTIES	POTENTIAL ADVANTAGES	POTENTIAL DISADVANTAGES
HUMAN DERMIS				
Alloderm	Lifecell	Non–cross-linked; Aseptic without irradiation	Preserved matrix; Large reported clinical experience	Freeze dried; Needs refrigeration; Small sizes
Flex HD	Musculoskeletal Transplant Foundation (MTF)/Ethicon	Non–cross linked; Aseptic	No refrigeration or rehydration	Small reported clinical experience
Allomax	Bard/Davol	Proprietary Tutoplast process to remove cells and preserve matrix	Low-dose gamma irradiation to sterilize	Small reported clinical experience; Requires hydration
PORCINE DERMIS				
Permacol	Covidien	Chemically cross-linked	Large sizes; No refrigeration or rehydration; Large reported clinical experience	Concern for increased foreign body reaction due to heavy cross-linking; Chemical odor and concern for inflammation
Strattice	LifeCell	Non–cross-linked; Terminally sterilized	Large sheets; No rehydration	Few clinical data
XenMatrix	Bard/Davol	Non–cross-linked; Electron beam sterilized	No rehydration; Large sheets	Few clinical data
PORCINE INTESTINE				
Surgisis	Cook	Modified intestinal submucosal matrix; Non–cross-linked	Long clinical experience; No refrigeration	Reports of enzymatic degradation; Requires rehydration
BOVINE				
Veritas	Synovis	Pericardium		Small clinical experience in ventral hernia
Tutopatch	Tutogen	Pericardium		Little data
SurgiMend	TEI Biosciences	Fetal dermis; Non–cross-linked	Favorable fetal collagen content; Long shelf life	Requires rehydration; Very little data

2. Tissue Sources for Biologic Mesh Materials (Table 18-1)

▲ The application of biologic materials to abdominal wall repair began with autologous source material. Tensor fascia lata (TFL) has the widest experience. De-epithelialized autologous dermis also has been used. Muscle flaps and now even composite tissue transfers, both pedicle based and free flaps, have been described. Autologous small bowel and omentum also are reported as tissue sources for abdominal wall repair. Donor site morbidity is the obvious limitation of autologous biologic tissue sources. There are no large studies of TFL or autologous dermis in abdominal wall repair, and the long-term durability, especially when used as bridging repair, is not known.

▲ The need for more readily available biologic reconstructive matrices and the limitation of autologous tissue donor site morbidity led to the development of off-the-shelf human allograft sources for abdominal wall reconstruction. To date, this has been dominated by human dermal allografts. Although early results have been good, there is an inherent limitation in the need for human tissue banking and the risk of transmission of infectious disease. Before processing, potential donors undergo screening that includes a medical and social history review, physical examination and serologic testing to minimize the risk of disease transmission. Donor tissue that passes rigorous screening then undergoes physical and chemical processing to further reduce the risk of disease transmission before implantation. Occasionally, social and cultural restrictions may preclude the application of human tissue sources to specific patient groups.

- ▲ The unique regulatory limitations of human tissue banking and the need for better processing quality control drove the introduction of xenografts as biologic materials for abdominal wall reconstruction. This also reduces the cost of xenografts that on the average are 50% less expensive than allografts. This trend has been dominated by porcine intestinal submucosa, porcine dermis, bovine fetal dermis, and bovine adult pericardium. One fundamental limitation of xenografts is the presence in humans of preformed anti-xenograft antibodies. The anti-galactose-alpha-1,3-galactose antibodies are the best described. There is also evidence for the induction of nonspecific inflammatory pathways as part of a generalized foreign body reaction. With xenografts as with allografts, social and cultural restrictions may apply.

3. Biologic Mesh Modification and Processing

- ▲ The use of biologic allografts and xenografts for soft tissue repair required the development of processing techniques that allowed for the removal of immunogenic cells, while preserving a functional biologic matrix. This remnant biologic matrix is constructed primarily of collagen, and depending on the degree of preservation of the native structure, maintains measurable biologic function even in the acellularized state.
- ▲ Porcine intestinal submucosa is a readily available source of biologic matrix. In its varied forms it maintains adequate mechanical qualities and has a recognized safety profile when applied for abdominal wall repair or reconstruction. The proprietary process for stripping and harvesting the intestinal submucosa results in modification of the original biologic structure. Intestinal submucosa also has been laminated to improve mechanical performance.
- ▲ The importance of preserving the native dermal matrix structure and to what degree is still debated. Cross-linking of dermal matrix xenografts was introduced as a method to increase mechanical strength and to protect the collagen-based implant against enzymatic degradation by collagenases. Cross-linking also is believed to reduce the immunogenic potential of the acellularized matrix, due mainly to expression of galactose-alpha-1,3-galactose molecular epitopes. In its simplest form, cross-linking causes molecular bonds to form between native collagen molecules. Several steps during biologic mesh processing can cause matrix cross-linking, as with the use of detergents, enzymes, or high-energy beams for sterilization. These steps, in addition to intentional chemical modification of the matrix or terminal sterilization, all induce varying degrees of matrix cross-linking. The level of matrix cross-linking can be quantified by measuring the mesh collagen melting point. Higher degrees of cross-linking result in higher matrix melting points. Examination by electron microscopy also can be used to look for the preservation of biologic matrix structure. If the goal of biologic mesh–based soft tissue reconstruction is to support the repopulation of the donor matrix with host cells, like endothelial cells and fibroblasts, it appears that high levels of cross-linking impair that recellularization process. The host may even recognize a highly cross-linked material as foreign and induce a foreign body capsule response. A balance must therefore be struck between biologic mesh durability and regenerative potential. The end result is observed to be varying degrees of incorporation, resorption, or encapsulation. It appears that the outcome depends on material source, material processing, host response, surgical technique, and the level of wound contamination or inflammation. Further experimental studies and well-designed clinical trials are needed to characterize the optimum materials and methods.
- ▲ Allografts and xenografts vary in the degree of terminal sterilization. Some methods limit terminal sterilization, using instead aseptic techniques. It is believed that this ensures preservation of extracellular matrix structure with improved biologic function following implantation. Other biologic mesh materials undergo true terminal sterilization, as with low-dose gamma irradiation. It is believed that this step may be important to minimizing infectious complications.

TABLE 18-2. Summary of Biologic Mesh Mechanisms of Action

TISSUE PROCESSING	IMMUNOLOGIC RESPONSE	BIOLOGIC RESPONSE	HOST RESPONSE/OUTCOME
Matrix preserved Block alpha-gal epitope	Relatively inert	Fibroblast ingrowth Angiogenesis Remodeling	Matrix tissue regeneration
Matrix structure significantly modified Exposure of foreign antigens Matrix heavily cross-linked	Immunologically active or inflammatory	Increased proteases Inflammation Scar formation Some cellular ingrowth Limited cellular ingrowth Inflammation Giant cell formation	Matrix resorption and potential scar plate Host foreign body encapsulation Contraction

4. Mechanism of Action of Biologic Meshes (Table 18-2)

▲ The primary function of soft tissue prostheses, whether synthetic or biologic meshes, is to provide immediate and long-term mechanical stability to the abdominal wall reconstruction. Level one evidence derived from a randomized, controlled trial found that the use of a reinforcing mesh prosthesis reduces the incisional hernia recurrence rate by 50%. The major risk of synthetic mesh implants is the permanent foreign body reaction, infection, encapsulation, extrusion, and erosion. There is now experimental and clinical evidence that biologic meshes may be repopulated with endothelial cells, revascularized and then incorporated into an abdominal wall reconstruction. It is the early establishment of a blood supply that is believed to establish improved resistance to infection. Further, as a blood supply is restored, other cells involved in tissue repair like inflammatory cells and fibroblasts may be recruited to promote more normal wound healing, and ideally, tissue regeneration.

▲ Biologic meshes provide the potential for extracellular matrix directed repair signaling. Preserved vascular channels, for example, may allow endothelial cells or their precursors to enter the matrix, supporting angiogenesis by the process of inosculation. Other matrix molecules like fibronectin and glycosaminoglycans, when preserved, may act as signals for fibroblast integration and host collagen synthesis. The amount of other matrix molecules also varies widely depending on the biologic mesh tissue source. Human dermis, for example, contains relatively more elastin than porcine dermis, rendering it more compliant.

5. Reported Clinical Results with Biologic Meshes

▲ The choice of biologic mesh material may be based on a variety of considerations, including characteristics of the patient and abdominal wall defect, surgeon familiarity with the material, and cost. The risk for surgical wound complication and subsequent infection may determine the selection of a synthetic versus a biologic repair material. On the balance, the biologic mesh material should provide sustained mechanical function resulting in an acceptable recurrence rate with resistance to wound infection, especially when compared to the synthetic counter parts.

- ▲ The majority of reports of surgeons' experience with biologic mesh repairs come from single center, retrospective reviews. A randomized controlled trial of biologic mesh-based repairs versus synthetic mesh–based repairs for ventral hernia has never been reported. Multi-institutional, single-arm studies suggesting a proof-in-principle for the safety and efficacy of biologic mesh–based repairs are now appearing. It is broadly concluded that biologic mesh–based abdominal wall reconstructions can be safe and effective. Like most new techniques and technologies, it also appears surgical technique and material choice in the application of biologic meshes together affect outcomes. Without high level evidence, the decision tree remains primarily driven by surgeon experience and expert opinion.
- ▲ The most frequent early application of biologic mesh for abdominal wall reconstruction was to manage complex ventral hernia repairs. This usually meant the need to perform an abdominal wall reconstruction in the setting of moderate or even significant contamination. Many surgeons reported the reliability of biologic mesh–based repairs, and the opportunity to avoid the technique of intentional, incisional ventral hernia. Numerous series now report the ability to safely salvage an abdominal wall repair when at increased risk for wound complication, with wound infection and recurrence rates that are acceptable when compared to more standard synthetic mesh–based repairs in lower risk settings. It was recognized that planned incisional hernia leads almost uniformly to progressive loss of domain; an increased risk of intestinal fistulization; and by definition, the requirement for further reconstructive procedures. Included was the frequent need for a skin graft with donor site morbidity.
- ▲ The increased use of decompressive laparotomies and damage control laparotomies resulted in an increased number of surgical patients with complex abdominal wall injuries. The ability to manage the open abdomen over a prolonged period of time supported this clinical approach. Often, at the time of abdominal wall repair, a reinforcing material was needed by the surgeon because of contamination and the risk of wound healing delay, hypotensive hypoperfusion of the abdominal wall, or other common comorbidities like obesity or immunosuppression. Biologic mesh reinforced abdominal wall repairs are reported as safe and reliable in this setting as well.
- ▲ Accumulating reports of the risk for the intraperitoneal placement of synthetic onlay meshes (IPOM) also drove the application of biologic meshes to abdominal wall reconstruction. The U.S. NSQuIP database and Dutch Hernia Registry found that reoperation in the presence of a prior synthetic mesh in the intraperitoneal position significantly increased the risk of unplanned bowel injury and resection from 3% to 23 % .
- ▲ Some surgeons and centers have reported recurrence rates for incisional hernia as high as 100% when using biologic meshes. A consensus is emerging that this is not the universal experience and that some of this is due to surgical technique and some of it is due to material properties. It appears that the use of biologic meshes to bridge a gap in the abdominal wall leads to a high incidence of "bulging" or recurrence. Regardless of the definition of recurrent incisional hernia, a bulging defect is visible, it may impair abdominal wall function as during a sit-up, and usually the patient is displeased with the result. Some of this may be an inherent biologic limitation of the biologic meshes, in that in order for revascularization and general recellularization to occur, the biologic implant must be in contact with well-perfused host tissue. It now appears that biologic meshes perform better when used as reinforcing materials to an already reconstructed abdominal wall, as after component separation. The human allograft dermis also contains more elastin that may result in more stretching, leading to a clinical bulge. It is not clear whether porcine dermis or intestinal submucosa does this less or should be held to the same limitations.

- Currently, biologic meshes are very compliant, especially when compared to most synthetic meshes. This can make handling more difficult and most surgeons experience a learning curve for understanding the unique material properties. This has resulted in limited adaptation to laparoscopic applications, for example. The concern for bulging following a bridging technique also has limited the development of laparoscopic ventral hernia repair using biologic meshes.
- No head-to-head comparative trials have been performed to date evaluating different biologic repair materials in incisional hernia repair, and differentiation between products is based on early reported findings with only a limited number of the available prostheses. Detailed human and animal data describing the qualities of biologic repair materials are only available for some of these prostheses.

Selected References

Breuing K, Butler CE, Ferzoco S, et al: Incisional ventral hernias: Review of the literature and recommendations regarding the grading and technique of repair, *Surgery* 148(3):544–558, 2010.

Diaz JJ Jr, Conquest AM, Ferzoco SJ, Vargo D, Miller P, Wu YC, et al: Multi-institutional experience using human acellular dermal matrix for ventral hernia repair in a compromised surgical field, *Arch Surg* 144(3):209–215, 2009 Mar.

Espinosa-de-Los-Monteros A, de la Torre JI, Marrero I, Andrades P, Davis MR, Vasconez LO: Utilization of human cadaveric acellular dermis for abdominal hernia reconstruction, *Ann Plast Surg* 58(3):264–267, 2007 Mar.

Franz MG: The biology of hernia formation, *Surg Clin North Am* 88(1):1–15, 2008 Feb:vii.

Gray SH, Vick CC, Graham LA, Finan KR, Neumayer LA, Hawn MT: Risk of complications from enterotomy or unplanned bowel resection during elective hernia repair, *Arch Surg* 143(6):582–586, 2008 Jun.

Halm JA, de Wall LL, Steyerberg EW, Jeekel J, Lange JF: Intraperitoneal polypropylene mesh hernia repair complicates subsequent abdominal surgery, *World J Surg* 31(2):423–429, 2007 Feb.

Luijendijk RW, Hop WCJ, van den Tol P, de Lange DCD, Braaksma MMJ, Ijzermans JNM, et al: A comparison of suture repair with mesh repair for incisional hernia, *New England Journal of Medicine* 343(6):392–398, 2000 Aug 10.

Synthetic Mesh Choices for Surgical Repair

Sean B. Orenstein, MD and Yuri W. Novitsky, MD, FACS

1. Introduction to Synthetic Mesh Materials

- Modern herniorrhaphy relies on the use of prosthetic implants to allow for tension-free repairs of hernia defects. Such widespread use of mesh implants has greatly reduced the incidence of hernia recurrence. Surgeons continuously seek the ideal mesh—pliable and durable with chemical inertness and limited immunogenicity. Synthetic meshes have been used for over half a century, since Dr. Francis Usher popularized the use of polypropylene in the late 1950s. However, only recently have there been any changes in their original design. Current manufacturing techniques involve modifications of mesh polymers, reduction in fiber density, increase in pore size, and combinations of the above in attempts to create an "ideal mesh" to replace native fascia during hernia repair.

2. Mesh Characteristics (Table 19-1)

1. Material

- Polypropylene constitutes the most common polymer used in surgical meshes. It is highly durable and has been proved successful in hernia repairs for over 50 years. Because of unraveling at the edges when cut, current meshes are typically knitted instead of woven. While still popular because of its strength, durability, and pliability, polypropylene meshes are not without their drawbacks. Traditional polypropylene induces a strong inflammatory reaction upon implantation. Such inflammation can lead to excessive fibrosis, loss of pliability, and chronic pain. Additionally, when exposed to bowel, uncoated polypropylene may lead to extensive adhesions and/or fistulas.
- Polyester is a hydrophilic polymer incorporated into meshes. It has been manufactured as a 2-dimensional (flat) sheet or a 3-dimensional sheet to allow for greater incorporation of host tissues. One of the advantages of polyester is its pliability, which allows the surgeon to easily manipulate and fixate the mesh to the conformations of the abdominopelvic walls. Polyester is unique in its hydrophilic nature; however, the clinical relevance of this feature remains unknown. Like polypropylene, unprotected polyester can lead to significant inflammatory reactions with ensuing fibrosis, adhesions, and fistulas.

Table 19-1 Synthetic Mesh Characteristics

MATERIAL	MESH PRODUCT	MANUFACTURER	MESH CHARACTERISTICS
Standard Meshes			
Polypropylene	Prolene	Ethicon	Heavyweight – 105 g/m^2
	Marlex	C.R. Bard	Heavyweight – 95 g/m^2 Microporous – 0.6 mm
	Trelex	Boston Scientific	Heavyweight – 95 g/m^2 Microporous – 0.6 mm
	ProLite	Atrium	Midweight – 85 g/m^2 Microporous – 0.8 mm
	ProLite Ultra	Atrium	Lightweight – 50 g/m^2 Microporous – 0.75 mm
	Prolene Soft	Ethicon	Lightweight – 45 g/m^2 Macroporous – 2.4 mm
	Soft Mesh	C.R. Bard	Lightweight – 44 g/m^2 Macroporous – 6.3 mm
	Visilex Mesh	C.R. Bard	Macroporous – 2.5 mm
Polyester	Parietex TET	Covidien	3-D mesh Midweight – 80 g/m^2 Macroporous – 1.8 × 1.5 mm
	Mersilene	Ethicon	2-D mesh Heavyweight, Macroporous
Polytetrafluoroethylene (PTFE)	Infinit	W.L. Gore	Macroporous
Standard Composite Meshes			
Polypropylene with poliglecaprone	Ultrapro	Ethicon	Lightweight – 28-40 g/m^2 Macroporous – 2.0-4.0 mm
Polypropylene with polyglactin	Vypro II	Ethicon	Lightweight – 35 g/m^2
Anti-adhesion Composite Meshes			
Expanded polytetrafluoroethylene (ePTFE)	Dualmesh	W.L. Gore	(solid laminar sheet) 2-sided: Micro- and macroporous*
	Dulex	C.R. Bard	(solid laminar sheet) 2-sided: Micro- and macroporous*
Polypropylene mesh and ePTFE	Composix E/X	C.R. Bard	Heavyweight, microporous polypropylene (abdominal wall surface) and microporous ePTFE (anti-adhesion)
	Composix L/P	C.R. Bard	Lightweight, macroporous polypropylene (abdominal wall surface) and microporous ePTFE (anti-adhesion)
	Ventralex	C.R. Bard	Mesh designed for small defects (e.g., umbilical, port site hernias)
Polypropylene mesh + poliglecaprone coating	Physiomesh	Ethicon	Lightweight* Macroporous – 3 mm
Polypropylene and polyglycolic acid (PGA) mesh + carboxymethylcellulose-sodium hyaluronate-polyethylene glycol (CMC-HA-PEG) coating	Sepramesh	C.R. Bard	Heavyweight – 101 g/m^2 Microporous – 0.35 mm
Polypropylene and polyglycolic acid (PGA) mesh + carboxymethylcellulose-sodium hyaluronate-polyethylene glycol (CMC-HA-PEG) coating	Ventralite	C.R. Bard	Lightweight – 54 g/m^2 Microporous – 0.4 mm
Polypropylene mesh with oxidized regenerated cellulose (ORC) coating	Proceed	Ethicon	Lightweight – 50 g/m^2 Macroporous – 2.5 mm
Polypropylene mesh + omega-3 fatty acid coating	C-Qur	Atrium	Midweight – 85 g/m^2 Microporous – 0.8 mm
	C-Qur Lite	Atrium	Lightweight – 50 g/m^2 Microporous – 0.75 mm
3-D Polyester + collagen-polyethylene glycol (PEG) coating	Parietex Composite	Covidien	Midweight – 80 g/m^2 Macroporous – 1.8 × 1.5 mm
Biodegradable Meshes			
Polyglycolic acid:trimethylene carbonate (PGA:TMC)	Bio-A	W.L. Gore	3D Matrix
Polyglactin	Vicryl	Ethicon	*

*Information not available.

▲ Polytetrafluoroethylene (PTFE) is a carbon and fluorine-based synthetic hydrophobic polymer most commonly recognized in nonstick cookware (Teflon). Laminar or "expanded" polytetrafluoroethylene (ePTFE) biomaterials for use in hernia repair (Dualmesh, W.L. Gore) were introduced in 1983. PTFE is a strong and relatively inert biomaterial; it is flexible and soft with resultant ease of handling of the mesh. Until recently, PTFE-based mesh has been manufactured as solid sheets of expanded PTFE with both microporous and macroporous (corrugated) surfaces to allow anti-adhesion and tissue ingrowth properties, respectively. Dualmesh also can be coated with a silver chlorhexadine layer (Dualmesh Plus, W.L. Gore) to impede mesh infectability.

▲ Newer PTFE-based monofilament mesh (Infinit, W.L. Gore) uses a knitted configuration instead of a solid laminar sheet. This modification was designed to promote tissue ingrowth and mesh integration during extraperitoneal implantation.

2. Weight and Density

▲ Studies have shown that traditional "heavyweight" meshes demonstrate four times the tensile and burst strength of the native abdominal wall. As a result, traditional meshes may be overengineered for use in most hernia repairs. The latest generation of meshes has been designed to reduce the amount of implanted prosthetic material. These so-called lightweight meshes are manufactured with thinner filaments and/or larger pore sizes resulting in markedly reduced mesh "weights," measured in grams per m^2. Such reduction (>50%) in prosthetic weight potentially allows for a reduced inflammatory reaction, more flexibility, and improved compliance, especially in the long-term.

3. Porosity

- ▲ In addition to reducing fiber caliber and density, increasing the distance between the mesh fibers also contributes to overall foreign body reduction. Following implantation, each mesh fiber is surrounded by some degree of inflammation and fibrosis. Microporous mesh induces significant perifilamentous fibrosis that tends to blend together, creating a scar plate. As pore size is increased between fibers, less bridging fibrosis may be observed, with subsequent reduced scar plate formation. This results in improved fluid transport across the mesh, theoretically lessening seroma formation. Marlex is considered a microporous mesh, with a pore size of 0.6 mm. Ultrapro, one of the most macroporous meshes, contains pore sizes ranging from 2 to 4 mm (diagonal-shaped pores).

4. Anti-adhesion Barrier

- ▲ The advent of laparoscopic surgery necessitated development of so-called *composite* meshes. The principal benefit of these meshes is the ability to strategically place them intraperitoneally to impede adhesion formation on one side while promoting tissue ingrowth on the other side. While most intraperitoneal meshes incorporate two layers of materials, Dualmesh (W.L. Gore and Associates, Flagstaff, AZ, USA) is manufactured by the fusion of two layers of ePTFE. A macroporous layer is corrugated and roughened to promote tissue ingrowth. This is paired with a microporous layer, which is best suited for the visceral surface by allowing for minimal and filmy adhesions. Accordingly, the smooth microporous layer is designed to face the peritoneal cavity and the rough macroporous side is to be placed against the abdominal wall to allow for tissue incorporation.
- ▲ The ability of ePTFE to resist adhesion formation is also used in Composix EX (C.R. Bard, Cranston, NJ, USA). This mesh type includes a smooth microporous layer of ePTFE under a layer of standard polypropylene. The smooth ePTFE surface is positioned toward the abdominal contents and serves as a protective interface against the bowel. The polypropylene side faces the abdominal wall to be incorporated into the native peritoneum and fascial tissue. Although it still remains popular, many surgeons have recently been reluctant to use this product because of fear of potential exposure of polypropylene to the abdominal viscera, stemming from technical errors at implantation or excessive shrinkage of the ePTFE layer, with resultant increase in adhesion formation and other serious intestinal complications.
- ▲ The layers of most other composite meshes consist of a synthetic material and an anti-adhesion polymer. The peritoneal layer (tissue ingrowth side) is composed of a typical polypropylene or polyester sheet. Visceral (nonadhesive) surfaces consist of various chemical polymer-based coatings. Today, such coatings include omega-3 fatty acids (C-Qur), poliglecaprone (Physiomesh), hyaluronic acid (Sepramesh), polyethylene glycol (Parietex), and oxidized regenerated cellulose (Proceed), among others. These coatings are intended to persist until neoperitoneum has covered the mesh, typically within 10 to 14 days after implantation. However, such absorbable adhesion barriers may be damaged by handling of the mesh during implantation, thus reducing its anti-adhesive properties.

5. Absorbable, Partially Absorbable, and Biodegradable Meshes

- ▲ The aforementioned meshes are composed of permanent polymers; however, varieties of permanent meshes contain absorbable materials. The addition of absorbable fibers such as polyglactin (Vicryl, Ethicon, Inc) in Vypro composite meshes (Ethicon, Inc) or poliglecaprone (Monocryl, Ethicon, Inc) in Ultrapro adds stiffness to the composite mesh. This feature is particularly important for the lighter weight meshes to improve mesh handling during implantation, while reducing the overall foreign material within the patient after complete resorption of the extra fibers occurs.
- ▲ Bio-A (W.L. Gore and Associates) represents the first biodegradable synthetic mesh sheet. Its intended function is more akin to a biologic mesh prosthetic than a typical knit synthetic mesh, as its biodegradable scaffold is gradually replaced by native collagen. Composed of polyglycolic acid and trimethylene carbonate (similar to a PDS suture material), it resorbs in approximately 3-6 months. Although this material has a proven record in staple/suture line reinforcement and hiatal repairs, its efficacy in reinforcement of tensile forces during abdominal wall reconstructions remains unclear.

3. Clinical Implications of Biomaterials

1. Material Type:

- ▲ Polyester, polypropylene, and PTFE remain the three most common synthetic substrates used for mesh. Although tissue reactions of biomaterials vary greatly in the literature, our recent experience in rodent experiments demonstrated that the polyester-based mesh was the greatest inducer of inflammation and appeared to impose a severe chronic foreign body reaction. While the polypropylene meshes displayed significant inflammation and some foreign body reaction, the severity was strikingly less when compared to polyester. Compared to the knit meshes in our study, integration of the laminar ePTFE mesh within tissues was met more with heavy fibrosis and encapsulation instead of integration. This has been seen in other in vivo studies and clinically, with excised samples of previously implanted ePTFE demonstrating significant fibrosis. In addition, decreased neovascularization seen in our study may have further predisposed ePTFE mesh to a diminished biocompatibility. Heavy fibrosis and encapsulation may lead to mesh shrinkage. Overall, we found polypropylene to exhibit the highest degree of tissue biocompatibility followed by ePTFE and, finally, polyester. The clinical implications of these findings are not entirely clear, and no randomized controlled trials have evaluated these materials in a comparative fashion.

2. Material Weight

- ▲ Most prosthetics, although chemically inert, generate an intense host inflammatory reaction. The host response to implanted prosthetic biomaterials follows a cascading sequence of events (coagulation, inflammation, angiogenesis, epithelialization, fibroplasia, matrix deposition, and contraction) with a resultant formation of dense connective tissue at the site of implantation. Although this may have an important positive role in mesh incorporation, the increased amount of connective tissue does not necessarily translate to strength and durability of the hernia repair. A rigid scar plate resulting from pronounced perifilamentous fibrosis and deposition of collagen fibers contributes to the loss of prosthetic pliability. In the long-term, such acquired stiffness of mesh products contributes to the changes in compliance of both the hernia site and the whole abdominal wall. Clinically, this decrease in compliance can lead to a sensation of stiffness and result in both physical discomfort and significant limitations in the activities of daily living in many patients. The deleterious foreign body effects of synthetic meshes have been linked to the amount of foreign body implanted. As a result, a goal of modern mesh manufacturers has been the development of prosthetic implants that are able to meet the tensile demands of the abdominal wall while limiting the foreign body burden at the site of the repair. Similar to our previous experience, as well as that of other investigators, our laboratory recently confirmed that lightweight and midweight polypropylene mesh displayed a marked reduction in fibrosis and foreign body reaction when compared to the heavyweight polypropylene. Beyond doubt, reduction of the overall "weight" of the mesh implant is associated with a significant increase in biocompatibility of the prosthetic.
- ▲ The clinical evidence for the benefits of this theoretical improvement is evolving. In a recent randomized trial of inguinal herniorrhaphies, the use of lightweight mesh reduced the foreign body sensation to less than half of that reported with standard densely woven polypropylene mesh. In addition, physically active patients reported significantly less pain on exercise. In another series of hernia patients, a reduction of paresthesia from 58% in the heavyweight group to 4% in the lightweight group was noted. More recently, the most compelling evidence for the benefits of lightweight mesh to date was published. In a double-blinded, prospective series of hernia patients with bilateral inguinal defects, both traditional and lightweight meshes were implanted with each patient being their own control. One hundred percent of patients were able to point out correctly the side with a lightweight mesh. The patients reported overall significant decrease in mesh sensation and pain at the site of implantation. Overall, it appears that the implantation of lightweight polypropylene mesh results in decreased chronic discomfort and reduced restriction of physical activities while providing more than adequate strength for the reinforcement of hernia repairs. It is important to point out, however, that the use of lightweight meshes as a "bridge" should probably be avoided as it may lead to excessive bulging and, rarely, central mesh failures. Therefore, we have adopted a policy of highly selective use of lightweight products. For laparoscopic ventral hernia repairs without defect closure, for rare cases of "bridging" of defects during open ventral herniorrhaphies, and during laparoscopic repairs of moderate to large *direct* inguinal hernias, we advocate the use of midweight or traditional meshes to ensure a durable repair.

3. Microporous vs. Macroporous mesh:

▲ Although the significance of mesh porosity has been suggested, until recently we found limited objective evidence linking pore size to biocompatibility. It does appear, however, that a great deal of importance lies with the fibrotic reactions that take place between the mesh fibers or fiber bundles. With smaller mesh pores, the fibrosis that surrounds each mesh fiber bridges with the fibrosis of adjacent mesh fibers. We found that macroporous meshes contain a "neutral zone" between mesh fibers free of any foreign body and resultant decrease in host inflammatory response and fibrosis. In fact, when comparing three different polypropylene meshes, we found that biocompatibility was clearly proportional to the pore size of the mesh. Additionally, the large pore "neutral zones" allow for local tissue ingrowth while reducing chronic inflammation across the entire mesh.

▲ Macroporous meshes appear to also demonstrate increased ability to resist infection. Recent European studies demonstrated safe use of macroporous meshes in clean-contaminated and even contaminated fields. Rapid mesh incorporation is likely a key contributor to these observations of decreased mesh infection. Additionally, larger pores may improve fluid transport across the mesh due to a decrease in flow resistance. This, in turn, leads to more efficient fluid removal, as well as nutrient and oxygen transport, possibly leading to a reduction in postoperative seromas and faster healing. Overall, there are markedly improved tissue reactions, decreased fibrosis, and likely decreased infectability in meshes with larger pore sizes.

4. Other Considerations

1. Anisotropy

▲ The material properties of meshes contribute to the overall mechanical behavior of the repair of hernia defects. While the differing elasticity of meshes when pulled in different directions (i.e. anisotropy) has not been well defined to date, ongoing studies show that many commonly used meshes have up to 20-fold differences in their stretchability when pulled in perpendicular directions. This may factor into the success of abdominal wall repairs, as the native abdominal wall is roughly twice as elastic in the vertical (craniocaudal) axis versus the horizontal axis. As a result, mesh implantation may need to be strategic in order to address the differences in both the textile properties of the prosthetic and the physiologic properties of the abdominal wall. However, proper mesh marking to guide surgeons in properly orienting mesh during implantation is lacking (nor is it required) in nearly all products on the market today.

2. Pre-shaped mesh

▲ In an effort to accommodate abdominopelvic contours during repair, preformed meshes are available. These meshes are typically used in inguinal repairs and assist surgeons to laparoscopically place a mesh over the myopectineal orifice without the buckling effect that may occur when using a flat piece of mesh. In addition, preformed plugs may be used to "occlude" an indirect inguinal defect. Clear-cut clinical benefits of preshaped meshes have not been established to date.

Selected References

Cobb WS, Kercher KW, Heniford BT: The argument for lightweight polypropylene mesh in hernia repair, *Surg Innov* 12:63–69, 2005.
Junge K, Klinge U, Rosch R, Klosterhalfen B, Schumpelick V: Functional and morphologic properties of a modified mesh for inguinal hernia repair, *World J Surg* 26:1472–1480, 2002.
Lichtenstein IL, Shulman AG, Amid PK, Montllor MM: The tension-free hernioplasty, *Am J Surg* 157:188–193, 1989.
Nilsson E, Haapaniemi S, Gruber G, Sandblom G: Methods of repair and risk for reoperation in Swedish hernia surgery from 1992 to 1996, *Br J Surg* 85:1686–1691, 1998.
Novitsky YW, Harrell AG, Hope WW, Kercher KW, Heniford BT: Meshes in hernia repair, *Surg Technol Int* 16:123–127, 2007.
Saberski ER, Orenstein SB, Novitsky YW: Anisotropic evaluation of synthetic surgical meshes, *Hernia* 15(1):47–52, 2011.
Usher FC, Ochsner J, Tuttle LL Jr: Use of marlex mesh in the repair of incisional hernias, *Am Surg* 24:969–974, 1958.

Index

A

Abdominal binders, postoperative use of, 38, 108, 137, 162
Abdominal compartment syndrome
   development of, 290
   monitoring for signs of, 312
Abdominal domain
   anterior, maintenance of, 294
   loss of, 244
      assessment of, 244–246, 245f
      physical examination determining, 246–247
      physiology associated with, 246
Abdominal wall anatomy, 2, 74, 75f
   anomalies of, 16–20
   deep fascial, 3f, 4–6
   lateral, 74
   muscular, 6–8
   neural, 14
   neurovascular, 8–10, 9f
   overview of, 2
   superficial fascial, 2–14, 3f
   vascular, 10–14
Abdominal wall expansion, 224–228. *See also* Tissue expansion
Abdominal wall musculature, 3f, 5f, 6–8
   functions of, 16
   preserving innervation and blood supply of, 140
Abdominal wall physiology, 14
   and muscular function, 16
   and respiratory function, 14–16
Abdominal wall skin
   preservation of blood supply and innervation to, 140. *See also* Perforator vessel preservation
   quality and reconstructive considerations
      in endoscopic component separation, 186
      in modified minimally invasive component separation, 173
Absorbable meshes, 326
Alloderm (Lifecell) mesh, 317t
Allograft sources
   development of, 317
   processing of, for surgical use, 318
   sterilization of, 318
Allomax (Bard/Davol), 317t
Angiosomes, concept of, 140
Anisotropy, of synthetic mesh, 328
Anterior external oblique fascia, components separation, 6, 7f
Anterior rectus sheath, 3f, 4–6, 5f, 206–208
   variations of, at different levels, 5f
Anterior superior iliac spine (ASIS), 3f, 262, 265f
Anterolateral thigh flap, 261t–262t, 284–288
   anatomy involved in, 284
   design of, 284
   marking and dissection of, 284–286, 285f, 287f
   variations of, 288
Anti-adhesive characteristics, of synthetic mesh, 325
Aponeurotic anatomy, 3f, 6–8, 206–208, 207f
Aquacel dressing (ConvaTec), 308

Arcuate line, 3f, 5f
   fascial layers above and below, 4–6
Atypical hernias, laparoscopic repair of, 42–59. *See also* Laparoscopic atypical hernia repair
Autologous source material, for mesh, 317

B

Balloon dissector, 186
Balloon-tipped trocar, 186
Barker technique, 294
Bio-A mesh (W.L. Gore), 323t, 326
Biodegradable meshes, 326
Biologic mesh, 316–321
   indications for, 128, 316
   mechanisms of action of, 319, 319t
   modification of, and processing, 318
   outcomes for, 319–321
      in abdominal wall reconstruction, 320
      comparative product studies in, 321
      in laparoscopic surgical repair, 321
      in open abdomen management, 320
      recurrent incisional hernia in, 320
   primary function of, 319
   surgeon experience and expert opinion on, 320
   tissue sources for, 317–318, 317t
Bovine mesh products, 317t, 318

C

Camper fascia, 2–14, 3f
Component separation, 6, 7f, 139
   endoscopic, 185–201. *See also* Endoscopic component separation
   modified minimally invasive, 171–184. *See also* Modified minimally invasive component separation
   open (conventional), 130–137. *See also* Open abdomen; Open component separation
   periumbilical perforator sparing, 139–170. *See also* Periumbilical perforator sparing (PUPS) component separation
   posterior. *See* Posterior component separation
Composite meshes, 323t, 325
Composix E/X mesh (C.R. Bard), 323t, 325
Composix L/X mesh (C.R. Bard), 323t
Congenital abdominal wall defects, 20, 302–304, 303f. *See also* Omphalocele
Costal margin, 3f
C-Qur Lite mesh (Atrium), 323t
C-Qur mesh (Atrium), 323t, 325
Cross-linking, of dermal matrices, 318

D

Deep circumflex iliac artery (DCIA), 276
Deep fascial layers, 3f, 4–6
   and anterior and posterior rectus sheath variations, 5f
Deep inferior epigastric artery(ies) (DIEA), 8, 9f, 10
   branching patterns of, 5f, 12
   dissected from rectus abdominis, 8, 17f
Deep inferior epigastric based flap, 261t–262t

Page numbers followed by b, t, and f indicate boxes, tables, and figures, respectively.

Deep superior epigastric arteries, 8, 9f
Dermal matrix structure, native, preservation of, 318
Double lay mesh placement, 156, 159f
Dualmesh (W.L. Gore), 64, 323t, 324
    anti-adhesive characteristics of, 325
Dulex mesh (C.R. Bard), 323t

E
Endoscopic component separation, 185–201
    anatomic considerations in, 185–186
    comorbidities and risk in, 185
    operative steps in, 188–196
        balloon dissector placement, 190, 191f
        balloon insufflation and orientation of oblique muscle fibers, 190, 191f
        balloon tipped trocar placement, 192
        blunt dissection of external oblique at costal margin, 192, 193f
        blunt dissection of inferior space, 192
        incision, 188
        LigaSure™ ultrasonic dissector placement, 194, 195f
        mesh placement and closure, 196
            intraperitoneal, 196–198, 197f, 199f
            retrorectus, 196
        mesh placement and closure in, 196
        plane development in oblique muscle, 188, 189f
        release of external oblique muscle, 192, 193f, 196, 197f
        retrorectus mesh placement and closure in, 196
        separation of external oblique from costal margin, 194, 195f
    pearls and pitfalls of, 200
    postoperative care in, 198
    preoperative considerations in, 185–198
        equipment, 186–198, 187f
        musculofascial anatomy, 186
        patient positioning, 188
        skin quality and reconstruction, 186
        trocar positioning and strategy, 188, 189f
Enteroatmospheric fistula, 300
Epigastric arcade, 8
Epigastric arteries, 9f, 10–14, 11f
    musculocutaneous perforators from, 10, 11f, 12
Epigastric vessels, branching patterns of, 5f, 12
ePTFE mesh, 64, 324
    anti-adhesive characteristics of, 30, 62–68
    clinical implications of, 326
Expanded polytetrafluoroethylene mesh. *See* ePTFE mesh
Extended deep inferior epigastric perforator flap, 280–282
    anatomy involved in, 280, 281f
    design of, 280
    marking and dissection of, 280–282
External oblique aponeurosis, 3f, 206–208
    identification of, 166
    incision and division of, 133, 134f, 137
        perforator sparing, 152, 153f
    release of, 176, 184
External oblique muscle, 3f, 4, 5f, 6
    endoscopic component separation of, 192, 193f, 196, 197f
        at costal margin, 194, 195f
        plane development in, 188, 189f
    innervation of, 14
    release of, 152, 153f
External oblique muscle flap, 261t–262t
Extracellular matrix directed repair
        signaling, 319

F
Fascia
    anterior wall, 6, 7f
    deep, 3f, 4–6
    superficial, 2–14, 3f
Fascial tissue expansion, 228, 236–240
    component separation procedure in, 236, 240, 243
    indications for, 225f, 228–229, 236, 237f
    operative steps in, 238–240
        excision of previous mesh, 238, 239f
        final, and closure, 240, 241f–242f
        hernia separation and mesh installation, 237f, 238
        sequence of, 238
    pearls and pitfalls of, 243
    skin necrosis prevention in, 243
    time line assessment in, 243
Fasciocutaneous flap(s), 261t–262t, 276–288, 277f
    anterolateral thigh, 284–288
    extended deep inferior epigastric perforator, 280–282
    groin, 276–280
    thoracoepigastric, 282–284
Fetal abdominal wall defects, discovery of, 314
Flank hernia repair, open, 97–109. *See also* Open flank hernia repair
Flank hernias, 97
Flap(s), types of, 261t–262t
Flap closure, of abdominal wall, 259–289
    comorbidity considerations in, 259
    defect assessment and flap selection in, 260–262, 261t–262t
    fasciocutaneous, 261t–262t, 276–288. *See also* Fasciocutaneous flap(s)
    muscle, 260–262, 261t–262t. *See also* Muscle flap(s)
    open wound management in, 259
    pearls and pitfalls of, 289
    postoperative care in, 288
    preoperative considerations in, 259–276
Fleur de lis incision pattern, 210, 211f
Flex HD (Musculoskeletal Transplant Foundation), 317t

G
Gastroschisis, 20, 302–304, 303f
    anatomy of, 305f
    developmental cause of, 304
    differentiation of, from omphalocele, 4, 12
Gastroschisis repair
    long-term outcome in, 312
    pearls and pitfalls of, 314
    postoperative care in, 312
    preoperative considerations in, 304
    primary closure in, 310, 311f
    staged closure in, 310, 311f
    sutureless, 312, 313f
Gore-Tex Dualmesh (W.L. Gore), 238
Gracilis muscle flap, 261t–262t
Groin flap, 261t–262t, 276–280
    anatomy involved in, 276, 277f
    design of, 278
    marking and dissection of, 278–280, 279f
Gross technique, staged closure in omphalocele surgery, 306, 307f

H
hands in pockets muscle fiber orientation, 190, 191f
hands on hips muscle fiber orientation, 190, 191f
Huger zones, of abdominal wall vascular anatomy, 8–14, 9f, 11f
    in planning component separation, 140
Human dermal mesh products, 317t
Human tissue banking, 317

I

Iliac crest, 3f
Iliolumbar flap, 261t–262t
Incisional hernia, 18, 19f
  physiology of, 18
  recurrence of, using biologic mesh, 320
Infinit mesh (W.L. Gore), 323t, 324
Inframammary fold (IMF), 282
Inguinal ligament, 3f
Internal oblique aponeurosis, 74
Internal oblique muscle, 4, 5f, 6
  innervation of, 14
  neurovascular bundles supplying, 14
Internal oblique muscle flap, 261t–262t
Inter-recti distance (IRD), 16, 17f
Interstitial parastomal hernia, 60, 61f
Intraperitoneal mesh placement, in PUPS component separation, 156, 157f–159f, 163f
Intraperitoneal onlay of mesh (IPOM) repair, 258, 320
Intrastomal parastomal hernia, 60, 61f

K

Keyhole technique, of mesh preparation, 62, 64, 65f

L

Laparoscopic atypical hernia repair, 42–44
  mesh overlap considerations in, 58
  operative steps in, 48–58
  patient position and trocar placement in, 46, 47f
  postoperative care in, 58
  preoperative considerations in, 44
  risk associated with, 58
Laparoscopic parastomal hernia repair, 62–68
  keyhole technique of mesh preparation in, 64, 65f
  lysis of adhesions in, 64
  mesh choice and preparation in, 64, 320
  mesh fixation in, 66–68, 67f, 69f
  mesh placement and closure in, 66–68, 67f, 69f
  operating room setup in, 62, 63f
  pearls and pitfalls of, 72
  Sugarbaker technique of, 70, 71f
  trocar placement in, 62, 63f
Laparoscopic ventral hernia repair, 22
  abdominal cavity insufflation in, 22, 23f
  contraindications to, 41
  mesh overlap required in, 22, 23f
  operative steps in, 24–38
    abdominal access, 26, 27f, 41
    adhesion lysis, 26–28, 27f
    mesh introduction and orientation, 30–32, 31f, 33f
    patient positioning, 24–26, 25f
    securing mesh, 34–38, 35f, 37f, 39f
    sizing hernia defect, 28, 29f, 41
  postoperative care in, 38–40
  postoperative complications in, 40
    mesh infection, 40
    persistent pain, 40
    seroma formation, 40
  postoperative follow-up visits in, 40
  preoperative considerations in, 24, 41
  previous mesh bowel adhesions in, 28, 29f
Laparotomy wound complications, risk of, 316
Lateral femoral circumflex artery
  ascending branch of, 266, 267f
  descending branch of, 272, 273f, 286, 287f
Lateral femoral cutaneous nerve (LFCN), 278

Lateral row perforators, 12
Latissimus dorsi muscle, 3f, 268–272, 269f
  innervation of, 268
Latissimus dorsi muscle flap, 261t–262t
  contraindications to, 270
  design of, 270
  free, 272
  marking and dissection of, 271–272, 273f
Light-weight synthetic meshes, 324
  improved clinical results in using, 327
Linea alba, 3f, 6, 7f, 206–208
Linea semilunaris, 3f, 6, 7f
Loss of abdominal domain, 244
  assessment of, 244–246, 245f
  physical examination determining, 246–247
  physiology associated with, 246
Lower intercostal arteries, 10, 11f, 12
Lumbar arteries, 10, 11f, 12
Lumbar hernia, 44, 45f
Lumbar hernia repair, 42–44
  mesh placement and fixation in, 58, 59f
  operative steps in, 54–58, 56f–57f

M

Marlex mesh (C.R. Bard), 323t
Medial row perforators, 12
Mercedes approach, to skin and fat excision, 216, 217f
Mersilene mesh (Ethicon), 323t
Mesh(es)
  biologic, 316–321. *See also* Biologic mesh
  synthetic, 322–329. *See also* Synthetic mesh
Midaxillary line, 3f
Minimally Invasive Component Separation with Inlay Bioprosthetic Mesh (MICSIB), 178, 179f, 180
Mitek bone anchors (Mitek Surgical Products), 104, 105f–107f
Modified minimally invasive component separation, 171–184
  anatomic considerations in, 171
  comorbidities and risk in, 171
  goals of, 171
  mesh placement and closure in, 178, 179f, 180, 184
  operative steps of, 173–182
    blunt dissection and tunnel creation, 176, 177f
    closure and drainage catheterization, 180, 182, 183f
    external oblique aponeurosis release, 176, 184
    fascial midline closure and mesh considerations, 178, 179f, 180, 184
    incision and adhesion lysis, 173
    preperitoneal fat dissection, 173–174
    retrorectus plane development, 174
    semilunar line access, 174, 175f
    subcutaneous fat dissection, 174
    surgical plane identification, 174, 175f
    suturing midline or mesh inlay, 180, 181f
  pearls and pitfalls of, 184
  postoperative care in, 182
  preoperative considerations in, 171–173, 184
    intraperitoneal, 172
    musculofascial, 172
    overall summary of, 173
    pain control in, 172
  skin quality and reconstructive considerations in, 173
Monocryl mesh (Ethicon), 326
Motor innervation, of abdominal wall, 14

Muscle flap(s), 260–262, 261t–262t
  latissimus dorsi, 268–272
  rectus femoris, 272–276
  tensor fascia lata, 262–266
Musculature, abdominal wall, 3f, 5f, 6–8
  functions of, 16
Musculocutaneous perforators, from epigastric arteries, 10, 11f, 12
Musculophrenic artery, 10, 11f, 12
Mutton chop flap, 261t–262t, 276

N
Negative pressure wound therapy, 135
  after panniculectomy, 218, 219f, 222
Neonatal abdominal wall defects, 302–304, 314. *See also* Gastroschisis; Omphalocele
Nerve supply, of abdominal wall, 14, 15f
Neuromas, formation of, and removal, 14

O
Oblique aponeurosis
  external, 3f, 206–208
    identification of, 166
    incision and division of, 133, 134f, 137
      perforator sparing, 152, 153f
    release of, 176, 184
  internal, 74
Oblique muscle
  external, 3f, 4, 5f, 6
    endoscopic separation of, 192, 193f, 196, 197f
      at costal margin, 194, 195f
      plane development in, 188, 189f
    innervation of, 14
    release of, 152, 153f
  internal, 4, 5f, 6
    innervation of, 14
    neurovascular bundles supplying, 14
Oblique muscle fibers, orientation of, 190, 191f
Omentum flap, 261t–262t
Omphalocele, 20, 302–304, 303f
  anatomy of, 304
  developmental cause of, 305f
  differentiation of, from gastroschisis, 4, 12
Omphalocele repair
  long-term outcome in, 312
  non-operative (escharotic), 308
  pearls and pitfalls of, 314
  postoperative care in, 312
  preoperative considerations in, 304
  primary closure in, 306, 307f
  staged closure in, 306
    Gross technique, 306, 307f
    Schuster technique, 308, 309f
    sequential sac ligation in, 308, 309f
    tissue expanders in, 308
Onlay mesh placement
  intraperitoneal, 258, 320
  in PUPS component separation, 160
Open abdomen, 290, 291f, 293–294
  acute, 290, 291f
  commercial visceral drape procedure in, 294, 296f–297f
  complications in, 300
  dressing application and maintenance in, 298, 300
  fascial closure in, 298, 299f
    component separation during, 301
  iodine impregnated visceral drape procedure in, 294, 295f–296f
  operative steps in, 293–298

Open abdomen (*continued*)
  pearls and pitfalls of, 300–301
  planned, 293
  postoperative care in, 298–300
  preoperative pharmacology in, 292
  preoperative resuscitation in, 290
  reoperation in, 298
  stable, 290, 291f
  visceral coverage without fascial closure in, 300–301
Open component separation, 130–137
  anatomic considerations in, 130
  comorbidities and risk in, 131
  mesh placement and closure in, 133, 135, 136f
  operative steps in
    adhesion lysis, 132
    external oblique fascia incision and division, 133, 134f, 137
    muscle fascia closure in, 133
    muscle fascia reinforcement in, 135, 136f
    musculofascial considerations, 132, 137
  pearls and pitfalls of, 137
  postoperative considerations in, 137
  preoperative considerations in, 130–131
  skin flap management in, 137
  wound complication prevention in, 135, 137
    negative pressure therapy in, 135
Open flank hernia repair, 97
  incision and dissection in, 98
  mesh choice in, 104
  mesh placement and fixation in, 104, 105f–107f, 109f
  patient positioning in, 98, 99f
  pearls and pitfalls of, 108
  postoperative care in, 108
  preoperative considerations in, 97
  preperitoneal dissection and adhesion lysis in, 98
  preperitoneal plane development in, 100, 101f–102f
Open parastomal hernia repair, 110–112
  comorbidity considerations in, 112, 128
  dissection planes in, 110–112, 111f, 128
  mesh options for, 128
  mesh stoma aperture options in, 125f
  operative options in, 114
  operative steps in, 114–126
    adhesion lysis and stomal mobilization, 114
    anterior component separation, 116, 117f
    midline laparotomy, 114, 115f
    previous stoma site closure, 122, 123f
    redundant skin excision, 126
    retrorectus mesh placement and securement, 122, 123f–125f
    retrorectus mobilization, 116, 117f–119f
    stoma pull through, 126, 127f
    stoma site transposition and posterior sheath closure, 120, 121f, 128
  ostomy site selection in, 110–112, 113f
  pearls and pitfalls of, 128
  postoperative care in, 126
  two-team approach in, 112
Open retromuscular ventral hernia repair, 74–95
  dietary considerations in, 92
  mesh considerations in, 77
  mesh placement and closure in, 88–91, 89f–90f, 94–95
  operative considerations in, 94
    technical, 94–95
  operative steps in, 77–91
    adhesion lysis and pre-existing mesh removal, 77
    incision planning, 77

Open retromuscular ventral hernia repair *(continued)*
  lateral dissection beyond linea semilunaris, 80–84. *See also* Posterior component separation
  linea alba reconstruction, 91
  mesh fixation, 88–91, 89f–90f
  posterior layer reconstruction, 86, 87f
  posterior rectus sheath incision, 78–80. *See also* Rives-Stoppa-Wantz technique
  outcomes of, 92–93
  pearls and pitfalls of, 93
  postoperative care in, 91–92, 95
  postoperative pain management in, 92
  preoperative considerations in, 76–77, 93
  preoperative imaging in, 76

P

Panniculectomy, 204–223
  abdominal wall anatomy in, 204–208
    adipocutaneous, 208
    aponeurotic, 206–208, 207f
    muscular, 204, 205f
    vascular, 204, 205f, 208, 209f
  operative steps in, 210–218
    closure techniques, 218, 219f
    incision choice, 210
    Mercedes approach to skin and fat excision, 216, 217f
    perforator vessel preservation, 209f, 212
    skin and fat excision, 212–216, 213f, 215f
  pearls and pitfalls of, 222
  postoperative care and management in, 218–220, 221f
    home care instructions, 220
    infection risk, 210
    negative pressure wound therapy, 222
  preoperative considerations in, 208–210
    imaging, 208, 209f
    prior incision patterns, 210
    risk factor assessment, 208–210
    surgical history, 210
  and ventral incisional hernia repair, 166–168, 167f, 169f
Parastomal hernia(s)
  characteristics of, 60
  types of, 60, 61f
Parastomal hernia repair
  laparoscopic, 60–72. *See also* Laparoscopic parastomal hernia repair
  open, 110–128. *See also* Open parastomal hernia repair
Parietex Composite mesh (Covidien), 323t, 325
Parietex TET (Covidien), 323t
Pectoralis major muscle, 3f
Perforator vessel preservation, 140, 141f
  in component separation, 185–201. *See also* Endoscopic component separation
  in panniculectomy, 209f, 212
  periumbilical, 140. *See also* Periumbilical perforator sparing component separation
Peristomal parastomal hernia, 60, 61f
Periumbilical perforator sparing (PUPS) component separation, 139–170
  external oblique fascia identification in, 166
  fascial advancement in, maximizing, 166
  fascial release achieved in, 145, 157f
  mesh choice in, 145
  mesh placement in, 156, 157f–159f, 163f
    onlay, 160
  mesh suturing in, appropriate tension, 166
  operative steps in, 146–162

Periumbilical perforator sparing (PUPS) component separation *(continued)*
    external oblique aponeurosis division, 152, 153f
    fascial approximation and tension assessment, 148, 149f
    fascial approximation and tension reassessment, 154
    fascial closure, 158f, 160
    hernia dissection and adhesion lysis, 148, 149f
    hernia examination, 146, 147f
    mesh placement, 156, 157f–159f, 163f
    onlay mesh placement, 160
    patient positioning, 146
    posterior rectus fascia division, 154, 155f
    preoperative markings, 146, 147f
    skin closure, 158f, 162, 163f
    subcutaneous drain placement, 160, 161f
    subcutaneous tunnel connection, 152, 153f
    subcutaneous tunnel creation, 150, 151f, 153f
  and panniculectomy, 166–168, 167f, 169f
  postoperative care in, 162
    abdominal binder, 162
    and wound complications, 168
  preoperative considerations in, 142–145
    abdominal CT scan, 142–144, 143f
    comorbidities, 142
    component separation technique, 144–145
    CT angiogram, 144
    mesh choice, 145
    physical examination, 142
  rationale for, 139–140
    preservation of cutaneous vessels and nerves, 140
    preservation of muscle vessels and nerves, 140
  in reoperative patients, 164
    with previous ventral hernia repair, 164
    with prior surgical scars, 164
    with stomas and stoma sites, 164, 165f
  wound complications in, 168
Permacol (Covidien), 317t
Physiomesh (Ethicon), 323t, 325, 328
Pneumoperitoneum. *See* Progressive preoperative pneumoperitoneum
Polyester mesh, 322, 323t
  clinical implications of, 326
Polymer substrates, of synthetic mesh, 322–324
  clinical implications of, 326
Polypropylene mesh, 322, 323t
  clinical implications of, 326
Polytetrafluoroethylene (PTFE) mesh, 323t, 324
  clinical implications of, 326
Porcine dermal mesh products, 128, 317t, 318
Porcine intestinal mesh product, 317t, 318
Porcine intestinal submucosa, 318
Porosity, of synthetic mesh, 325
  and clinical implications, 328
Posterior component separation
  with intramuscular dissection, 80, 81f.
  and repair, outcomes of, 93
  in Rives-Stoppa retromuscular hernia repair, 254, 255f–257f
  with transversus abdominis release (TAR), 82–84, 83f, 85f
Posterior layer reconstruction, 86, 87f
Posterior rectus fascia/sheath, 3f, 4, 206–208
  division of, in PUPS component separation, 154, 155f
  incision of, 78–80. *See also* Rives-Stoppa-Wantz technique
  medial advancement of, 84, 85f
  neurovascular bundles supplying, 93
  variations of, at different levels, 5f
Preformed synthetic mesh, 329

Preperitoneal plane development, 80, 100, 101f–102f
Proceed mesh (Ethicon), 323t, 325
Progressive preoperative pneumoperitoneum, 246
   operative stages in, 248–258
      abdominal wall reconstruction, 252
         intraperitoneal onlay of mesh (IPOM), 258
         Rives-Stoppa with PSCT, 254
      computed tomography scan and observations, 252, 253f
      percutaneous intraperitoneal catheter placement, 248–250, 249f, 251f
      percutaneous vena cava filter placement, 248
      peritoneal insufflation, 250, 251f
   patient care plan in, 250
   pearls and pitfalls of, 258
   physiologic collapse during, 258
   postoperative care in, 258
   preoperative steps in
      computed axial tomography, 247
      physical examination, 246–247
      stoma and mesh removal considerations, 248
      weight loss, 247
Prolene mesh (Ethicon), 323t
Prolene Soft mesh (Ethicon), 323t
ProLite mesh (Atrium), 323t
ProLite Ultra mesh (Atrium), 323t
Pubic tubercle, 3f
PUPS component separation technique. See Periumbilical perforator sparing (PUPS) component separation
Pyramidalis muscle, 3f, 8

R
Rectus abdominis muscle(s), 3f, 5f, 6, 74
   blood supply of, patterns, 5f, 12
   diastasis of, 16–18
   functional loss in removal of, 8
   functions of, 16
   innervation of, 14, 15f, 74
   versatility of, in flap procedures, 8
Rectus abdominis muscle flap, 261t–262t
Rectus diastasis, 16–18, 17f
Rectus femoris muscle, anatomy of, 272–274, 273f
Rectus femoris muscle flap, 261t–262t, 272–276
   design of, 274
   extended, 276
   marking and dissection of, 274–276, 275f
Rectus sheath, 4, 5f, 74
   anterior, 3f, 4–6, 5f
      variations of, at different levels, 5f
   posterior, 3f, 4
      variations of, at different levels, 5f
Repair signaling, extracellular matrix directed, 319
Respiratory function, of abdominal wall, 14–16
Retromuscular plane, techniques for lateral extension, 80–84
Retromuscular ventral hernia repair, open, 74–95
   dietary considerations in, 92
   mesh choices in, 77
   operative considerations in, 94
      technical, 94–95
   operative steps in, 77–91
      adhesion lysis and previous mesh removal, 77
      incision planning, 77
      lateral dissection beyond linea semilunaris, 80–84. See also Posterior component separation
      linea alba reconstruction, 91
      mesh fixation, 88–91, 89f–90f

Retromuscular ventral hernia repair, open, (continued)
      posterior layer reconstruction, 86, 87f
      posterior rectus sheath incision, 78–80. See also Rives-Stoppa-Wantz technique
   outcomes of, 92–93
   pearls and pitfalls of, 93
   postoperative care in, 91–92, 95
   postoperative pain management in, 92
   preoperative considerations in, 76–77, 93
   preoperative imaging in, 76
Retrorectus mesh placement
   for parastomal and midline hernias, 122, 123f–125f
   in PUPS component separation, 156, 157f–159f, 163f
Retrorectus plane development, 174
Reverdin needle suturing, 88, 89f–90f, 104, 105f, 122, 124f
Rives-Stoppa retromuscular hernia repair, 252
   with posterior component separation, 254, 255f–257f
Rives-Stoppa-Wantz technique, 78–80
   dissection of retromuscular space in, 78, 79f
   exposure of Cooper's ligaments/pubis in, 80, 81f
   exposure of subxiphoid space in, 80, 81f
   outcomes of repair surgery with, 92–93

S
Scarpa fascia, 2–14, 3f
Schuster technique, in ruptured omphalocele surgery, 308, 309f
Scroll technique, 62, 72
Semilunar lines, 8
Sensory innervation, of abdominal wall, 14
Sepramesh (C.R. Bard), 323t, 325
Seroma formation, in laparoscopic ventral hernia repair, 40
Serratus anterior muscles, 3f
Sizing hernia defect, 28, 29f, 41
Skin, abdominal wall, preservation of blood supply and innervation to, 140. See also Perforator vessel preservation
Skin flap management, in open component separation, 137
Skin tissue expansion, 224
   adequate, estimating, 236
   expander inflation in, 232, 233f
   expander removal in, and closure of skin defect, 234, 235f
   indications for, 224–226, 225f, 229
   operative steps of, 230–234
      expander insertion, 227f, 230
      expander placement and wound closure, 231f, 232
      incisions, 227f, 230, 231f
      patient preparation, 230
Soft Mesh (C.R. Bard), 323t
Soft tissue defects
   analysis of, 229
   fascial, 225f, 228, 237f, 239f, 242f. See also Fascial tissue expansion
   skin, 224–226, 225f, 227f. See also Skin tissue expansion
Strattice (LifeCell), 317t
Subcutaneous emphysema, 258
Subcutaneous parastomal hernia, 60, 61f
Subxiphoid hernia, 42, 43f
Subxiphoid hernia repair, 42–44
   mesh placement and fixation in, 54, 55f–56f
   operative steps in, 54, 55f
Sugarbaker technique, laparoscopic, 62, 70, 71f
Superficial circumflex iliac artery (SCIA), 8, 9f, 276, 277f, 279f
Superficial epigastric artery (SEA), 276
Superficial external pudendal artery, 8, 9f
Superficial fascial layers, 2–14, 3f
Superficial inferior epigastric artery (SIEA), 8, 9f, 12, 276
Superficial inferior epigastric flap, 261t–262t

Superficial inferior epigastric vein (SIEV), 266
Superior epigastric artery, 10, 282
Suprapubic hernia, 42, 43f
Suprapubic hernia repair, 42–44
   mesh placement and fixation in, 52, 53f
   operative steps in, 48–52, 49f, 51f
   preperitoneal space mobilization in, 58
SurgiMend (TEI Biosciences), 317t
Surgisis (Cook), 317t
Symphysis pubis, 3f
Synthetic mesh, 322
   anti-adhesive composite, 323t
   biodegradable, 323t
   characteristics of, 322–326, 323t
      absorbable and biodegradable, 326
      anti-adhesive, 325
      polymeric substrate, 322–324
      porosity, 325
      weight and density, 324
   clinical implications of, 326–328
      anisotropy and, 328
      polymer substrates and, 326
      porosity and, 328
      preformation and, 329
      weight and foreign body effect in, 327
   standard composite, 323t

T

Tegaderm dressing (3M), 312
Tendinous inscriptions, 6, 7f
Tensor fascia lata, as source of mesh, 317
Tensor fascia lata muscle, anatomy of, 262–264, 265f
Tensor fascia lata muscle flap, 261t–262t, 262–266
   design of, 264, 265f
   marking and dissection of, 266, 267f
   pitfalls of, 266
   postoperative steps for, 266
   variations of, 266
Thigh muscles, and cross-sectional anatomy, 263f
Thoracodorsal artery, 268, 269f
Thoracoepigastric flap(s), 261t–262t, 282–284
   anatomy involved in, 282, 283f
   design of, 282, 283f
   marking and dissection of, 284
Tisseel (Baxter Corp.), 52
Tissue banking, human, 317
Tissue expander(s)
   choice of, 229
   pneumoperitoneal, 246. *See also* Progressive preoperative pneumoperitoneum
Tissue expansion, 224, 229
   of abdominal wall fascia, 228
      indications for, 225f, 229
      operative steps of, 236–240. *See also* Fascial tissue expansion
   of abdominal wall skin, 224–226
      indications for, 225f, 229
      operative steps of, 230–234. *See also* Skin tissue expansion
      midline abdominal hernia amenable to, 224–226, 225f, 227f, 235f
   in staged closure of omphalocele, 308
Tissue prostheses. *See* Biologic mesh; Synthetic mesh
Tissue repair signaling, extracellular matrix directed, 319

Transversalis fascia, 4, 5f
Transverse rectus abdominis myocutaneous (TRAM) flap
   abdominal wall function after, 16
   subcostal scars and, 10
Transversus abdominis muscle, 4, 5f, 6, 74, 75f
   innervation of, 14
   neurovascular bundles supplying, 14
Transversus abdominis release (TAR), in posterior component separation, 82–84, 83f, 85f
   cautions regarding, 93
Trelex mesh (Boston Scientific), 323t
Tutopatch (Tutogen), 317t

U

Ultrapro mesh (Ethicon), 323t, 325–326
Ultrasonic dissector (LigaSure™), 186
Umbilicus, 3f

V

Vascular supply, of abdominal wall, 10–14, 204, 205f
   deep inferior epigastric arterial patterns in, 5f, 10, 12
   musculocutaneous perforators in, 10, 11f, 12
   veins in, 12, 13f
   zones in, 9f, 11f
Vastus lateralis muscle flap, 261t–262t
Venous drainage, of abdominal wall, 12, 13f
Ventral hernia, 18, 19f
   and loss of abdominal domain, 246
   physiology of, 18
Ventral hernia repair
   component separation rationale in, 139. *See also* Component separation
   component separation technique in, 6, 7f. *See also* Component separation
   open retromuscular, 74–95. *See also* Open retromuscular ventral hernia repair
   progressive preoperative pneumoperitoneum in, 246
   standard laparoscopic, 22–41. *See also* Laparoscopic ventral hernia repair
Ventralex mesh (C.R. Bard), 323t
Ventralite mesh (C.R. Bard), 323t
Veritas (Synovis), 317t
Vicryl mesh (Ethicon), 323t, 326
Visceral drapes, for open abdomen
   commercial, 294, 296f–297f
   iodine impregnated, 294, 295f–296f
Visilex Mesh (C.R. Bard), 323t
Vypro II mesh (Ethicon), 323t, 326

W

Weight, of synthetic mesh
   and density, 324
   and foreign body effect, 327
Wound healing, mesh comparisons in, 316

X

XenMatrix (Bard/Davol), 317t
Xenograft sources, 318
   processing of, for surgical use, 318
   sterilization of, 318
Xiphoid process, 3f